System Dynamics Models for Public Health and Health Care Policy

System Dynamics Models for Public Health and Health Care Policy

Editors

Jack Homer
Gary B. Hirsch

MDPI • Basel • Beijing • Wuhan • Barcelona • Belgrade • Manchester • Tokyo • Cluj • Tianjin

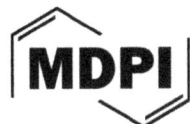

Editors
Jack Homer
Sloan School
MIT
Cambridge, MA
United States

Gary B. Hirsch
Creator of Learning
Environments
SB/SM, MIT
Wayland, MA
United States

Editorial Office
MDPI
St. Alban-Anlage 66
4052 Basel, Switzerland

This is a reprint of articles from the Special Issue published online in the open access journal *Systems* (ISSN 2079-8954) (available at: www.mdpi.com/journal/systems/special_issues/dmhd).

For citation purposes, cite each article independently as indicated on the article page online and as indicated below:

LastName, A.A.; LastName, B.B.; LastName, C.C. Article Title. *Journal Name* **Year**, *Volume Number*, Page Range.

ISBN 978-3-0365-7841-5 (Hbk)
ISBN 978-3-0365-7840-8 (PDF)

© 2023 by the authors. Articles in this book are Open Access and distributed under the Creative Commons Attribution (CC BY) license, which allows users to download, copy and build upon published articles, as long as the author and publisher are properly credited, which ensures maximum dissemination and a wider impact of our publications.
The book as a whole is distributed by MDPI under the terms and conditions of the Creative Commons license CC BY-NC-ND.

Contents

About the Editors vii

Preface to "System Dynamics Models for Public Health and Health Care Policy" ix

Morgan Clennin, Jack Homer, Alex Erkenbeck and Cheryl Kelly
Evaluating Public Health Efforts to Prevent and Control Chronic Disease: A Systems Modeling Approach
Reprinted from: *Systems* **2022**, *10*, 89, doi:10.3390/systems10040089 1

Estee Vermeulen-Miltz, Jai Kumar Clifford-Holmes, Bernadette Snow and Amanda Talita Lombard
Exploring the Impacts of COVID-19 on Coastal Tourism to Inform Recovery Strategies in Nelson Mandela Bay, South Africa
Reprinted from: *Systems* **2022**, *10*, 120, doi:10.3390/systems10040120 15

Eric Frank Wolstenholme
Using Cascaded and Interlocking Generic System Archetypes to Communicate Policy Insights—The Case for Justifying Integrated Health Care Systems in Terms of Reducing Hospital Congestion
Reprinted from: *Systems* **2022**, *10*, 135, doi:10.3390/systems10050135 33

Bobby Milstein, Jack Homer and Chris Soderquist
How Can a Community Pursue Equitable Health and Well-Being after a Severe Shock? Ideas from an Exploratory Simulation Model
Reprinted from: *Systems* **2022**, *10*, 158, doi:10.3390/systems10050158 49

Ke Zhou and Mengru Zhang
Resilience Development in Multiple Shocks: Lessons in Mental Health and Well-Being Deterioration during COVID-19
Reprinted from: *Systems* **2022**, *10*, 183, doi:10.3390/systems10050183 61

Wayne Wakeland and Jack Homer
Addressing Parameter Uncertainty in a Health Policy Simulation Model Using Monte Carlo Sensitivity Methods
Reprinted from: *Systems* **2022**, *10*, 225, doi:10.3390/systems10060225 91

Jefferson K. Rajah, William Chernicoff, Christopher J. Hutchison, Paulo Gonçalves and Birgit Kopainsky
Enabling Mobility: A Simulation Model of the Health Care System for Major Lower-Limb Amputees to Assess the Impact of Digital Prosthetics Services
Reprinted from: *Systems* **2023**, *11*, 22, doi:10.3390/systems11010022 109

Gary B. Hirsch and Heather I. Mosher
Using a System Dynamics Simulation Model to Identify Leverage Points for Reducing Youth Homelessness in Connecticut
Reprinted from: *Systems* **2023**, *11*, 163, doi:10.3390/systems11030163 137

Abraham George, Padmanabhan Badrinath, Peter Lacey, Chris Harwood, Alex Gray and Paul Turner et al.
Use of System Dynamics Modelling for Evidence-Based Decision Making in Public Health Practice
Reprinted from: *Systems* **2023**, *11*, 247, doi:10.3390/systems11050247 157

Özge Karanfil
Dynamics of Medical Screening: A Simulation Model of PSA Screening for Early Detection of Prostate Cancer
Reprinted from: *Systems* **2023**, *11*, 252, doi:10.3390/systems11050252 . . . . **175**

About the Editors

Jack Homer

Jack Homer is an expert in system dynamics simulation modeling, a former faculty member at the University of Southern California, and has been a full-time consultant to private and public organizations since 1989. He is also a Research Affiliate with the Sloan School at MIT. His articles on modeling applications and methodology are frequently cited, and many are published in the books entitled "Models That Matter" (2012) and "More Models That Matter" (2017).

In the health sector, Dr. Homer has carried out modeling projects for federal agencies including CDC, NIH, CMS, FDA, and VHA. This includes multiple projects for the CDC from 2001 to 2019, including as lead modeler on the Diabetes System Model and the "PRISM" cardiovascular risk model. He has also carried out projects for many foundations, think tanks, and state and county agencies. Notable among these is his work on health and well-being systems' transformation for the Rippel Foundation's ReThink Health initiative since its inception in 2011.

Dr. Homer is the recipient of several awards from the International System Dynamics Society, the CDC, AcademyHealth, and the Applied Systems Thinking Institute. He has a PhD from MIT, where he studied system dynamics and economics and wrote his dissertation on the adoption and evolution of new medical technologies.

Gary B. Hirsch

Gary Hirsch has been consulting with organizations on management strategy and organizational change for the past 50 years, working with clients in diverse areas such as health care, human services, education, microfinance, and news media. He specializes in applying system dynamics and systems thinking and creating simulation-based learning environments that help clients understand the complex problems they are dealing with. He is a leader in promoting systemic approaches to health problems and health care delivery at the regional and national levels.

Mr. Hirsch received SB and SM degrees from MIT's Sloan School of Management with concentrations in System Dynamics and Public Sector Management. He is the author of three books and numerous journal and magazine articles, book chapters, and conference presentations. Mr. Hirsch is also a founder and leader of a free medical program that provides care to a low-income population in towns west of Boston.

Mr. Hirsch has worked with health providers in the US, the Netherlands, Pakistan, Vietnam, and East Africa. His work has focused on community-level delivery systems, health status improvement for communities, the care of chronic illnesses such as cardiovascular disease and diabetes, health workforce policies, public policy problems such as addiction to heroin and other opioids, emergency preparedness, youth homelessness, and assisting a state children's services agency in the creation of a new system of care. Mr. Hirsch has also carried out work on the control of influenza pandemics and HIV/AIDS, programs for improving the oral health of young children, and a systemic study of the factors affecting donor availability for organ transplantation.

Preface to "System Dynamics Models for Public Health and Health Care Policy"

System dynamics (SD) is a simulation modeling discipline first developed by MIT's Jay Forrester in the late 1950s, and it has been applied to medical and health care issues since the 1960s. Its emphasis is on analyzing complex issues by quantitatively representing their inherent stocks and flows, behavioral feedback loops, delays, and nonlinearities. Applications to public health and health care have increased greatly in number over the years, and since 2017, they have accounted for 10-20% of the hundreds of papers presented each year at the International SD Conference. The advent of COVID-19 recently boosted the number of SD health applications, but the upward trend has been evident since the 1990s. As of this writing, the bibliography of the SD Society includes about 750 published health applications, of which, nearly 80% were published after 2000 and 60% after 2010. Dozens of journals and books have featured SD health applications over the years. Many health organizations at the local, national, and international levels—including the US CDC and the World Health Organization—have been long-time sponsors of SD studies. By any measure, health-related modeling is a very active part of the SD field.

Yet, many people (both systems methodologists and health researchers and policymakers) are only dimly aware of this good and important work. We gladly accepted the invitation to guest edit a Special Issue in *Systems* as an opportunity to highlight innovative new work, concentrate it in a single supportive journal, and bring it to a broader audience. We solicited papers on all aspects of public health and health care policy. We stipulated that all submitted papers needed to base their findings on strong evidence and solid methodology and be written in a clear, straightforward style. We oversaw a rigorous review process, supported by the always helpful editorial team at *Systems*, with special thanks to Managing Editors Margie Wang and Janie Zhang. Thanks also to all of the anonymous paper reviewers whose constructive comments ensured that the papers would be of the highest quality.

The result was the collection of ten excellent articles in this reprint. Arranged here in order of their publication dates (from June 2022 to May 2023), they cover a wide variety of topics in the field of public health (including chronic disease, COVID-19, youth homelessness, and community health and well-being), medicine (lower-limb prosthetics and prostate cancer screening), and modeling methodology (the use of cascaded system archetypes and Monte Carlo sensitivity analysis).

We hope you will get as much out of reading these papers as we did in their development.

Jack Homer and Gary B. Hirsch
Editors

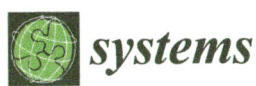

Article

Evaluating Public Health Efforts to Prevent and Control Chronic Disease: A Systems Modeling Approach

Morgan Clennin [1,*], Jack Homer [2], Alex Erkenbeck [1] and Cheryl Kelly [1]

[1] Kaiser Permanente Colorado, Institute for Health Research, Aurora, CO 80014, USA; alex.erkenbeck@kp.org (A.E.); cheryl.kelly@kp.org (C.K.)

[2] Homer Consulting and MIT Research Affiliate, Barrytown, NY 12507, USA; jack@homerconsulting.com

* Correspondence: morgan.n.clennin@kp.org

Abstract: The growing burden of chronic disease represents a complex challenge to public health. Innovative approaches, such as system dynamics simulation modeling, can aid public health professionals in understanding such complex issues and identifying effective solutions. This paper describes a system dynamics model and its application in projecting the impacts of evidence-based interventions on chronic disease for the state of Colorado. The development of the model was guided by data and input from subject matter expertise, peer-reviewed literature, and surveillance data. The model includes 28 intervention levers for chronic disease prevention, screening, and management. Interventions were simulated from 2020 to 2050 to project their impact on ten preventable causes of death. The simulations indicated the 6 most impactful interventions by 2050 to be adult smoking prevention, diabetes prevention, smoking cessation, blood pressure management, adult physical activity promotion, and colorectal cancer screening. Together, these 6 interventions could reduce preventable deaths by 7.1%, or 74% of the 9.6% reduction from all 28 interventions combined. This system dynamics model is a flexible tool that could be adapted or extended to include other populations or preventable chronic diseases. Prioritization and wide-scale implementation of the most impactful interventions could significantly reduce preventable deaths resulting from chronic disease.

Keywords: simulation model; public health practice; chronic disease; prevention; cardiovascular diseases; cancer

Citation: Clennin, M.; Homer, J.; Erkenbeck, A.; Kelly, C. Evaluating Public Health Efforts to Prevent and Control Chronic Disease: A Systems Modeling Approach. *Systems* **2022**, *10*, 89. https://doi.org/10.3390/systems10040089

Academic Editor: Oz Sahin

Received: 6 June 2022
Accepted: 27 June 2022
Published: 28 June 2022

Publisher's Note: MDPI stays neutral with regard to jurisdictional claims in published maps and institutional affiliations.

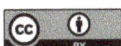

Copyright: © 2022 by the authors. Licensee MDPI, Basel, Switzerland. This article is an open access article distributed under the terms and conditions of the Creative Commons Attribution (CC BY) license (https:// creativecommons.org/licenses/by/ 4.0/).

1. Introduction

Despite significant efforts to understand complex health problems, such as chronic disease, public health professionals still face a difficult challenge in the prioritization of interventions. Well-designed experiments have provided important information about the effect sizes of single interventions over short follow-up periods. However, the existing literature cannot tell us what is likely to happen over longer periods of time, or how multiple interventions (clinical and population-wide) might interact to influence population health. The most pressing public health problems of the 21st century are the result of complex interactions between multiple interrelated factors. Hence, public health must supplement traditional analytic tools with systems approaches that can explicitly consider such complexities [1–7].

One such systems approach is system dynamics (SD) simulation modeling. Unlike some other approaches, SD models realistically represent complex causal pathways with intermediate variables, delays, nonlinearities, and feedback loops [6–9]. SD models of populations are typically compartmental, meaning they specify population subgroup categories rather than modeling each individual in the population separately. Since the 1970s, SD has been increasingly used to model many public health and health care issues such as chronic diseases [10–12]. One of the best-known SD applications is the Center for Disease Control and Prevention's Prevention Impacts Simulation Model (PRISM) of cardiovascular disease (CVD) risks and outcomes [13–19].

Building on previous work, our purpose is two-fold: (i) to describe a state-level SD model of CVD, cancer, and chronic pulmonary disease inspired by and in the general style of PRISM; and (ii) to demonstrate how this simulation model can be used to estimate the impacts of state-level public health efforts to prevent and control multiple chronic diseases over a period of 30 years. With these impact estimates, we can identify the evidence-based public health interventions (or combinations of interventions) that have the greatest potential to influence population health outcomes.

2. Materials and Methods

2.1. Model Development

The SD model was developed through a collaborative effort with key partners and subject matter experts across Colorado. Several meetings and conversations were held to (a) discuss the mechanisms by which specified interventions impact health outcomes, (b) identify peer-reviewed literature documenting the association between interventions and health outcomes, and (c) review the existing data sources to identify the best available state and national-level data for model inputs. The feedback received guided the development of a preliminary draft of the simulation model. The model was updated on an ongoing basis to reflect emerging evidence-based literature and/or new surveillance data through the end of the contract. Kaiser Permanente Colorado's Institutional Review Board deemed the study to be non-human subjects research.

2.2. Model Overview

This SD model is broader in disease scope than the PRISM model, detailing the primary risk factors and development pathways not only for CVD, but also for five types of preventable cancer (namely, colorectal, breast, cervical, oral, and respiratory), as well as asthma and chronic obstructive pulmonary disease (COPD). The model contains 28 intervention levers that were designed to reflect risk reduction strategies identified in Colorado's Chronic Disease State Plan 2018–2020 (https://cdphe.colorado.gov/chronicdisease (accessed on 1 June 2022)). These intervention levers are evidence-based strategies for the prevention, early detection, and treatment of cardiovascular disease, cancer, and chronic pulmonary disease. The long-term goal of such strategies is to reduce the burden of morbidity and mortality associated with the reference chronic disease outcomes.

Figure 1 presents an overview of the model's structural logic. The arrows depict causal chains of risk factors, interventions, disease conditions, and causes of death. The model covers the entire Colorado population, changing over time with births, net in-migration, deaths, and aging. Youth are represented in two age groups of 0–11 and 12–17, and adults in three age groups of 18–39, 40–64, and 65-plus. The model's chronic (controllable but not reversible) prevalent conditions include diabetes, hypertension, high cholesterol, CVD, asthma, and COPD. All five cancers are modeled from risk factors through latency periods to rates of incidence and then mortality, based on five-year mortality rates. Interventions affecting diet and physical activity may affect youth and/or adults, and these behavioral factors cascade to impact obesity, diabetes, hypertension, high cholesterol, CVD, asthma control, and two types of cancer (i.e., colorectal and breast). Smoking prevalence has similarly wide-ranging effects, impacting diabetes, CVD, asthma, COPD, and four types of cancer (i.e., respiratory, oral, colorectal, and breast).

The shaded boxes in Figure 1 show the 10 causes of death (aside from all-causes deaths) calculated in the model and Colorado's 2015 death count for each. Cause of death is defined as the first cause listed on the death certificate [20]. The total number of deaths across all 10 preventable causes of death (hereafter 'Combo10') represented 36.5% of all 2015 deaths in Colorado (or 13,270 of 36,352 deaths). Among the Combo10 deaths, CVD was the largest cause of death across the 10 preventable causes (6527 of 13,270 deaths, 49.2%), followed by COPD (2576 deaths, 19.4%), and respiratory cancers (1543 deaths, 11.6%).

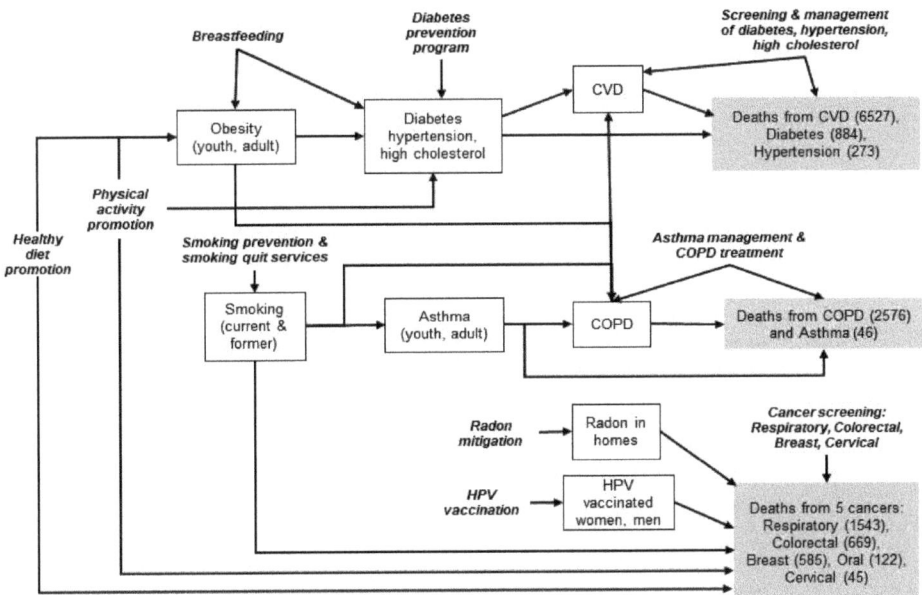

Figure 1. Model's structural logic. All conditions were calibrated based on state-level surveys, with detailed age group breakouts based on national data from NHANES and NHIS. Numbers in bold are Colorado deaths in 2015 for 10 specified causes of death, which together account for 13,270 out of Colorado's 36,352 total deaths in 2015. Key: bold italic = intervention; box = prevalent condition; shaded = cause of death.

The model was implemented using Vensim™ software (Ventana Systems Inc., Harvard, MA, USA) and contains more than 1600 interacting equations and parameters (detailed documentation of the model, in the form of an extensive reference guide, is available upon request from the authors). The model is initialized in 2000 and simulates forward by increments of one-quarter of a year through 2050; all output variables are recalculated at every increment. The model's base run, which closely matches historical data through 2019, assumes no change in exogenous inputs after 2020. Interventions can be ramped up at any time starting in 2020 and can be tested individually or in any combination.

2.3. Model Inputs

Data sources that included historical metrics of the specified disease types and associated risk factors were identified to calibrate the model. Table 1 presents the publicly available longitudinal data sources that were used for calibrating and validating the model. The identified data sources provide data inputs over the period of 1999–2019. The last column of the table presents calculated ratios (e.g., Colorado vs. national BRFSS, and national BRFSS vs. national NHANES) that were helpful for synthetic data extrapolations to fill in gaps in Colorado's historical records.

Table 1. Publicly available Colorado and US overall data sources used for calibrating the state-level system dynamics model.

Variable	Colorado	US Overall	Ratios [1]
Adult obesity	BR 1999–2018	BR 1999–2016, NH 1999–2008	CO vs. US: 0.73; BR vs. NH: 0.76
Youth obesity	NSCH 2003–2011 (age 10–17)	NH 1999–2008 (age 12–17)	CO vs. US: 0.72
Adult healthy diet	BR 1999–2009 (fruit-veg 5×/day)	BR 1999–2009 (fruit-veg 5×/day)	CO vs. US: 1.05
Youth healthy diet (high school)	HKCS 2015 (veg 2×/day)	(n/a)	(n/a)
Adult healthy drinks	BR 2009–2017 (sugary < 1/day)	(n/a)	(n/a)
Youth healthy drinks (age 1–14)	CCHS 2004–2014 (sugary < 1/day)	(n/a)	(n/a)
Adult physical activity	BR 2001–2009 (per guideline)	BR 2001–2009 (per guideline)	CO vs. US: 1.13
Youth physical activity (high school)	HKCS 2013–2015 (per guideline)	(n/a)	(n/a)
Breastfeeding (6 months+)	NIS 2001–2016	NIS 2001–2015	CO vs. US: 1.17
Adult current smoking	BR 1999–2019	BR 1999–2019, NH 1999–2008	CO vs. US: 0.91; BR vs. NH: 0.935
Adult former smoking	BR 2011–2019	BR 2011–2019, NH 1999–2008	CO vs. US: 1.04; BR vs. NH: 1.09
Youth smoking (high school)	YR 2005–2019	YR 1999–2019	CO vs. US: 0.85
Adult prediabetes	(n/a)	NH 1999–2008	(n/a)
Adult diabetes	BR 1999–2018	BR 1999–2016, NH 1999–2008	CO vs. US: 0.70; BR vs. NH: 0.74
Diabetes self-management education (DSME) or control	BR 2000–2017 (DSME)	BR 2011–2015 (DSME), NH 2005–2008 (control)	CO vs. US: 1.08; BR vs. NH: 0.98
Adult high blood pressure	BR 1999–2015	BR 1999–2015, NH 1999–2008	CO vs. US: 0.81; BR vs. NH: 0.825
Adult high cholesterol	BR 1999–2015	BR 1999–2015, NH 1999–2008	CO vs. US: 0.92; BR vs. NH: 0.715
Cardiovasc. disease (ever event)	BR 2005–2018	BR 2005–2016, NH 1999–2008	CO vs. US: 0.69; BR vs. NH: 0.99
Adult asthma	BR 2000–2016	BR 2000–2016, NHIS 2001–2016	CO vs. US: 0.99; BR vs. NHIS: 1.11
Youth asthma (0–17)	(n/a)	NHIS 2001–2016	(n/a)
Adult COPD	BR 2011–2016, NHIS 1999–2011	BR 2011–2016, NHIS 1999–2011	CO vs. US: 0.71 (BR), 0.78 (NHIS)
HPV vaccination female (age 13–17)	NIS 2008–2017 (2+ doses)	NIS 2012–2016 (2+ doses)	CO vs. US: 1.05
HPV vaccination male (age 13–17)	NIS 2013–2017 (2+ doses)	NIS 2012–2016 (2+ doses)	CO vs. US: 1.13

Table 1. Cont.

Variable	Colorado	US Overall	Ratios [1]
Colorectal cancer screen (age 50–85)	BR 2014–2016	BR 2014–2016	CO vs. US: 1.00
Mammography past 2 years (age 50–74)	BR 2014–2016	BR 2014–2016	CO vs. US: 0.95
Pap test past 3 years (age 21–65)	BR 2014–2016	BR 2014–2016	CO vs. US: 1.02
Cancer incidence over 5 years	USCS 2011–2015	(n/a)	(n/a)
Deaths by 5-or-10 year age group	CDPHE VSP 1999–2017 annual	(n/a)	(n/a)

[1] Ratios were used to fill in gaps in Colorado's historical records. Key: BR (BRFSS): Behavioral Risk Factor Surveillance System (CO and US); NIS: National Immunization Survey (CO and US); NH (NHANES): National Health and Nutrition Examination Survey (US); YR (YRBSS): Youth Risk Behavior Surveillance System (CO and US); NSCH: National Survey of Children's Health (CO and US); USCS: United States Cancer Statistics (CO and US); HKCS: Healthy Kids Colorado Survey (CO); CDPHE VSP: CO Dept of Public Health and Environment, Vital Statistics Program (CO); CCHS: Colorado Child Health Survey (CO); NHIS: National Health Interview Survey (CO and US); 5 cancer types: respiratory, colorectal, breast, oral, cervical; 11 death causes: diabetes, hypertension, CVD, asthma, COPD, 5 cancers, all-cause; (n/a): not available or not needed for CO model calibration. Adult refers to those 18+ years old.

Table 2 shows the 28 types of interventions represented in the model, divided into four categories. The 11 population health interventions primarily target population approaches to improve healthy behaviors and involve no clinical visits. The 4 clinical prevention interventions are similarly preventive but do involve clinical resources. The 7 clinical screening interventions improve the detection of prevalent disease conditions so that they can be better managed or treated. The 6 clinical management interventions help bring diagnosed disease conditions under control. As shown in the table, each intervention has a corresponding target subpopulation ('target description'), performance metric for which improvement in a health behavior or outcome is sought ('performance definition'), and estimated performance levels for the baseline year of 2018—prior to any intervention implemented in the model ('2018 value'). For example, success for the 'healthy food—adults' intervention was defined by the percentage of all Colorado adults reporting the consumption of five or more fruits and vegetables per day, which was reported to be 25% of the population in 2018.

Table 2. Evidence-based interventions (n = 28) included in the system dynamics simulation model [1].

Intervention Types	Target Description	Performance Definition (Data Source)	2018 Value
Population health			
Healthy food—adults	Adults age 18+	Fruits/vegetables 5× per day (BRFSS)	25%
Healthy food—youth	Youth age 0–17	Vegetables 2× per day, high school (HKCS)	30.5%
Healthy beverage—adults	Adults age 18+	Less than 1 sugary drink per day (BRFSS)	74%
Healthy beverage—youth	Youth age 0–17	Less than 1 sugary drink per day, ages 1–14 (CCHS)	85%
Physical activity—adults	Adults age 18+	Exercise per national guidelines (BRFSS)	57%
Physical activity—youth	Youth age 0–17	Exercise per national guidelines, high school (HKCS)	52%
Breastfeeding	New mothers	Breastfeed non-exclusive for 6 months (NIS for CO)	67%
Antismoking—adults	Adults age 18+	Smoking initiation below 2018 level, ages 18+ (NHIS)	0%
Antismoking—youth	Youth age 0–17	Smoking rate below 2018 level, high school (YRBSS)	0%
Radon in new homes	New housing units	Radon mitigation beyond 2018 level (CDPHE)	0%
Radon in resales	Housing unit resales	Radon mitigation beyond 2018 level (CDPHE)	0%

Table 2. Cont.

Intervention Types	Target Description	Performance Definition (Data Source)	2018 Value
Clinical prevention			
Diabetes prevention program	Diagnosed (or high risk for) prediabetes	Completion of NDPP program (CDC for CO)	0.1%
Female HPV vaccination	Females age 13–26	At least 2 doses (NIS for CO)	55%
Male HPV vaccination	Males age 13–26	At least 2 doses (NIS for CO)	55%
Smoking quit services	Adults age 18+	Successful quit rate above 2018 level (NHIS)	0%
Clinical screening			
Blood glucose	Adults age 18+	Checked past 2 years (BRFSS)	74%
Blood pressure	Adults age 18+	Checked past 2 years (BRFSS)	83%
Cholesterol	Adults age 18+	Checked past 2 years (BRFSS)	81%
Lung CT scan	Smokers age 50–80	Per national guidelines (NHIS for US)	4.4%
Colorectal cancer	Adults age 50–84	Per national guidelines (BRFSS)	68%
Mammography	Females age 50–74	Per national guidelines (BRFSS)	74%
Pap test	Females age 21+	Per national guidelines (BRFSS)	81%
Clinical management			
Diabetes	Diagnosed diabetes	Completion of diabetes self-mgmt class (BRFSS)	60%
Hypertension	Diagnosed hypertension	Control per guidelines (NHANES for US)	65%
High cholesterol	Diagnosed high cholesterol	Control per guidelines (NHANES for US)	60%
Asthma—youth	Diagnosed asthma age 0–17	No past year attack (NHIS for US)	47%
Asthma—adults	Diagnosed asthma age 18+	No past year attack (NHIS for US)	55%
COPD	Diagnosed COPD	Daily treatment (BRFSS for selected states)	50%

[1] Shown for each intervention is the corresponding target population, baseline performance metric, data source, and value of the metric in 2018.

2.4. Model Testing and Analysis

To test the model, each intervention was initiated in January 2020 and ramped up to a specified final dose or yield by January 2021. The dose refers to the fraction of the targeted population (see Table 2) that is (a) not meeting the performance metric at baseline; and (b) would successfully and permanently meet the performance metric after exposure to the intervention [21]. For model testing, the dose remained in effect until the end of the simulation in 2050.

To demonstrate how this SD model could be applied in public health, each intervention was first tested individually at a representative dose based on (a) the implementation literature; or (b) a corresponding national Healthy People 2030 (HP2030) goal (n = 18 interventions) [22]. For example, one HP2030 goal (HDS-05) calls for increasing the proportion of hypertensive adults whose blood pressure is under control from 47.8% to 60.8% nationally, which corresponds to a dose of 25% (=(0.608 − 0.478)/(1 − 0.478)). Next, we used the model to test 27 different combinations of interventions, performed by layering in interventions (at their representative doses) one by one in order of their individual impact on Combo10 deaths in 2050. That is, we first tested a combination of the most impactful (#1 ranking) intervention with the second most impactful (#2); for the next test we added #3, and so forth, until all 28 interventions were combined in the final test.

3. Results

Table 3 reports the independent and cumulative impacts of the 28 interventions included in the model on the simulated death rates per 100,000 adults as of 2050. For each intervention, its independent impact on the Combo10 deaths is reported as the rate (i.e., death rate per 100,000) and percent (%) change relative to the base run. Next, the cumulative impact on Combo10 deaths is reported as the summative rate and percent change relative to the base run (e.g., top ranked intervention only, top intervention and second ranked intervention, and so on). Finally, the last column reports the proportion of the total cumulative impact across all 28 interventions that is accounted for by the corresponding ranked interventions. For example, when the top 3 ranked interventions are combined, the result is a 4.86% reduction in the Combo10 death rate, which represents 50.7% of the cumulative 9.58% reduction in Combo10 death rate from combining all 28 interventions.

Table 3. Independent and cumulative intervention impact on simulated death rates per 100,000 adults as of 2050 (across 10 preventable causes of death, 'Combo10') and percentage reduction relative to the base run.

Intervention_Dose % [1]	Rank [2]	Independent Impact		Cumulative Impact		Proportion of Total Cumulative Impact
		Death Rate per 100,000	% Change	Death Rate per 100,000	% Change	
Base run	0	411.098	0.00%	411.098	0.00%	0.0%
Smoking Prevention_23	1	402.391	2.12%	402.391	2.12%	22.1%
Diabetes Prevention_18	2	404.690	1.56%	396.066	3.66%	38.2%
Smoking Cessation_16.5	3	405.258	1.42%	391.119	4.86%	50.7%
Blood Pressure Management_25	4	406.856	1.03%	387.019	5.86%	61.1%
Physical Activity_11	5	407.652	0.84%	383.876	6.62%	69.1%
Colorectal Cancer Screening_26.5	6	409.220	0.46%	382.029	7.07%	73.8%
Diabetes Screening_20	7	409.494	0.39%	380.604	7.42%	77.4%
Asthma Control_16	8	409.605	0.36%	379.371	7.72%	80.6%
Cholesterol Management_18	9	409.766	0.32%	378.140	8.02%	83.7%
Blood Pressure Screening_20	10	409.806	0.31%	376.764	8.35%	87.2%
Fruit and Vegetable Consumption_5	11	409.934	0.28%	375.771	8.59%	89.7%
Diabetes Management_7	12	410.033	0.26%	374.768	8.84%	92.2%
Radon Reduction, Housing Resale_100	13	410.138	0.23%	374.009	9.02%	94.2%
Cholesterol Screening_20	14	410.577	0.13%	373.480	9.15%	95.5%
Radon Reduction, New Construction_100	15	410.704	0.10%	373.249	9.21%	96.1%
Respiratory Cancer Screening_10.5	16	410.789	0.08%	372.986	9.27%	96.8%
Smoking Prevention, Youth_23	17	410.805	0.07%	372.765	9.32%	97.3%
Asthma Control, Youth_16	18	410.876	0.05%	372.605	9.36%	97.7%
COPD Treatment_3.9	19	410.884	0.05%	372.409	9.41%	98.2%
Mammograms_16	20	410.924	0.04%	372.239	9.45%	98.7%
HPV Vaccination, Females_61.5	21	410.977	0.03%	372.119	9.48%	99.0%
Sugar Sweetened Beverage Policy_5	22	410.997	0.02%	372.036	9.50%	99.2%
Physical Activity Youth_6	23	410.999	0.02%	371.960	9.52%	99.4%
Breastfeeding Iniatives_23	24	411.007	0.02%	371.873	9.54%	99.6%
Pap Smears_19.5	25	411.028	0.02%	371.810	9.56%	99.8%
HPV Vaccination, Male_61.5	26	411.035	0.02%	371.750	9.57%	99.9%
Fruit/Vegetable Consumption Youth_5	27	411.052	0.01%	371.714	9.58%	100.0%
Sugar Sweetened Beverage Policy Youth_5	28	411.096	0.00%	371.712	9.58%	100.0%

[1] Interventions target adults population unless youth denoted. [2] Interventions are ranked from highest to lowest based on their individual impact.

3.1. Base Run

In the base run (which assumes no interventions implemented), the annualized Combo10 death rate per 100,000 adults rises from 341.3 (2025) to 411.1 (2050). This is due to increases over time in per-capita deaths from diabetes, hypertension, CVD, colorectal and breast cancer, and COPD. These death rates increase due to aging of the population and reflect the legacy of the substantial rise in obesity over the past decades [23,24].

3.2. Individual Intervention Testing Results

Interventions (assuming the representative doses) were ranked from most to least impactful in terms of their ability to reduce the Combo10 death rate by the end of the simulation in 2050. The single-intervention results are shown in the 'independent impact; columns in Table 3, with the base run result shown at the top for comparison purposes. Three distinct clusters of interventions were distinguished based on magnitude of impact. The first cluster included top-ranking interventions 1 to 5 with impacts in the range of 2.12% down to 0.84%. The second cluster encompassed interventions 6 to 13 with impacts ranging from 0.46% down to 0.23%. The last cluster included interventions 14 to 28 with impacts of 0.13% or less. We find that reasonable uncertainties about assumptions (e.g., intervention dose) could lead to changes in the order of ranking within each cluster, but they are unlikely to move an intervention out of one cluster and into another.

Figure 2 presents the single-intervention testing results for the six most impactful interventions as a graph over time from 2020 to 2050. The outcomes are expressed as a percent reduction from the base run in the Combo10 death rate. Taken together, these six most impactful interventions include at least one intervention from each of the four general categories (i.e., population health, clinical prevention, clinical screening, or clinical management); differ in terms of which causes of death they avert (collectively averting all of the Combo10 types except cervical cancer); and vary in the speed and strength of their impacts.

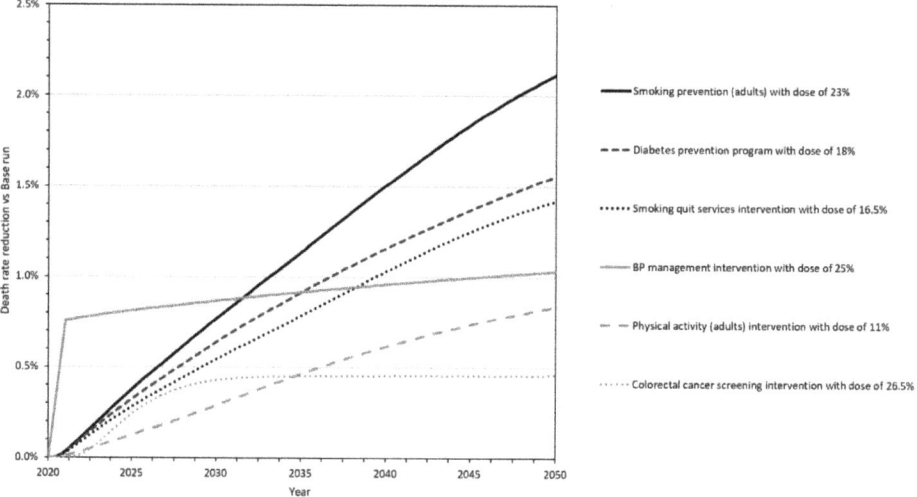

Figure 2. Simulated Combo10 death rate reduction over time relative to the base run for the six top interventions tested individually, 2020–2050; 'Combo10' first-listed causes of death: diabetes, hypertension, CVD, asthma, COPD, and 5 types of cancer. All interventions started in January 2020, ramped up to the indicated dose by January 2021. Top six interventions: (i) SmokePrev_adult23: smoking prevention (adults) intervention with a dose of 23%; (ii) DPP18: diabetes prevention program with a dose of 18%; (iii) SmokeQuit16.5: smoking quitting services intervention with a dose of 16.5%; (iv) BPmgmt25: BP management intervention with a dose of 25%; (v) PA_adult11: physical activity (adults) intervention with a dose of 11%; (vi) CRCscreen26.5: colorectal cancer screening intervention with a dose of 26.5%. For additional information, see Supplemental File Table S1.

In particular:
1. Smoking prevention for adults (Smoking Prevention_23) is a population health intervention that averts eight of the Combo10 causes of death (see Figure 1 to trace this and other interventions to impacted deaths). The dose was estimated to be 23% based on HP2030 goal TU-02. The death reduction is rapid for CVD but delayed for other causes of death as the intervention effects traverse changes in the incidence and prevalence of diabetes, cancer, asthma, and COPD before gaining strength throughout the simulation. It is the second-most impactful intervention through 2030, and the single most impactful by 2040 and 2050.
2. The National Diabetes Prevention Program (Diabetes Prevention_18) is a clinical prevention intervention that ultimately averts 4 of the 10 specified causes of death. The dose was estimated at 18% based on HP2030 goal D-01. The death reduction is delayed (traversing the incidence and gradual progression of diabetes) but gains strength throughout the simulation to make this the second-most impactful intervention by 2040 and 2050.
3. Smoking cessation services and products (Smoke Cessation_16.5) represent a clinical prevention intervention that averts eight causes of death. The dose is estimated at 16.5% based on HP2030 goal TU-14. Its effects are similar to those of the smoking prevention intervention above, only not as strong. It is the third-most impactful intervention by 2040 and 2050.
4. Blood pressure management (Blood Pressure Management_25) is a clinical management intervention that averts deaths from hypertension and CVD. The dose is estimated at 25% based on HP2030 goal HDS-05. The death reduction starts quickly and strongly, making this the most impactful of the six interventions through 2030 and the fourth-most impactful in 2040 and 2050.
5. Adult physical activity (Physical Activity_11) is a population health intervention that averts seven causes of death. The dose is estimated at 11% based on HP2030 goal PA-02. The death reduction is delayed (traversing changes in the prevalence of obesity, diabetes, hypertension, high cholesterol, and COPD) but grows rapidly after 2030 to make this the fifth-most impactful intervention by 2040 and 2050.
6. Colorectal cancer screening (Colorectal Cancer Screening_26.5) is a clinical screening intervention that averts deaths from CRC. The dose is estimated at 26.5% based on HP2030 goal C-07. The death reduction is delayed by several years (traversing the progression of colorectal cancer) but is substantial by 2030, making this the sixth-most impactful intervention by 2040 and 2050.

3.3. Combination Intervention Testing Results

The 'cumulative impact' columns of Table 3 present the results of combination testing and show how the addition of each subsequent intervention contributes to a reduction in the Combo10 death rate in 2050. All 28 interventions combined produce a Combo10 death rate reduction of 9.6% by 2050. A small number of top interventions are responsible for a majority of the combined potential. For example, the first 3 interventions together produce a reduction of 4.9%, which is 51% of the full combination; and the top 6 interventions together produce a reduction of 7.1%, which is 74% of the full combination of 28.

4. Discussion

4.1. Findings

Here, we have described and demonstrated a SD simulation model of CVD, cancer, and pulmonary disease using publicly available data for the state of Colorado. The model was initialized in 2000 and closely matches historical data through 2019. The model simulates 28 evidence-based interventions individually or in combination from 2020 to 2050 across four public health domains (i.e., population health, clinical prevention, clinical screening, and clinical disease management). The interventions were tested individually at representative doses, and the six interventions with the largest projected impact by 2050 on the combined 10 causes of death (5 types of cancer plus CVD, hypertension, diabetes, asthma, and COPD) were identified. These top six interventions were adult smoking prevention, diabetes prevention, smoking cessation, blood pressure management, adult physical activity promotion, and colorectal cancer screening.

We have compared these six interventions to the others with a lower impact to look for differentiating characteristics. The top interventions were found to share the following characteristics: (a) significant room for improvement in performance; (b) significant intervention dose; (c) significantly affecting at least one of the six leading causes of death—CVD, COPD, respiratory cancer, diabetes, colorectal cancer, or breast cancer; and (d) a shorter lead time from behavioral change to impact on deaths. Less impactful interventions lacked at least one of these characteristics. These characteristics should be considered by public health decision-makers weighing alternative interventions to improve population health.

In combination testing, we found that a small number of the top interventions could together deliver a majority of the potential impact on deaths from all 28 evidence-based interventions combined. In particular, the top 6 interventions (6/28 = 21% of all interventions) produced a combined simulated impact equal to 74% of that of all interventions combined. This result is reminiscent of the well-known 80/20 rule, or more generally the Pareto principle or Zipf's law, observed in many fields of study, in which a relatively small subset of contributing elements are responsible for the great majority of the total combined contribution [25].

4.2. Next Steps and Future Applications

The next steps and future applications of the model include incorporating data from state-level implementation of the sorts of interventions we have identified here. Incorporating real-world data would enable users of this SD model to test actual doses that were achieved during intervention implementation in a specific state. The model could be used to prospectively evaluate the long-term impacts of such efforts and provide realistic expectations for impacts on population health over the course of three decades. This would likely include exploring various strategic combinations of interventions, such as those sharing a particular public health approach (e.g., population health) or focusing on a particular set of diseases (e.g., cancers). Additionally, the model can be used to identify the evidence-based public health interventions (or combinations of interventions) that have the greatest potential to influence population health outcomes. Such prospective evaluations can help to guide the prioritization and implementation of diverse public health approaches that will be required to alleviate the burden of chronic disease.

Future extensions of the model could further improve its usefulness. First, the model could be adapted to other U.S. states and/or extended to include other chronic diseases for which a strong enough evidence base exists. Second, the model could be supplemented with additional outcome metrics of interest to researchers and decision-makers. The PRISM model, for example, calculates disease impacts on life years, disability-adjusted life years, quality-adjusted life years, and work productivity. It also includes estimates of intervention implementation cost, but these can be difficult to estimate and may vary widely depending on the assumed specifics of implementation [13,14]. Finally, the model could be extended to address questions of health inequity by characteristics such as race, education, income, and urbanicity. Toward this end, we have done some preliminary disaggregation of the model, making it possible to explore the implications (for disparity as well as total impact) of interventions targeted toward subgroups that have higher risks but also higher barriers to intervention adoption.

4.3. Strengths and Limitations

SD is an attractive approach for chronic disease modeling and has proven its value over the years, as the PRISM model attests. However, such models are only as strong as the quality of data inputted into the model. To continually improve the model efficacy, the best available data should be continually monitored and updated. For example, future iterations of this model might adjust doses for each intervention based on their impact during the COVID-19 pandemic. Because of their compartmental nature (in contrast with individual-level microsimulations), SD models can be quite broad in scope, and alternative scenarios can be set up and run in a matter of seconds. However, compartmental models such as PRISM and the newer one described here do have a limitation: they cannot easily identify and quantify emergent clinical phenomena and distributions at the individual level, such as co-morbidity patterns. For such focused analysis, excellent microsimulations have been built, including single-disease models of particular cancers, CVD, and COPD [26–30]. For the purposes of public health decision-making, however, SD models can provide a practical yet rigorous approach to projecting population-level intervention impacts into the near and longer terms.

5. Conclusions

The SD simulation model discussed here can help public health decision-makers to systematically evaluate the short- and long-term impacts of diverse approaches to improving population health. In our Colorado application, the six top interventions for reducing projected deaths were adult smoking prevention, diabetes prevention, smoking cessation, blood pressure management, adult physical activity promotion, and colorectal cancer screening. These six interventions address 9 of the 10 specified types of preventable death (all but cervical cancer, which causes the fewest deaths of the 10 types) and encompass four public health domains. Together, they would make a powerful and relatively compact package of interventions for reducing deaths from chronic disease, potentially delivering 74% of the impact of 28 evidence-based interventions combined.

Supplementary Materials: The following supporting information can be downloaded at: https://www.mdpi.com/article/10.3390/systems10040089/s1, Table S1: Simulated Combo10 death rate reduction over time relative to the base run for the six top interventions tested individually, 2020–2050 (supporting Figure 2).

Author Contributions: All authors have met authorship requirements. Specifically, all authors substantially contributed across the following inputs for manuscript development: conception and design (M.C. and C.K.), acquisition of data (J.H. and A.E.), analysis (J.H.) and interpretation of data (J.H., M.C., A.E. and C.K.), drafting the article (M.C. and J.H.), data visualization (A.E. and J.H.), and reviewing the article and revising it critically (A.E., C.K. and J.H.). All authors have read and agreed to the published version of the manuscript.

Funding: This work was supported by funding from the Colorado Department of Public Health and Environment's Cancer, Cardiovascular, and Chronic Pulmonary Disease Grants Program. All data presented in this article were extracted from publicly available data sources.

Institutional Review Board Statement: This study was deemed non-human subjects research by Kaiser Permanente Colorado's Institutional Review Board.

Informed Consent Statement: Not applicable.

Data Availability Statement: All data presented in this article were extracted from publicly available data sources. See Table 1 for data sources.

Conflicts of Interest: The authors declare no conflict of interest.

References

1. Academy of Medical Sciences. *Improving the Health of the Public by 2040: Optimizing the Research Environment for a Healthier, Fairer Future*; Academy of Medical Sciences: London, UK, 2016.
2. Gerhardus, A.; Becher, H.; Groenewegen, P.; Mansmann, U.; Meyer, T.; Pfaff, H.; Puhan, M.; Razum, O.; Rehfuess, E.; Sauerborn, R.; et al. Applying for, reviewing and funding public health research in Germany and beyond. *Health Res. Policy Syst.* **2016**, *14*, 43. [CrossRef] [PubMed]
3. Rutter, H.; Savona, N.; Glonti, K.; Bibby, J.; Cummins, S.; Finegood, D.; Greaves, F.; Harpe, L.; Hawe, P.; Moore, L.; et al. The need for a complex systems model of evidence for public health. *Lancet* **2017**, *390*, 2602–2604. [CrossRef]

4. Diez Roux, A.V. Complex systems thinking and current impasses in health disparities research. *Am. J. Public Health.* **2011**, *101*, 1627–1634. [CrossRef] [PubMed]
5. Fink, D.S.; Keyes, K.M. Wrong answers: When simple interpretations create complex problems. In *Systems Science and Population Health*; El-Sayed, A.M., Galea, S., Eds.; Oxford U Press: New York, NY, USA, 2017; Chapter 3.
6. Sterman, J.D. Learning from evidence in a complex world. *Am. J. Public Health* **2006**, *96*, 505–514. [CrossRef] [PubMed]
7. Sterman, J.D. *Business Dynamics: Systems Thinking and Modeling for a Complex World*; Irwin McGraw-Hill: Boston, MA, USA, 2000.
8. Homer, J. Levels of evidence in system dynamics modeling. *Sys. Dyn. Rev.* **2014**, *30*, 75–80. [CrossRef]
9. Homer, J. Best practices in system dynamics modeling, revisited: A practitioner's view. *Sys. Dyn. Rev.* **2019**, *35*, 177–181. [CrossRef]
10. Homer, J.; Hirsch, G. System dynamics modeling for public health: Background and opportunities. *Am. J. Public Health* **2006**, *96*, 452–458. [CrossRef] [PubMed]
11. Hirsch, G.; Homer, J.; Tomoaia-Cotisel, A. (Eds.) System dynamics applications to health and health care. 15 previously published articles with new introduction and extended bibliography. *Sys. Dyn. Rev.* **2015**. Available online: http://onlinelibrary.wiley.com/journal/10.1002/(ISSN)1099-1727/homepage/VirtualIssuesPage.html (accessed on 1 June 2022).
12. Darabi, N.; Hosseinichimeh, N. System dynamics modeling in health and medicine: A systematic literature review. *Sys. Dyn. Rev.* **2020**, *36*, 29–73. [CrossRef]
13. Yarnoff, B.; Honeycutt, A.; Khavjou, O.; Bradley, C.; Bates, L.; Homer, J. *PRISM: The Prevention Impacts Simulation Model*; Reference Guide for Model Version 3s; RTI International: Research Triangle Park, NC, USA, 2020; Available online: https://prism-simulation.cdc.gov/app/cdc/prism/#/ (accessed on 1 June 2022).
14. Yarnoff, B.; Honeycutt, A.; Bradley, C.; Khavjou, O.; Bates, L.; Bass, S.; Kaufmann, R.; Barker, L.; Briss, P. Validation of the Prevention Impacts Simulation Model (PRISM). *Prev. Chron. Dis.* **2021**, *18*, E09. Available online: www.cdc.gov/pcd/issues/2021/20_0225.htm (accessed on 1 June 2022).
15. Homer, J.; Milstein, B.; Wile, K.; Trogdon, J.; Huang, P.; Labarthe, D.; Orenstein, D. Simulating and evaluating local interventions to improve cardiovascular health. *Prev. Chron. Dis.* **2010**, *7*, A18. Available online: http://www.cdc.gov/pcd/issues/2010/jan/08_0231.htm (accessed on 1 June 2022).
16. Hirsch, G.; Homer, J.; Wile, K.; Trogdon, J.G.; Orenstein, D. Using simulation to compare 4 categories of intervention for reducing cardiovascular risks. *Am. J. Public Health* **2014**, *104*, 1187–1195. [CrossRef] [PubMed]
17. Homer, J.; Wile, K.; Yarnoff, B.; Trogdon, J.G.; Hirsch, G.; Cooper, L.; Soler, R.; Orenstein, D. Using simulation to compare established and emerging interventions to reduce cardiovascular disease risks in the United States. *Prev. Chron. Dis.* **2014**, *11*, E195. Available online: http://www.cdc.gov/pcd/issues/2014/14_0130.htm (accessed on 1 June 2022).
18. Honeycutt, A.A.; Wile, K.; Dove, C.; Hawkins, J.; Orenstein, D. Strategic planning for chronic disease prevention in rural America: Looking through a PRISM lens. *J. Public Health Mgmt. Pract.* **2015**, *21*, 392–399. [CrossRef] [PubMed]
19. Soler, R.; Orenstein, D.; Honeycutt, A.; Bradley, C.; Trogdon, J.; Kent, C.K.; Wile, K.; Haddix, A.; O'Neil, D.; Bunnell, R. Community-based interventions to decrease obesity and tobacco exposure and reduce health care costs: Outcome estimates from Communities Putting Prevention to Work for 2010–2020. *Prev. Chron. Dis.* **2016**, *13*, e47. Available online: http:///www.cdc.gov/pcd/issues/2016/15_0272.htm (accessed on 1 June 2022).
20. Colorado Department of Public Health and Environment. CoHID: Colorado Health Information Dataset. 2021. Available online: https://cdphe.colorado.gov/cohid (accessed on 1 June 2022).
21. Harner, L.T.; Kuo, E.S.; Cheadle, A.; Rauzon, S.; Schwartz, P.M.; Parnell, B.; Kelly, C.; Solomon, L. Using population dose to evaluate community-level health initiatives. *Am. J. Prev. Med.* **2018**, *54*, S117–S123. [CrossRef] [PubMed]
22. Office of Disease Prevention and Health Promotion. Healthy People 2030. U.S. Department of Health and Human Services. 2020. Available online: https://health.gov/healthypeople/objectives-and-data/browse-objectives (accessed on 1 June 2022).
23. Hales, C.M.; Carroll, M.D.; Fryar, C.D.; Ogden, C.L. Prevalence of obesity and severe obesity among adults: United States, 2017–2018. In *National Center for Health Statistics Data Brief*; No. 360; Centers for Disease Control and Prevention: Atlanta, GA, USA, 2020; p. 7.
24. Wang, Y.C.; McPherson, K.; Marsh, T.; Gortmaker, S.L.; Brown, M. Health and economic burden of the projected obesity trends in the USA and the UK. *Lancet* **2011**, *378*, 815–825. [CrossRef]
25. Newman, M.E.J. Power laws, Pareto distributions and Zipf's law. *Contemp. Phys.* **2005**, *46*, 323–351. [CrossRef]
26. Knudsen, A.B.; Zauber, A.G.; Rutter, C.M.; Naber, S.K.; Doria-Rose, V.P.; Pabiniak, C.; Johanson, C.; Fischer, S.E.; Lansdorp-Vogelaar, I.; Kuntz, K.M.; et al. Estimation of benefits, burden, and harms of colorectal cancer screening strategies: Modeling study for the US Preventive Services Task Force. *JAMA* **2016**, *315*, 2595–2609. [CrossRef] [PubMed]
27. Moolgavkar, S.H.; Holford, T.R.; Levy, D.T.; Long, C.Y.; Foy, M.; Clarke, L.; Jeon, J.; Hazelton, W.D.; Meza, R.; Schultz, F.; et al. Impact of reduced tobacco smoking on lung cancer mortality in the United States during 1975–2000. *J. Natl. Cancer Inst.* **2012**, *104*, 541–548. [CrossRef] [PubMed]
28. Plevritis, S.K.; Munoz, D.; Kurian, A.W.; Stout, N.K.; Alagoz, O.; Near, A.M.; Lee, S.J.; van den Broek, J.J.; Huang, X.; Schechter, C.B.; et al. Association of screening and treatment with breast cancer mortality by molecular subtype in US women, 2000–2012. *JAMA* **2018**, *319*, 154–164. [CrossRef] [PubMed]

29. Bibbins-Domingo, K.; Coxson, P.; Pletcher, M.J.; Lightwood, J.; Goldman, L. Adolescent overweight and future adult coronary heart disease. *New Eng. J. Med.* **2007**, *357*, 2371–2379. [CrossRef]
30. Najafzadeh, M.; Marra, C.A.; Lynd, L.D.; Sadatsafavi, M.; FitzGerald, J.M.; McManus, B.; Sin, D. Future impact of various interventions on the burden of COPD in Canada: A dynamic population model. *PLoS ONE* **2012**, *7*, e46746. [CrossRef]

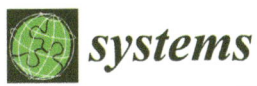

Article

Exploring the Impacts of COVID-19 on Coastal Tourism to Inform Recovery Strategies in Nelson Mandela Bay, South Africa

Estee Vermeulen-Miltz [1,2,*], Jai Kumar Clifford-Holmes [1,3], Bernadette Snow [1,2] and Amanda Talita Lombard [1]

1 Institute for Coastal and Marine Research, Nelson Mandela University, Gqeberha 6001, South Africa
2 One Ocean Hub, University of Strathclyde, Glasgow G1 1XQ, UK
3 Institute for Water Research, Rhodes University, Makhanda 6139, South Africa
* Correspondence: esteever01@gmail.com

Abstract: Globally, the COVID-19 pandemic bought devastating impacts to multiple economic sectors, with a major downfall observed in the tourism sector owing to explicit travel bans on foreign and domestic tourism. In Nelson Mandela Bay (NMB), South Africa, tourism plays an important role; however, negative effects from the pandemic and resulting restrictions has left the sector dwindling and in need of a path to recovery. Working together with local government and stakeholders, this study applied system dynamics modelling to investigate the impacts of COVID-19 on coastal tourism in NMB to provide decision-support and inform tourism recovery strategies. Through model analysis, a suite of management interventions was tested under two 'what-if' scenarios, with reference to the business-as-usual governance response scenario. Scenario one specifically aimed to investigate a desirable tourism recovery strategy assuming governance control, whereas scenario two investigated a scenario where the effects of governance responses were impeded on by the exogenous effects from the virus. Results suggest that uncertainty remained prevalent in the trajectory of the infection rate as well as in associated trends in tourism; however, through the lifting of travel restrictions and the continual administration of vaccines, a path to recovery was shown to be evident.

Keywords: COVID-19; tourism recovery; public policy; system dynamics; participatory modelling

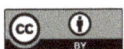

1. Introduction

The COVID-19 pandemic, and its subsequent lockdowns, was a severe shock to the global economy. After the initial spread of the virus from its origin in China, governments around the world started to respond, some more cautiously and hastily than others, in an effort to combat the spread of the virus. Despite interventions, a continual rise in infection rates led to the declaration of a global pandemic by the World Health Organisation (WHO) in March 2020. Thereafter, stricter government interventions through national lockdowns were introduced to assist in 'flattening the infection curve'. Though the national lockdowns were introduced with good intent to help 'save lives', the strict restrictions caused devastating impacts on the global economy. This effect was exacerbated in South Africa (SA) and locally in Nelson Mandela Bay (NMB), the focus area of this study, where the economy was previously strained by slow economic growth and social imbalances [1]. Multiple sectors have been devasted by the impacts of COVID-19, with many countries experiencing large contractions in Gross Domestic Product (GDP) and a consequential decline in employment levels [2]. It has been projected that the tourism sector will be one of the most affected by the pandemic, with devastating impacts that have never been observed before. Globally, COVID-19 caused a ~70% decrease in international tourism, return to the levels of 30 years ago, a significantly greater reduction than what was observed during the SARS virus in 2003 or the global economic recession in 2009, which resulted in contractions of ~0.4% and ~4%, respectively [2,3]. Economies slowly started to recover in 2021 owing to the lift of 'lockdown' restrictions in response to the administration of vaccines; however, sectors such as tourism, that were less resilient to the exogenous shock of the pandemic, are still experiencing negative effects, with remaining uncertainty concerning the rate of recovery to pre-pandemic levels.

In SA, and at a local scale, in NMB, uncertainty around recovery has manifested throughout in the tourism sector. Tourism plays an important role in the metro, with a total economic contribution (direct and induced) of ~R14 billion in 2019 (~11% of GDP), and employs a total of 98,000 persons, with the largest contribution coming from domestic tourism [4]. As a result of the pandemic, in reference to 2019, the metro experienced a 72% and 45% contraction in foreign and domestic tourists, respectively, followed by a 61% decrease in bednight sales and a 37% decline in direct tourism spend [4]. To 'control' COVID-19 transmission in SA, the government adopted an adaptive risk reduction strategy based on a five-level alert system, with level five corresponding to the strictest level of restrictions (i.e., national lockdown). The restrictions, particularly those associated with public movement, drastically impacted domestic and foreign tourism, where provincial travel was only permitted for levels one and two, and foreign travel only at level one, notwithstanding individual country's travel ban thresholds. Additional restrictions including beach closures and accommodation capacity limitations further affected coastal tourism in the bay. Moreover, the trajectory of COVID-19 infections influenced travelers' behaviour patterns through changes in the perception of the susceptibility and severity of the situation [5]. This study therefore highlights the need for tourism stakeholders and related government authorities to understand the knock-on effects arising from COVID-19 and associated feedback processes to facilitate and enable sustainable tourism recovery.

The temporal nature underlying the impacts of COVID-19 on tourism, and the associated uncertainty regarding tourism recovery, makes it particularly amenable to the method of system dynamics modelling (SDM). SDM is a structured approach to systems thinking that involves mapping, modelling, and managing complex and dynamic problems [6]. The method has proven to be advantageous for policy makers to gain a holistic overview of the problem and recognise key feedback effects and time delays through analytical decision support. SDM has been widely applied in the field of epidemiology [7] and recently used to explore questions related to COVID-19 and the underlying social responses and consequential impacts. Different models have been applied to different regions and contexts and to address different questions. For example, SDM was applied to investigate the evolution of COVID-19 infection waves and societal responses at a global scale [8,9]. Similarly, Ibarra-Vega [10] and Sy et al. [11] assessed COVID-19 outbreak responses to various containment policies. SDM as a method has also been proven suitable for application in tourism management and planning [12–15]. In combination, a few simulation-based studies have been applied to explore tourism re-opening strategies amid COVID-19 [16,17] and specifically to investigate the impacts on coastal tourism [18]. The application of SDM has therefore proven to be particularly useful to explore the complex infection dynamics and to understand impacts on tourism over time by providing a virtual environment to simulate and test recovery strategies.

This study aimed to develop a system dynamics model to simulate the impacts of COVID-19 on coastal tourism in NMB, in order to provide decision-support and to inform recovery strategies. This entailed:

- Exploring the implications of COVID-19 on the tourism sector by **mapping the cause-and-effect** problem dynamics;
- Identifying **key model variables** that could serve as **leverage points** for potential management interventions;
- Simulating **scenarios** of how different management interventions can facilitate sustainable recovery of the tourism sector.

2. Methods: System Analysis and Simulation Design

System dynamics modelling (SDM) was applied in this study. Model development consisted of conceptualisation, model formulation, and model testing, in line with SDM best practices [19,20]. Model conceptualisation involved desktop research and stakeholder engagement, where Causal Loop Diagramming (CLD) was applied as a tool to facilitate stakeholder engagement and to capture multiple perspectives. The stakeholders involved in the process included representatives from the tourism sector, local government, accommodation groups, and local tourism operators. The meeting process was divided into three stages held between September 2021 and February 2022. The processes consisted of individual stakeholder meetings (to capture stakeholders' 'mental models') and two group modelling workshops: the first aimed at presenting the model results and discussing relevant scenarios and the second focused on discussing leverage points and management interventions from the stance of the local municipality. A more comprehensive overview of the stakeholder engagement process is available in [21]. Thereafter, model formulation entailed formulating the stock–flow diagrams (SFDs) with associated algebraic equations and parameters values. Finally, model testing was performed through a series of validation tests to build confidence in the model structure and behaviour (see Section 2.3).

2.1. Model Boundary

The model boundary was drawn by collating information from the literature and stakeholder conversations into a holistic CLD. This included identifying and mapping the common causal links that capture the dynamics associated with the impacts of COVID-19 on coastal tourism in the bay. The boundary map shows the causal links and feedback loops between the key model variables. These feedback loops are described in more detail below (Figure 1 and Table 1).

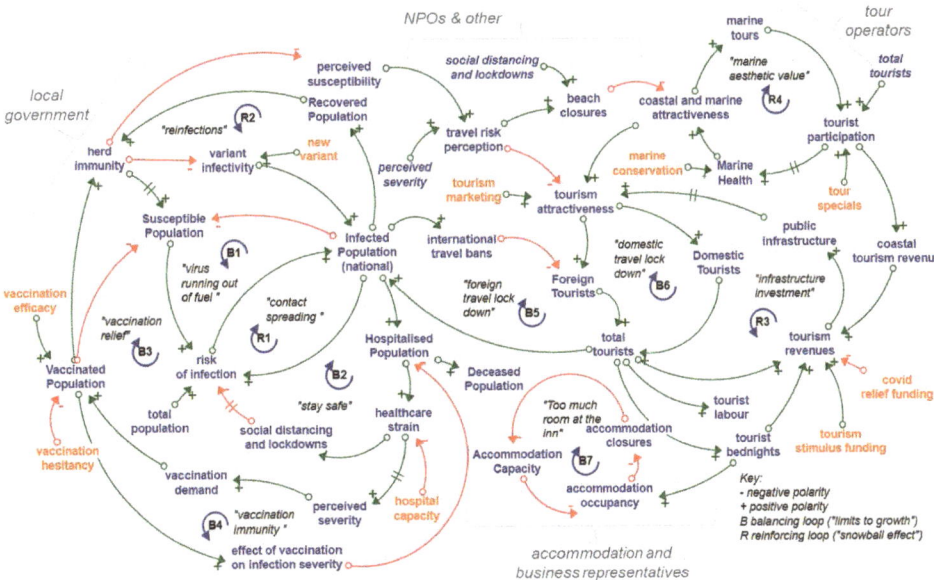

Figure 1. Casual map (or Casual-Loop-Diagram) illustrating the key model variables and feedback loops making up the model structure. Positive arrows (in green) represent a positive polarity and negative arrows (in red) represent a negative polarity; 'B' represents a balancing (negative) loop and 'R' represents a reinforcing (positive) loop. Orange variables show the suggested leverage points. Grey boxes illustrate areas of input from different stakeholder groups.

Table 1. Description of the balancing and reinforcing feedback loops affecting model behaviour. The sequence of variables in each loop is described, where a plus corresponds to a positive polarity and a minus a negative polarity.

Feedback Loop	Feedback Loop Description
Balancing Feedback Loops	
B1 "virus running out of fuel" *(infected − susceptible + risk of infection + infected)*	The "virus running out of fuel" balancing loop explains how the infection population decreases as the susceptible population decreases, thus limiting the number of infection cases. More susceptible persons, more infections, more infections, less susceptible people.
B2 "stay safe" *(infected + hospitalised + healthcare strain + social restrictions − risk of infection + infected)*	"Stay safe" demonstrates how a reduction in social contacts through lockdown and social distancing regulations reduces the risk of infection, which decreases the infected population. More infections, more social restrictions, lower risk of infection, lower infected population.
B3 "vaccination relief" *(infected + hospitalised + healthcare strain + perceived severity +vaccination demand + vaccinated − susceptible + risk of infection + infected)*	This loop shows that more infected cases result in a higher vaccination demand, which in turn may increase the number of vaccinated persons, which reduces the susceptible population vulnerable to being infected.
B4 "vaccination immunity" *(hospitalised + healthcare strain + perceived severity + vaccination demand + vaccinated − infection severity + hospitalised)*	The "vaccination immunity loop" captures the effects of decreased severity and hospitalisations as the vaccinated population increases.
B5 "foreign travel lock-down" *(infected + international travel ban − foreign tourists + infected)*	The foreign and domestic tourism lockdown loops explain how the number of infected cases decreases the number of foreign and domestic tourists due to various travel restrictions. This results in less movement from tourists and, hence, the risk of infection transmission.
B6 "domestic travel lock-down" *(infected + perceived severity + travel risk − tourism attractiveness + domestic tourists + infected)*	
B7 "too much room at the inn" *(accommodation occupancy − closures − capacity − occupancy)*	This loop explains how a low accommodation occupancy can result in more accommodation closures, which in turn decreases tourism accommodation capacity, which increases the accommodation occupancy fraction across the metro.
Reinforcing feedback loops	
R1 "contact spreading" *(infected + risk of infection + infected)*	Contact spreading explains that more infected persons can increase the risk of infection, transmission of the infection, and, hence, the number of infections. However, this loop is counteracted on by the 'virus running out of fuel' balancing loop.
R2 "reinfections" *(infected + recovered + herd immunity + susceptible + risk of infection + infected)*	The "reinfections loop" shows the reinforcing effect, where those who have recovered from infection or who were vaccinated become susceptible again after the assumed immunity delay.
R3 "tourism infrastructure investment" *(tourism attractiveness + tourists + revenues + public infrastructure + tourism attractiveness)*	The tourism infrastructure investment loop shows that an increase in tourism can increase the tourism budget, which can result in higher investment in public and tourism infrastructure, which can increase the attractiveness of tourism and hence the number of tourists.
R4 "marine aesthetic beauty" *(coastal and marine attractiveness + marine tours + tourist participation + marine health awareness + marine health + attractiveness)*	"Nature showing off" explains how a healthy marine environment can increase the level of participation in coastal and marine activities, which can result in a higher awareness of the natural value of the bay and a greater awareness of the need to protect this natural value.

2.2. Model Structure

The model is divided into three sub-models: (1) COVID-19 infection dynamics; (2) tourism dynamics of NMB; (3) coastal tourism impacts (Figure 2). Figure 2 shows that COVID-19 affects tourism, which in turn affects COVID-19 infection dynamics. Similarly, tourism affects coastal tourism activities, which in turn affects the attractiveness of tourism in NMB. A simplified overview of the sub-model structures is shown below (Figures 3–5). The model was built in Stella® Architect software [22]. It simulates the dynamics over a five-year period, from January 2019 to December 2023, using a daily time scale and the Euler integration method. The model was parameterised with data and information obtained from scientific literature, news articles, and stakeholders. Additional information on model documentation is available in the supplementary materials (Tables S1 and File S1).

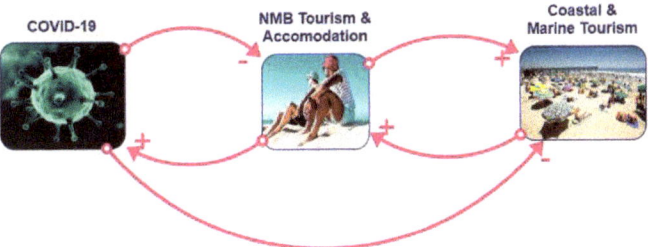

Figure 2. Holistic model structure showing the links between the three submodels.

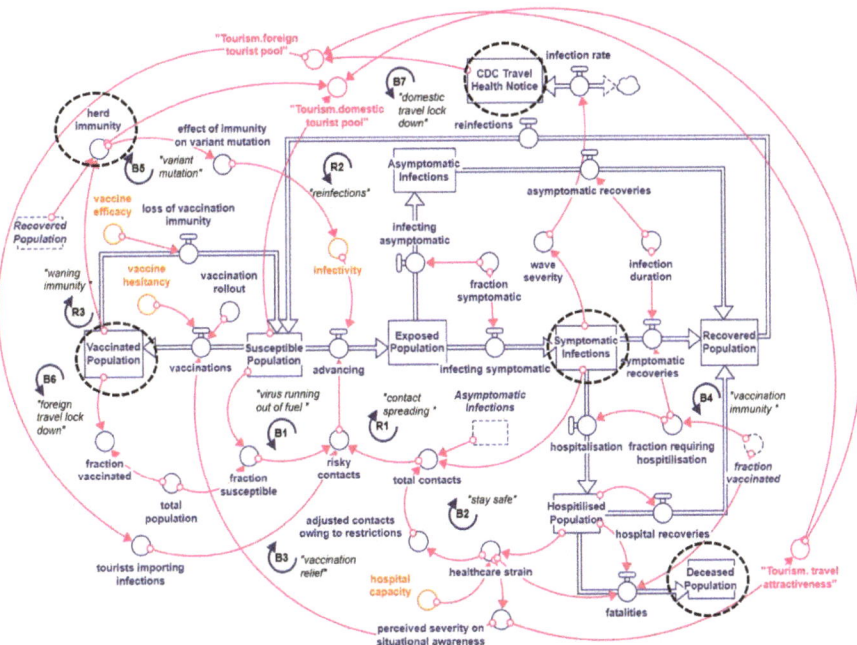

Figure 3. Simplified stock–flow diagram showing the main model variables that were formulated to simulate the COVID-19 infection dynamics at a national scale. Encircled variables represent the key output variables of interest, which were chosen based on their importance for decision-making and policy analysis. Variables in pink are those connected to another sub-model, and orange variables are applied in scenario analysis or in the visual user interface. This structure also applies to Figures 4 and 6 below.

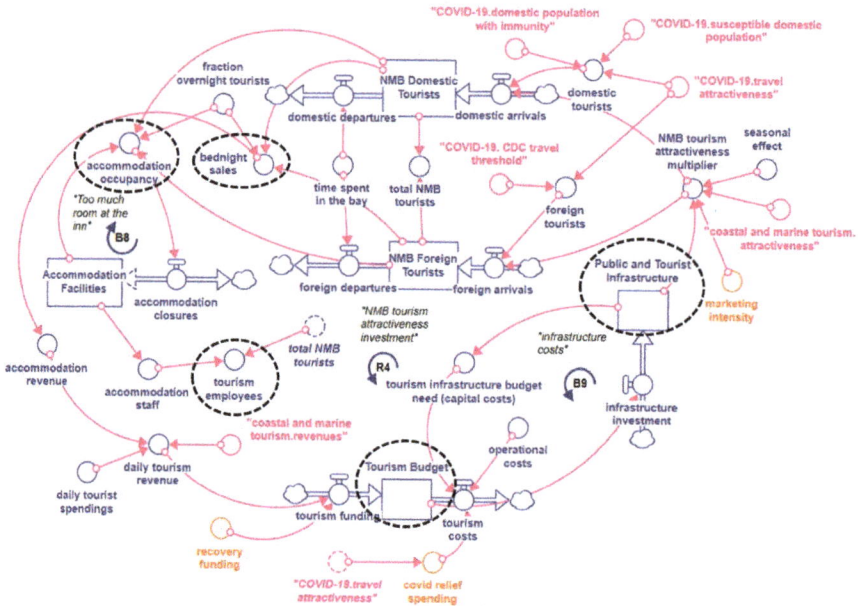

Figure 4. Stock–flow diagram showing the main model variables that were formulated to capture the impacts of COVID-19 on tourism in Nelson Mandela Bay (NMB).

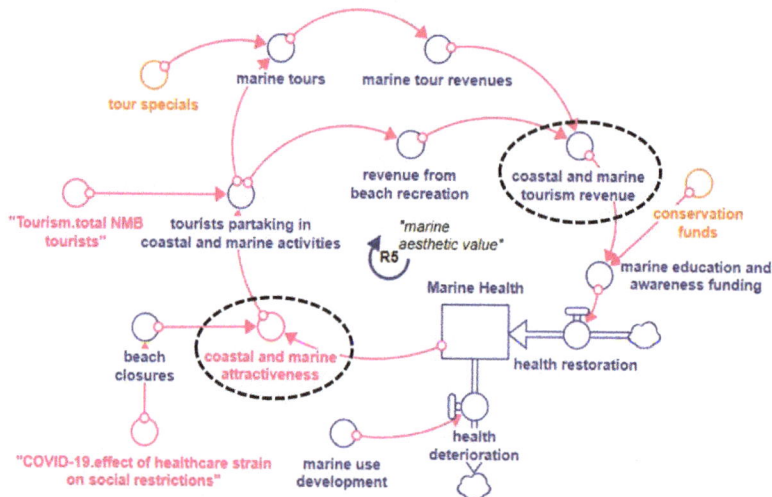

Figure 5. Stock–flow diagram showing the main model variables that were formulated to capture the impacts of COVID-19 on coastal and marine tourism activities.

2.2.1. COVID-19 Sub-Model Structure

COVID-19 Infection Dynamics

The COVID-19 sub-model captures the infection dynamics at a national scale, given that government decisions regarding the pandemic were initially based on country-level statistics, which in turn were enforced in provincial and local regions (Figure 3). The model is based on the Susceptible–Exposed–Infected–Recovered (SEIR) structure, which is commonly applied in epidemiology [7–9]. The COVID-19 infection is initiated by an imported infection at the beginning of 2020 through foreign tourists. Thereafter, the infection dynamics are formulated such that the *Susceptible Population* (60 million persons) flows into the *Exposed Population* depending on the *infectivity* of the virus, which can depend on the variant of the virus. In the model, the infectivity is estimated to be 0.0125 dmnl, so as to obtain a reproduction factor between 3 and 5 dmnl, depending on the number of social contacts (~14 persons/person/day) and duration of the infection (~14 days) [23]. After an incubation delay of approximately ~5 days [8,10], the exposed population then becomes either *symptomatically* or *asymptomatically* infectious. According to [24], it has been found, based on seroprevalence estimates (i.e., SARS-CoV-2 antibody positivity among the population), that, for every reported, case there are approximately nine asymptomatic cases (and hence unreported). This has particularly increased uncertainty regarding transmission of the virus among asymptomatic infectious and susceptible persons. Depending on the *infection duration*, asymptomatic and symptomatic persons recover, except for the severe symptomatic cases (~15–20% [25]) that are admitted to hospital. Further, depending on the fatality of the virus (~3–5% [10]), the *hospitalised population* can recover or become deceased, where the *fatality fraction* is subject to the level of healthcare strain, defined by hospital capacity (i.e., intensive care (ICU) beds = 3000 persons; [1,26]). Based on the level of health care strain, decisions are made based on the severity of the infection trend and hence the level of social restrictions, which, in turn, are intended to decrease the number of social contacts to slow transmission of the virus. In order to 'control' infection trends in the model (i.e., decrease transmission), the process of *vaccination* is introduced, which ultimately 'drains' the *susceptible population* stock, at least for the period of vaccine efficacy. The model does not differentiate between different types of vaccines or differences in vaccine efficacy, though this may be important to consider for future work. Nor does the model differentiate between the effectiveness of infection-induced immunity against vaccination immunity, as suggested in [27], but rather assumes that the recovered and vaccinated population may become susceptible again after 180 days (6 months) [28,29] in the absence of an immune-escaping variant. Therefore, the effects of vaccination are formulated with the purpose of decreasing the level of hospitalisations and fatalities, and to achieve 'heard immunity' (i.e., ~70% of the population with immune response either from vaccination or recovery from previous infection as defined by WHO) such that the likelihood of mutation and infection is decreased. The rate of vaccination is affected by a daily (initial) vaccination goal of ~300,000 persons/day [30], which is formulated through a step function starting in March 2021 and changes depending on *vaccination demand*, which is dependent on the *perceived severity* induced through the level of *healthcare strain*. Lastly, the rate of vaccination is constrained by *vaccination hesitancy*, which has been shown to range between 50 and 70% [31] on the basis of cultural grounds, or from being unaware, apathetic, or misinformed [32].

Effects of COVID-19 on Tourism Behaviour

The national infection trends and wave severity further impact tourism demand in NMB, with different effects for foreign and domestic tourism behaviour (Figures 3 and 5). Foreign travel risk is formulated by applying the formula that was developed by the Centres for Disease Control and Prevention (CDC). This calculates the *travel health threshold*, which is based on the cumulative infection incidence per 100,000 individuals of the population over a consecutive 28-day period [33]. Then, according to the four-level system criteria of the CDC, reported numbers above 500 persons categorise countries on the red list and prohibit travel, whereas reported figures below 500 gradually lowers restrictions. Therefore, in the model, *foreign tourism* depends on the number of tourists that normally visit SA per year (10.2 million in 2019 [34]), subject to the current travel restriction level. In contrast, *domestic tourism* in SA is formulated through a *domestic tourism pool*, which is represented by the populations that are assumed to have 'herd immunity', as they are assumed to be more willing to travel. The portion of the population that are less likely to travel are those that remain susceptible and are therefore still affected by the perceived risk of travel emanating from trends in healthcare strain, which is expected to delay travel decisions by ~365 days. This logic was derived from an investigation conducted by [5], whereby changes in the infection rate directly affected the perceived severity of the situation, hence decreasing attractiveness of travel, whereas, understanding the chances of contracting the virus affected perceived susceptibility and the willingness to travel. This theory is in line with the concept of "risk habituation" by [35], whereby perceived risk decreases as threats decrease or becoming increasingly familiar. Variables associated with the effects of socio-economic uncertainty on one's willingness to travel are additionally considered to be relevant to the problem context but have been excluded from the model boundary during the current analysis and can be considered for future adaptations.

2.2.2. Tourism Sub-Model Structure

NMB Tourism and Accommodation

In NMB, there are two stocks of tourists, namely *domestic* and *foreign tourists*, initialised to 2019 data (Figure 4). The number of tourists, both foreign and domestic, is dependent on the attractiveness of NMB as a tourist destination, which depends on factors such as seasonality, tourism infrastructure, the attractiveness of coastal and marine activities, and, finally, the effects on travel emanating from the COVID-19 infection rate (Figures 3 and 4). Regardless of the purpose for travel, tourists are typically in the bay for short trips (~3 days for domestic tourists and ~2 days for foreigners [36]). The number of tourists staying in paid accommodation at any time (~36% for domestic tourists and 50% for foreign tourists), relative to the number of accommodation facilities (~400 facilities) and accommodation capacity (~15,000 persons), determines the level of *accommodation occupancy*. The number of bednights sold multiplied by the average rate per night (~R600 person/day) further contributes to local tourism revenue, in addition to those obtained from daily tourist spending (~R800–R1500/person/day [36]) and revenue from coastal and marine activities. It is then assumed that a fraction of total tourism revenues (~20%), collected through tourist taxes and levies, contributes towards the local municipal tourism budget. A higher tourism budget is required to increase tourism attractiveness through local investments in public and tourism infrastructure; however, degrading infrastructure simultaneously increases expenditure, in addition to operational costs and costs associated with COVID-relief funding during the periods of travel restriction. Lastly, tourism labour is assumed to increase in relation to the number of tourists visiting the bay, assuming 1 employee for every 40 tourists, calculated according to the number of employees in the sector obtained from [37,38]. In the tourism sub-model, the main variables of interest are the total number of *bednights sold*; *accommodation occupancy*; the *total number of tourists*; the *tourism budget*; *tourism employees*; and the state of *tourist infrastructure*. These variables have been identified in the literature, as well as by stakeholders, to be particularly important as indicators with which to measure the impacts of COVID-19 on the tourism sector (Figure 4).

Coastal Tourism Dynamics

The coastal tourism sub-model specifically aims to capture the knock-on effects on beach recreation and marine tour participation and associated revenues (Figure 5). As reported in [38,39], coastal and marine tourism attracts approximately 55% of visiting tourists through beach recreation alone. The normal coastal and marine attractiveness factor is largely dependent on the marine aesthetic value of the bay, which is formulated through a stock variable "*Marine health*". Marine health is, however, subject to changes in the rate of cumulative pressure from other marine developments in the bay [40] (Figure 5). Next, marine wildlife tours are considered an attractive marine activity [41], with the number of tour participants affected by the *attractiveness of marine wildlife tours* [42] and *tour costs*. The number of tourists engaging in coastal and marine activities and a portion of the revenues obtained can be considered valuable in creating marine awareness and funding conservation activities aimed at conserving *marine health*. All the same, the impacts that arose directly from the pandemic included beach closures and the closure of beach establishments [43]. This decreased the overall attractiveness of coastal and marine tourism, largely decreasing the number of tourists visiting the bay, with consequences on tourism accommodation, revenue, and labour (Figure 5).

2.3. Model Testing

As the study was undertaken simultaneous to the evolving dynamics of the COVID-19 pandemic, model validation was a continuous and iterative process. This involved comparing the model data to available observational data to determine the 'goodness of fit' and assisted in manually calibrating the model to verify the estimated model parameters. To verify the model behaviour, infection data for South Africa were sourced from Johns Hopkins University and compared to model results (Figure 6a). To calculate the 'goodness of fit' between the observed and model data, the model data were exported and the coefficient of determination, a measure of the data variance, was calculated in Microsoft Excel. According to the final baseline run, the model explains 73% of the data variance of the observed COVID-19 infections, measured according to the seven-day-moving average (Figure 6a). The model was first validated in October 2021, before the onset of the fourth wave associated with the Omicron variant. According to the outdated model run (October version), the projected simulation suggested that SA may experience a fourth wave over the December 2021 holiday period, albeit with a smaller amplitude (Figure 6b). This projection was consistent with the projection from the SA COVID-19 Ministerial Advisory Committee, which reported that "the fourth wave will likely be a small mini wave", and that the severity of the fourth wave depends on a balance between the prospects of a new immune-escaping variant versus vs. the rate of vaccination by this time [24]. After observing changes in the reported infections during the fourth wave, the model structure and assumptions were re-evaluated and adjusted accordingly.

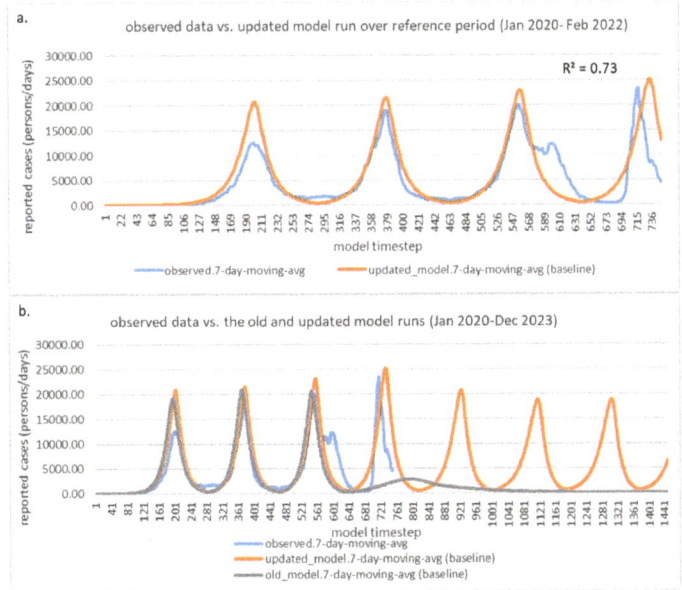

Figure 6. Behaviour over time graphs of the seven-day-moving average of infections in South Africa (persons/days) over the reference period (January 2020–November 2021 or 664 days) (**a**) and for the projected model period (December 2023 or 1444 days) (**b**). Model results are shown in orange and observed data obtained from Our World in Data are shown in blue.

To validate trends in tourism at a local scale, observed data in accommodation occupancy from 2019 to 2021 were compared with the modelled occupancy data. Stakeholders specifically suggested the validation of trends in tourism one-year prior to the onset of the pandemic to verify the model against trends observed 'normally'. The data were made available to the study by the Nelson Mandela Bay Municipality (NMBM), the Department of Economic Development, Tourism and Agriculture, and were recommended as an effective indicator with which to measure tourism variability at a local scale [4].

Baseline results show that the modelled accommodation occupancy captures 71% of the variance of the observed data (Figure 7). Additional testing included running extreme parameter tests and ensuring that the model was dimensionally consistent and structurally robust. Finally, a multivariate sensitivity analyses, using the Latin Hypercube Sampling method, was performed over 50 runs to investigate changes in model behaviour under a combination of parameter values. The parameter values of the included model variables were varied by 50% of the baseline value, as suggested in [19] (Table A1). Results of the multivariate sensitivity analysis are shown in Appendix A (Figure A1). As expected, the extreme conditions tests and multivariate sensitivity analysis revealed variability in the model results, though the results remained robust and behaviourally sound.

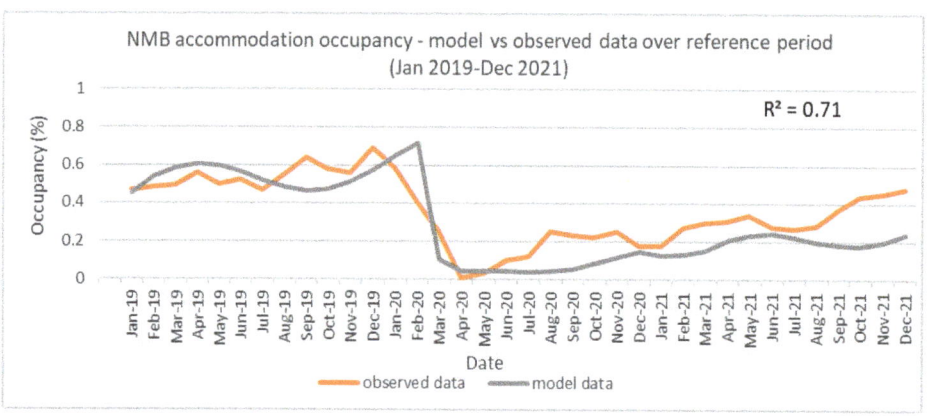

Figure 7. Nelson Mandela Bay accommodation occupancy levels as observed (in orange) and simulated in the model (in grey) from January 2019 to December 2021.

3. Results

3.1. Model Scenarios

Once the model was considered to be sufficiently robust (i.e., it performed the right behaviour for the right reasons), scenario planning was performed. This consisted of testing the model results under two scenarios compared to the baseline (or business-as-usual (BAU)) scenario. The BAU scenario captures the infection trends and projected tourism recovery under current governance decision-making strategies as formulated in the model. As for the two exploratory scenarios, scenario one investigates a desirable tourism recovery strategy, assuming that the government has control of the situation, through enabling a rapid vaccination rollout process, securing efficacious vaccines, and ensuring effective tourism management. In contrast, scenario two portrays a situation of governance instability, whereby uncertainty regarding the infection trajectory, owing to high levels of vaccination hesitancy, risks of an immune-escaping variants, and a lax tourism response strategy leads to a less desirable recovery trajectory.

Table 2 shows the variables and associated parameter values that were varied during the scenario analysis. 'Vaccination acceptance' corresponds to the fraction of the population accepting the vaccination, and 'vaccination efficacy' corresponds to the probability of losing immunity after the assumed period of 180 days (or 6 months) [28]. The intervention 'government response time' corresponds to the time delay for government to respond to the severity of the pandemic and implement social restrictions, and changes to the 'ICU capacity' can affect the level of healthcare strain and, ultimately, fatalities. In the tourism sub-model, the 'CDC travel limit' corresponds to the threshold by which foreign travel becomes prohibited, and 'marketing intensity' refers to a change in marketing campaigns. Then, the 'fraction of funds to COVID relief' is the portion of the tourism budget that is diverted towards COVID-related costs, implementation, and business support and, lastly, 'infrastructure upgrade costs' refers to the minimum costs associated to small infrastructure upgrades that can contribute towards tourism attractiveness.

Table 2. Key variables and associated parameter values applied in the scenario analysis.

Model Parameter and Unit	Base Value–Business as Usual	Scenario 1–Governance Control	Scenario 2–Governance Instability
COVID-19 Interventions			
Vaccination acceptance (dmnl) (opposite to hesitancy)	0.50	0.80	0.40
Vaccination efficacy (immunity duration) (dmnl)	180	270	90
Government response time (days)	30	15	40
ICU capacity (persons)	3000	4000	2500
Tourism Interventions			
CDC travel limit (persons)	500	1000	800
Marketing intensity (%)	1	1.2	1
Fraction of tourism budget to COVID relief (%)	1	0.3	0.4
Infrastructure upgrade costs (R)	3×10^6	2×10^6	4×10^6

For the COVID-19 sub-model, the results of the scenario analysis were specifically investigated in terms of the COVID-19 infection rate and the number of vaccinated persons in SA (Figure 8). Furthermore, to investigate the impacts of COVID-19 on coastal tourism, results were analysed in terms of the total number of bednights sold in NMB, accommodation occupancy, tourism infrastructure condition, and coastal tourism attractiveness (Figure 9). Though other indicators such as tourism revenues and tourism employment are also important, these results are not shown; however, it is expected that changes in these indicators are primarily driven through changes in the number of tourists. Under the baseline simulation, the model shows three consecutive infection peaks corresponding to the results showed in the observed data, in addition to a fourth peak around December 2021, with a maximum of ~25,000 persons/days (Figures 6 and 8a). Moreover, Figure 8b shows the number of vaccinated persons (assuming full vaccination) to reach approximately 18 million by February 2022, though this tends to level off, as the portion of the population that is willing to accept the vaccine becomes vaccinated and, due to decreasing vaccination demand.

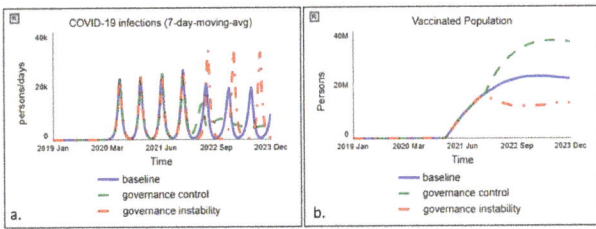

Figure 8. Model results of the infectious cases (persons/days) (a) and vaccinated population (persons) (b) under three scenarios. The baseline run (or business-as-usual scenario) is shown in solid blue, scenario one in dashed green lines, and scenario two in dot-dashed red.

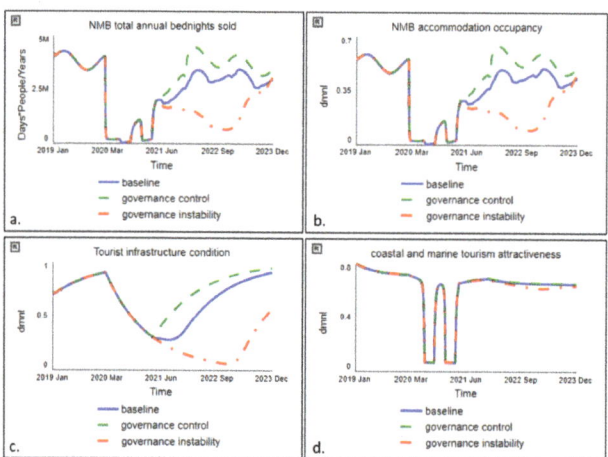

Figure 9. Model results of the total number of tourist bednight sales in NMB (people.days/years) (**a**) and associated tourism indicators: accommodation occupancy (dmnl) (**b**), tourist infrastructure condition (dmnl) (**c**) and coastal marine attractiveness (dmnl) (**d**) under three model scenarios. The baseline run (or business-as-usual scenario) is shown in solid-blue, scenario one in dashed green lines and two in dot-dashed red.

Trends in NMB tourism show a sharp decrease in the numbers of bednights sold during the 'midst' of the pandemic, when foreign and domestic travel was prohibited, as well as when NMB was declared a national COVID-19 hotspot in December 2020, leading to subsequent beach closures (Figure 9a) [44]. Similarly, the trend in accommodation occupancy decreased to as low as 1% in April 2020 and is slowly recovering to levels around 35–40% from mid-2021, in line with observed results and stakeholder perspectives (Figures 7 and 9b). Figure 9c,d shows the projected impacts of the pandemic on public and tourism infrastructure condition, which is shown to decreases over the period of the pandemic owing to a lack of tourism revenue and a diminishing tourism budget. The condition of tourist infrastructure is, however, projected to increase as tourists slowly return; however, this is dependent on the magnitude of upgrades, associated costs, and delays in initiating upgrades. Lastly, Figure 9d shows the level of participation in coastal tourism, with two evident dips in attractiveness corresponding to the time of beach closures, which drastically reduced the attractiveness of beach recreation during this time.

Results from scenario 1 illustrate a more desirable recovery trajectory, as shown in terms of the infection rate as well as in NMB tourism, with the former showing smaller infection peaks from February 2022 to December 2023 and the latter showing a visible increase in the number of tourists and bednights sold from October 2021 onwards, with trends in occupancy recovering to pre-pandemic levels in early 2022 (Figures 8 and 9a,b). Figure 9c,d show that tourist infrastructure condition is also expected to recover with the return of tourists, and that no more beach closures can be expected, possibly owing to the adaptations to the levels of social restrictions due to increasing immunity. The results from scenario 2,show an increase in wave peaks, with a fifth peak expected over June 2022, followed by additional waves owed to low levels of immunity among the population as well an increased risk of breakthrough infections (Figure 8a,b). Trends in NMB tourism and accommodation concurrently take a longer time to recover to levels observed in 2019 in this scenario, with projected knock-on effects on the state of local tourism infrastructure further inhibiting future tourism growth (Figure 9a–d). Both scenarios show how the beach closures drastically impacted coastal tourism attractiveness during the periods of infection peaks; however, as social restrictions were relaxed, coastal and marine tourism attractiveness recovered (Figure 9d). Furthermore, the effect of marine health on coastal tourism attractiveness is less evident in the results, owing to a longer delay associated with changes in marine health.

3.2. Model Interface

An additional output from the study is the model visual user interface (VUI) (Figure 10), which provides a 'user-friendly' portal to engage with the model. Decision-makers or stakeholders can unravel the cause-and-effect model structure and explore model scenarios by adjusting the model variables through 'levers' on the interface. Additional variables (e.g., variant infectivity, variant introduction time) are additionally included to investigate the impacts of future variants on the resilience of tourism recovery strategies. The VUI can additionally be used in a collaborative stakeholder setting, whereby stakeholders representing different institutions or areas of the problem can implement alternative management interventions to investigate tourism recovery strategies in NMB, similar to what was demonstrated during the group stakeholder workshops.

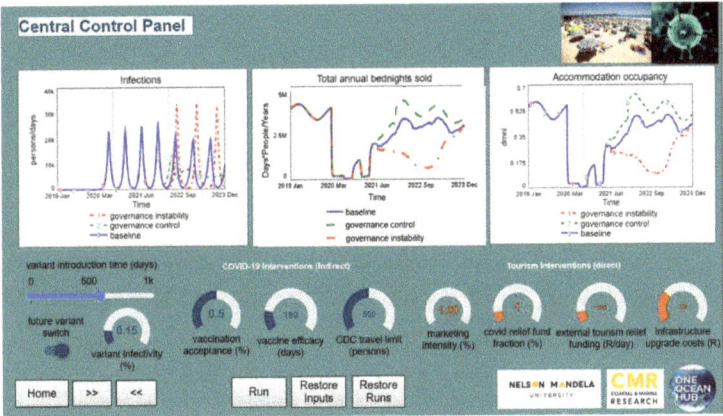

Figure 10. Central control panel in the visual user interface to enable additional scenario analyses. The interface is accessible through the following link: https://exchange.iseesystems.com/public/esteevermeulen/nelson-mandela-bay-covid-19---coastal-and-marine-tourism-recovery-tool (accessed on 8 July 2022).

4. Discussion: Recommendations and Policy Design

The scenario analysis that was performed to investigate the impacts of COVID-19 on coastal tourism in NMB highlighted the complexity and uncertainty that existed, and remains to exist, around projected infection trends, recovery delays, and vulnerabilities of the tourism sector to the effects of the COVID-19 pandemic (Figures 8 and 9). During the time of writing, the baseline simulation suggested that, under current governance response and vaccination rates, subsequent waves are expected with lower infection peaks and levels of severity in terms of healthcare strain and fatalities (Figures 8 and 9). While this may be logical, the projection relies on the assumption that current vaccinations are sufficiently effective against existing variants, though skepticism exists regarding the length of the immunity of current vaccinations (i.e., waning immunity) [45], as well as existing controversy surrounding mandatory vaccination protocols to overcome vaccination hesitancy [32,46]. Moreover, the analysis reveals that, even though government can adopt different means to respond, there can be scenarios where even strong response strategies may be weakened by factors beyond their control, such as by breakthrough infections owing to the introduction of immune-escaping variants, as shown by the recent Omicron variant [47].

Nonetheless, the model is an analytical tool with which to investigate uncertainty, such that governments could 'test' their strategies through 'what-if' scenarios in order to evaluate the resilience of their responses and, hence, the knock-on effects on the tourism sector. Moreover, the model demonstrated how the rate of tourism recovery is dependent on various feedback effects and the effectiveness of management interventions under alternative governance scenarios. The analysis has additionally highlighted that there is not necessarily only one response with which to assist in the recovery of coastal tourism in NMB, but rather multiple interventions, each with a different degree of leverage that could simultaneously be applied to achieve a more desirable trajectory. Such interventions could include, but are not limited to, the following:

- Rapid vaccination procurement and administration;
- Vaccination awareness and campaigns to address vaccination hesitancy;
- Research and development into vaccination efficacy;
- Adaptations to international travel limit thresholds recognising the need for personal responsibility and well-being relative to situational awareness;
- Allowing tourists to return to enhance tourism cash flow and the recovery of the tourism budget;
- Redirecting and possibly increasing the tourism budget towards public and tourism infrastructure to increase tourism attractiveness;
- Funding diversion towards tourism marketing to stimulate demand;
- Collaboration among local government directorates (tourism, public health, safety and security, infrastructure and engineering) to establish a consensus regarding departments' recovery mandates.

Lastly, there has been confusion regarding the levels of restrictions, which has contributed to the levels of social and sectoral adherence fatigue. Though the government has opted towards adaptive, risk-adverse strategies (as is required for a rapid response), adverse and sudden changes to COVID-19 regulations and decision-making thresholds has made it difficult for sectors to adapt. Therefore, governments should remain transparent about their decision-making criteria and develop decision frameworks that are informed through scientifically robust models and datasets.

5. Conclusions

This study highlights the importance of exploratory simulation to support decision-making. Using system dynamics modelling, this study investigated the impacts of COVID-19 on coastal tourism in Nelson Mandela Bay (NMB), South Africa, with the aim to devise and simulate the effects of potential recovery pathways. The model provided the means to simulate stakeholder's mental models under alternative scenarios to demonstrate how feedback behaviour and time delays can affect tourism recovery. Though the model boundary may be limited to this specific problem, the boundary may be adapted, and the assumptions adjusted, to explore similar policy questions in the future. This can include downscaling the model to investigate infection trends at a more local scale and the transmission of COVID-19 among tourists and the local population in NMB, as well as incorporating localised socio-economic impacts into the model boundary. Additional scenarios can also be tested to investigate the effectivity of recommended tourism policies to future variants. Finally, additional behavioural validation with updated tourism data could further improve the analysis. This study concludes that there are various levels of uncertainty that need to be considered during the development of a recovery plan for the tourism sector or any other economic sector in this regard, but that small changes in multiple interventions could result in more sustainable recovery pathways.

Supplementary Materials: The following supporting information can be downloaded at: https://www.mdpi.com/article/10.3390/systems10040120/s1. Table S1. Model Documentation. File S1. Model Equations.

Author Contributions: E.V.-M. was the lead modeler and author on this paper. J.K.C.-H. assisted in model development, stakeholder engagement and writing. A.T.L. and B.S. contributed to writing, editing and providing financial support. All authors have read and agreed to the published version of the manuscript.

Funding: This research was funded by the One Ocean Hub GCRF UKRI grant NE/S008950/1. Additional support and the APC was provided by the South African Research Chairs Initiative through the South African National Department of Science and Innovation/National Research Foundation, by a Community of Practice grant (UID: 110612).

Institutional Review Board Statement: The study was conducted in accordance with the Declaration of Helsinki and approved by the Ethics Committee of Nelson Mandela University (H20-BES-DEV-003) for studies involving stakeholder engagement.

Informed Consent Statement: Informed consent was obtained from all participants involved in the study.

Data Availability Statement: All data used in this study can be found at https://ourworldindata.org/explorers/coronavirus-data-explorer (accessed on 15 February 2022), and [48] or in indicated references. The model interface is accessible at https://exchange.iseesystems.com/public/esteevermeulen/nelson-mandela-bay-covid-19---coastal-and-marine-tourism-recovery-tool (accessed on 8 July 2022).

Acknowledgments: The authors wish to thank all involved stakeholder institutions for their participation in the study.

Conflicts of Interest: The authors declare no conflict of interest.

Appendix A

Table A1. Model variables and associated parameter values applied in the multivariate sensitivity analysis. Parameter values were varied by ±50% of the base value and simulated using a UNIFORM distribution.

COVID-19 Sub-Model	
Asymptomatic contacts	[7; 14; 21]
Infectivity	[0.00625; 0.0125; 0.01875]
Immunity duration	[90; 180; 270]
Vaccination hesitancy	[0.50; 0.70; 0.80]
Hospital capacity (change for scenarios)	[1500; 3000; 4500]
ICU fraction	[0.10; 0.20; 0.30]
Travel risk perception delay	[180; 365; 545]
Governance reaction time (time to perceive severity)	[15; 30; 45]
NMB Tourism & Accommodation Sub-Model	
Fraction of tourism revenues to NMB tourism budget	[0.10; 0.20; 0.30]
Operational costs fraction	[0.15; 0.3; 0.45]
Public and Tourist Infrastructure costs	[1.5×10^6; 3×10^6; 4.5×10^6]
Public and Tourist Infrastructure condition (t0)	[0.6; 0.8; 1]
Fraction of tourism budget to COVID-relief	[0.25; 0.5; 0.75]
Coastal Tourism Sub-Model	
Marine heath (t0)	[0.6; 0.8; 1]

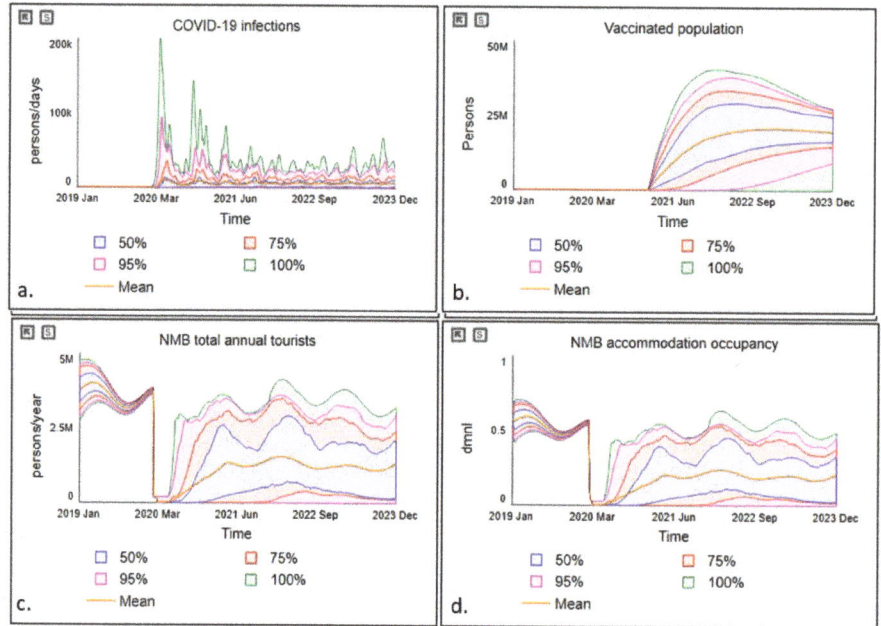

Figure A1. Outputs from the multivariate sensitivity analysis showing the variability in trends of infectious cases (persons/days) (**a**), vaccinated persons (persons) (**b**), the number of tourists visiting Nelson Mandela Bay (persons/year) (**c**), and accommodation occupancy levels (dmnl) (**d**). The confidence intervals represent the spread of uncertainty with 50% in blue, 75% in red, 95% in magenta, 100% in green, and the mean result in orange.

References

1. Schröder, M.; Bossert, A.; Kersting, M.; Aeffner, S.; Coetzee, J.; Timme, M.; Schlüter, J. COVID-19 in South Africa: Outbreak despite Interventions. *Nature Sci. Rep.* **2021**, *11*, 4956. [CrossRef] [PubMed]
2. UNCTAD. *COVID-19 and Tourism: Assessing the Economic Consequences*; UNCTAD: Geneva, Switzerland, 2020; Volume 9.
3. UNWTO. *COVID-19 and Tourism 2020: A Year in Review*; UNWTO: Madrid, Spain, 2020.
4. NMBM EDTA. *Nelson Mandela Bay Municipality—Economic Development, Tourism and Agriculture: Tourism Master Plan 2021–2030*; Gqeberha, South Africa, 2021. Available online: https://www.nelsonmandelabay.gov.za/DataRepository/Documents/2021-22-idp-adopted_6Mb5j.pdf (accessed on 25 February 2022).
5. Naseer, K.; Qazi, J.; Qazi, A.; Avuglah, B.K.; Tahir, R.; Rasheed, R.A.; Khan, S.K.; Khan, B.A.; Zeeshan, M.; Humayun, M.A.; et al. Travel Behaviour Prediction amid COVID-19 Underlaying Situational Awareness Theory and Health Belief Model. *Behav. Inf. Technol.* **2021**, 1–11. [CrossRef]
6. Richmond, B. Systems Thinking: Critical Thinking Skills for the 1990s and Beyond. *Syst. Dyn. Rev.* **1993**, *9*, 113–133. [CrossRef]
7. Homer, J.B.; Hirsch, G.B. System Dynamics Modeling for Public Health: Background and Opportunities. *Am. J. Public Health* **2006**, *96*, 452–458. [CrossRef] [PubMed]
8. Rahmandad, H.; Lim, T.Y.; Sterman, J. Behavioral Dynamics of COVID-19: Estimating Underreporting, Multiple Waves, and Adherence Fatigue across 92 Nations. *Syst. Dyn. Rev.* **2021**, *37*, 5–31. [CrossRef] [PubMed]
9. Struben, J. The Coronavirus Disease (COVID-19) Pandemic: Simulation-Based Assessment of Outbreak Responses and Postpeak Strategies. *Syst. Dyn. Rev.* **2020**, *36*, 247–293. [CrossRef]
10. Ibarra-Vega, D. Lockdown, One, Two, None, or Smart. Modeling Containing COVID-19 Infection. A Conceptual Model. *Sci. Total Environ.* **2020**, *730*, 138917. [CrossRef]
11. Sy, C.; Ching, P.M.; San Juan, J.L.; Bernardo, E.; Miguel, A.; Mayol, A.P.; Culaba, A.; Ubando, A.; Mutuc, J.E. Systems Dynamics Modeling of Pandemic Influenza for Strategic Policy Development: A Simulation-Based Analysis of the COVID-19 Case. *Process Integr. Optim. Sustain.* **2021**, *5*, 461–474. [CrossRef]
12. Sedarati, P.; Santos, S.; Pintassilgo, P. System Dynamics in Tourism Planning and Development. *Tour. Plan. Dev.* **2019**, *16*, 256–280. [CrossRef]
13. Kapmeier, F.; Gonçalves, P. Wasted Paradise? Policies for Small Island States to Manage Tourism-Driven Growth While Controlling Waste Generation: The Case of the Maldives. *Syst. Dyn. Rev.* **2018**, *34*, 172–221. [CrossRef]

14. Mai, T.; Smith, C. Scenario-Based Planning for Tourism Development Using System Dynamic Modelling: A Case Study of Cat Ba Island, Vietnam. *Tour. Manag.* **2018**, *68*, 336–354. [CrossRef]
15. Pizzitutti, F.; Walsh, S.J.; Rindfuss, R.R.; Gunter, R.; Quiroga, D.; Tippett, R.; Mena, C.F. Scenario Planning for Tourism Management: A Participatory and System Dynamics Model Applied to the Galapagos Islands of Ecuador. *J. Sustain. Tour.* **2017**, *25*, 1117–1137. [CrossRef]
16. Škare, M.; Soriano, D.R.; Porada-Rochoń, M. Impact of COVID-19 on the Travel and Tourism Industry. *Technol. Forecast. Soc. Change* **2021**, *163*, 120469. [CrossRef] [PubMed]
17. Zhong, L. A Dynamic Pandemic Model Evaluating Reopening Strategies amid COVID-19. *PLoS ONE* **2021**, *16*, e0248302. [CrossRef] [PubMed]
18. Gu, Y.; Onggo, B.S.; Kunc, M.H.; Bayer, S.; Gu, Y.; Onggo, B.S.; Kunc, M.H.; Bayer, S. Current Issues in Tourism Small Island Developing States (SIDS) COVID-19 Post-Pandemic Tourism Recovery: A System Dynamics Approach Small Island Developing States (SIDS) COVID-19 Post-Pandemic. *Curr. Issues Tour.* **2021**, *25*, 1481–1508. [CrossRef]
19. Ford, A. *Modelling the Environment*, 2nd ed.; Island Press: Washington, DC, USA, 2009.
20. Sterman, J.D. *Business Dynamics: Systems Thinking and Modeling for a Complex World*; McGraw-Hill Education: New York, NY, USA, 2010; ISBN 007238915X.
21. Vermeulen-Miltz, E.; Clifford-Holmes, J.K.; Snow, B.; Lombard, A.T. COVID-19 and Tourism Recovery in Nelson Mandela Bay, South Africa: A Participatory System Dynamics Approach. *J. Sustain. Tour.* **2022**. in review.
22. Richmond, B.; Peterson, S. *An Introduction to Systems Thinking, STELLA*; High Performing Systems, Inc.: Watkinsville, GA, USA, 2001; ISBN 0970492111.
23. Khairulbahri, M. Modeling the Effect of Asymptomatic Cases, Social Distancing, and Lockdowns in the First and Second Waves of the COVID-19 Pandemic: A Case Study of Italy. *SciMed. J.* **2021**, *3*, 265–273. [CrossRef]
24. Grant, L.; Otter, A.; Malan, M. How Do We Know If SA Is in a Third COVID-19 Wave—And Could There Be a Fourth? Mail Guardian. 9 June 2021. Available online: https://mg.co.za/coronavirus-essentials/2021-06-09-how-do-we-know-if-sa-is-in-a-third-covid-19-wave-and-could-there-be-a-fourth/ (accessed on 31 August 2021).
25. Li, Q.; Guan, X.; Wu, P.; Wang, X.; Zhou, L.; Tong, Y.; Ren, R.; Leung, K.S.M.; Lau, E.H.Y.; Wong, J.Y.; et al. Early Transmission Dynamics in Wuhan, China, of Novel Coronavirus–Infected Pneumonia. *N. Engl. J. Med.* **2020**, *382*, 1199–1207. [CrossRef]
26. Naidoo, R.; Naidoo, K. Prioritising 'Already-Scarce' Intensive Care Unit Resources in the Midst of COVID-19: A Call for Regional Triage Committees in South Africa. *BMC Med. Ethics* **2021**, *22*, 28. [CrossRef]
27. Brereton, C.; Pedercini, M. COVID-19 Case Rates in the UK: Modelling Uncertainties as Lockdown Lifts. *Systems* **2021**, *9*, 60. [CrossRef]
28. SAT, South African Tourism. *The Road to Recovery Report: South Africa Tourism*; SAT, South African Tourism: Johannesburg, South Africa, 2021; Volume 2.
29. Goldberg, Y.; Mandel, M.; Bar-On, Y.M.; Bodenheimer, O.; Freedman, L.; Haas, E.J.; Milo, R.; Alroy-Preis, S.; Ash, N.; Huppert, A. Waning Immunity after the BNT162b2 Vaccine in Israel. *N. Engl. J. Med.* **2021**, *385*, e85. [CrossRef] [PubMed]
30. Merten, M. South Africa Shifts the COVID-19 Vaccination Goal Posts to 70% of Adults by Christmas. Daily Maverick. 9 September 2021. Available online: https://www.dailymaverick.co.za/article/2021-09-09-south-africa-shifts-the-covid-19-vaccination-goal-posts-to-70-of-adults-by-christmas/ (accessed on 25 February 2022).
31. Ebrahim, Z. COVID-19: Three SA Experts Weigh in on Breakthrough Infections, Immunity, and Vaccine Hestiancy. News24 Health 2021. Available online: https://www.news24.com/health24/medical/infectious-diseases/coronavirus/to-vaccinate-or-not-to-vaccinate-against-covid-19-three-sa-experts-weigh-in-20210920-2 (accessed on 20 September 2021).
32. Mumtaz, N.; Green, C.; Duggan, J. Exploring the Effect of Misinformation on Infectious Disease Transmission. *Systems* **2022**, *10*, 50. [CrossRef]
33. CDC. *How CDC Determines the Level for COVID-19 Travel Health Notices*; CDC: Atlanta, GA, USA, 2021.
34. Stats, S.A. Tourism 2020. In *Report No. 03-51-02*; 2020; Volume 2. Available online: http://www.statssa.gov.za/publications/Report-03-51-02/Report-03-51-022020.pdf (accessed on 25 February 2022).
35. Raude, J.; MCColl, K.; Flamand, C.; Apostolidis, T. Understanding Health Behaviour Changes in Response to Outbreaks: Findings from a Longitudinal Study of a Large Epidemic of Mosquito-Borne Disease. *Soc. Sci. Med.* **2019**, *230*, 184–193. [CrossRef] [PubMed]
36. *NMBM EDTA Nelson Mandela Bay Tourism Statistics 2013–2019*; 2019. Available online: https://www.statssa.gov.za/ (accessed on 25 February 2022).
37. Myles, P.; Louw, E. *Nelson Mandela Bay 2011 Annual Tourism Research Report*. 2011. Available online: https://www.nmbt.co.za/uploads/1/files/doc_2011_annual_tourism_research_report.pdf (accessed on 25 February 2022).
38. Myles, P.; Louw, E. *Nelson Mandela Bay 2014 Annual Tourism Research Report*. 2014. Available online: https://www.nmbt.co.za/uploads/1/files/doc_2014_annual_tourism_research_report.pdf (accessed on 25 February 2022).
39. DEDEAT. *Eastern Cape Tourism State of Play Study*; Report Compiled for Eastern Cape Department of Economic Development, Environmental Affairs and Tourism by Grant Thornton; Eastern Cape Department of Economic Development, Environmental Affairs and Tourism: Bisho, South Africa, 2013.
40. Vermeulen-Miltz, E.; Clifford-Holmes, J.K.; Scharler, U.M.; Lombard, A.T. A System Dynamics Model to Support Marine Spatial Planning in Algoa Bay, South Africa. *Environ. Model. Softw.* **2022**. in review.

41. Gary, K. *"Know Your Bay" A Guide to the Features and Creatures of Our Algoa Bay Hope Spot*; WESSA: Cape Town, South African, 2018.
42. Judge, C.; Penry, G.S.; Brown, M.; Witteveen, M. Clear Waters: Assessing Regulation Transparency of Website Advertising in South Africa's Boat-Based Whale-Watching Industry. *J. Sustain. Tour.* **2020**, *29*, 964–980. [CrossRef]
43. Zielinski, S.; Botero, C.M. Beach Tourism in Times of COVID-19 Pandemic: Critical Issues, Knowledge Gaps and Research Opportunities. *Int. J. Environ. Res. Public Health* **2020**, *17*, 7288. [CrossRef]
44. Ellis, E. How Nelson Mandela Bay Went from 349 to 3092 Cases in Two Weeks. Daily Maverick. 7 November 2020. Available online: https://www.dailymaverick.co.za/article/2020-11-07-how-nelson-mandela-bay-went-from-349-to-3092-cases-in-two-weeks/ (accessed on 6 July 2021).
45. Gregory, A. Pfizer Covid Jab "90% Effective against Hospitalisation for at Least 6 Months". Guardian. 5 October 2021. Available online: https://www.theguardian.com/world/2021/oct/05/pfizer-covid-jab-90-effective-against-hospitalisation-for-at-least-6-months? (accessed on 16 November 2021).
46. World Health Organisation. *COVID-19 and Mandatory Vaccination: Ethical Considerations and Caveats*; Policy Brief; WHO: Geneva, Switzerland, 2021; pp. 13–17.
47. Schmidt, C. Why Is Omicron So Contagious? Scientific American. 17 December 2021. Available online: https://www.scientificamerican.com/article/why-is-omicron-so-contagious/ (accessed on 25 January 2022).
48. Dong, E.; Du, H.; Gardner, L. An Interactive Web-Based Dashboard to Track COVID-19 in Real Time. *Lancet Infect. Dis.* **2020**, *20*, 533–534. [CrossRef]

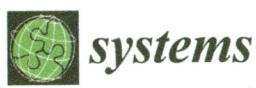

Article

Using Cascaded and Interlocking Generic System Archetypes to Communicate Policy Insights—The Case for Justifying Integrated Health Care Systems in Terms of Reducing Hospital Congestion

Eric Frank Wolstenholme

Symmetric Scenarios, Edinburgh EH8 8DL, UK; eric@symmetriclab.com

Citation: Wolstenholme, E.F. Using Cascaded and Interlocking Generic System Archetypes to Communicate Policy Insights—The Case for Justifying Integrated Health Care Systems in Terms of Reducing Hospital Congestion. *Systems* **2022**, *10*, 135. https://doi.org/10.3390/systems10050135

Academic Editor: Khalid Saeed

Received: 29 July 2022
Accepted: 30 August 2022
Published: 1 September 2022

Publisher's Note: MDPI stays neutral with regard to jurisdictional claims in published maps and institutional affiliations.

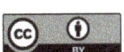

Copyright: © 2022 by the author. Licensee MDPI, Basel, Switzerland. This article is an open access article distributed under the terms and conditions of the Creative Commons Attribution (CC BY) license (https://creativecommons.org/licenses/by/4.0/).

Abstract: A persistent problem in UK hospitals is that of delayed discharges, where patients who are fit for discharge continue to occupy beds whilst awaiting care packages from Social Care. Integrated Care Systems (ICSs) in which Health and Social Care collaborate are now a major NHS initiative, the thinking being that such spending will have direct cost savings to health by freeing up expensive beds. The premise of this paper is that the benefits to health of assisting Social Care could also reduce a number of serious indirect costs and provide wide-ranging benefits to hospital patients, staff and budgets. This is accomplished by reducing the congestion arising from the use of many painful internal coping strategies and unintended consequences, which hospitals have to resort to when constrained by a lack of discharge solutions. The paper explores new and novel ways of using generic systems archetypes to create a hypothesis linking general Integrated Care Systems to congestion reduction throughout hospitals. Rather than use archetypes individually, they are applied here collectively in tandem. These are named 'cascaded archetypes', where the unintended consequence of one archetype becomes the driver for the next and are useful where fundamental solutions to problems are difficult to implement and unintended consequences must be dealt with.

Keywords: health; social care; integrated care; hospital; delayed hospital discharges; strategy; congestion; capacity; archetypes; unintended consequences

1. Introduction

For many years, hospitals in the UK and other government-funded health systems have struggled with the problem of delayed discharges. Typically, a relatively small number of usually older patients cannot be discharged due to a lack of continuing Health and Social Care capacity (care packages) although they have been declared as "medically fit" for discharge. The problem has been well documented [1–3] but despite many attempts at rectification it remains [4–6].

This paper builds on two very recent developments in Health and Systems Thinking, which have the potential to help the problem. The first is the formation of Integrated Care Systems (ICSs) within Health and Social Care [7], and the second is the development of new methods for communicating complex feedback structure.

1.1. Developments in Health—Integrated Care Systems

Integrated Care Systems denotes ways of coordinating the delivery of diverse health and social care services to the same person, based on the belief that services should be centred on the person, not the provider [8]. Within the UK, there are now different variations in each of England, Scotland, Wales, and Northern Ireland [9], mainly aimed at interventions to keep people out of hospital to reduce delayed hospital discharges. Rather than wait for government action to improve the funding of Social Care, trials are underway in places for health to both subsidise domiciliary social care wages and 'discharge to assess' facilities [10–12]. The benefits to health of these trials are being assessed mainly in terms of their direct benefits, such as maintaining the viability of Social Care delivery in the face of government spending cuts and saving the costs of expensive hospital beds. The flow of patients through health and social care is analogous to a supply chain and it seems logical that the most powerful actor in the chain (health) should subsidise the weakest for a win/win outcome.

However, it is the premise of this paper that the potential savings to health from integrated care initiatives are being significantly underestimated by not taking into account their potential to reduce many indirect costs associated with delayed discharges. These costs result from congestion which builds up at both the front and rear end of hospitals pathways. Delayed discharges reduce hospital capacity and admissions and increase patient waiting times. However, more damagingly, they cause hospitals to resort to numerous unofficial coping strategies to maintain patient throughput, each of which have numerous and serious unintended consequences for patients, staff and costs and which, ultimately, tend to defeat their purpose. These strategies are becoming so necessary and common that that they have become embedded in hospital practice and their unintended consequences, by necessity, overlooked.

Increases in congestion in hospital accident and emergency departments and wards is undoubtably due in part to increases in population aging and there are ongoing attempts to reduce demand by such things as same day emergency care, urgent treatment centres and primary care networks. However, it is too easy to blame all congestion on external demand and a cornerstone of system dynamics is to look for internal system drivers of problems. It is suggested here that hospital congestion is significantly compounded by the use of internal coping strategies. Indeed, as shown later the use of coping strategies can cause both health service supply problems as well as latent demand surges.

1.2. Developments in Systems Thinking

Determining and communication of complex feedback structure to facilitate system change is one of the axioms of system dynamics and this paper uses a new and novel approach which represents the cumulation of work over many years by the author to trace and demonstrate feedback connections between Health and Social Care [13–20]. One of the cornerstones of this work has been the judicial blend of qualitative and quantitative system dynamics, with qualitative hypotheses leading to testing with quantitative models and to further qualitative hypotheses. Numerous early models were quantitative and embedded the benefits to health of eliminating elements of coping strategies and individual generic archetypes were often used to explain unintended consequences. Discussions of the early quantitative work with health care staff have led over time to the surfacing of a much wider range of coping strategies with multiple unintended consequences. System dynamics has proven to be a valuable tool in teasing out the way in which organisations really work in response to the stress of capacity constraints. These coping strategies are all embodied in the next stage of qualitative analysis described in this paper. The resultant hypothesis is an amalgam of knowledge captured from health and social care professionals and from the modeler. A modeler who is also a domain expert, may be able to trace interconnections that those inside the field can sometimes miss and to link them to new initiatives such as ICSs.

The medium for communicating the hypothesis is to use generic systems archetypes collectively in tandem, rather than the more conventional approach of using them individually. These collective archetypes are named cascaded archetypes, where the unintended consequence of one archetype becomes the driver for the next and they are particularly useful in communicating situations where solutions are difficult to implement, and unintended consequences must be dealt with. The approach provides a balance between the use of individual system archetypes and the use of full causal loop diagrams. Some interesting choices must be made between keeping each archetype free-standing for simplicity, whilst showing important interlocking between them. The generic nature of the method could have wide application in other systems where capacity constraints inhibit achievement and informal strategies need to be surfaced.

1.3. The Aims, Impact and Shape of the Paper

It is hoped that approach described herein will communicate better the need to balance Health and Social Care capacities, lead to hospitals working more within their design capacities and justify further specific ICS initiatives to reduce the costs of internal coping strategies and congestion. Whilst no specific integrated care initiatives are defined in the paper, it is postulated that linking Integrated Care Systems generally to hospital congestion and communicating the wider benefits in a succinct and compelling manor could boost the case for and number and shape of specific initiatives.

Indeed, the use of cascading archetypes is already making a significant impact on Health policy within the NHS and will be subject to further quantification studies:

> 'We have found the thinking in this paper tremendously useful. It is a revelation and my favourite new idea. It provides a new way of thinking about the problems of Health and Social Care and how to improve our justification of Integrated Care Systems'.
>
> Steven Wyatt, Head of Research and Policy,
> NHS Strategy Unit

The paper will:
1. Restate and recast the essence of coping strategies,
2. Review generic system archetypes and introduce cascaded archetypes
3. Apply cascaded archetypes to tracing the linkages between delayed discharges and hospital congestion, together with the role of ICSs in reducing negative outcomes.
4. Reflect on the benefits and limitations of cascaded archetypes as a tool of system dynamics

2. A Brief Summary and Clustering of Hospital Coping Strategies

Five hospital internal coping strategies have been identified that are becoming permanent features of hospital practice (This list of hospital coping strategies first appeared in Chapter 10 in The Dynamics of Care. Springer, Cham, and is published here with the permission of Springer). These are effectively complex 'unofficial' pathways into, through and out of hospital. A summary of the literature on these strategies has been presented elsewhere [19].

A new way of thinking about these coping strategies introduced here is to cluster them into two groups. The first group is entitled 'patient absorption'. It is suggested that this group is usually employed in the first instance as capacity becomes constrained. The second is entitled 'patient expulsion and exclusion' and it is suggested that this group is usually employed as a last resort when hospital space, costs and congestion are approaching breaking point. The strategies are:

2.1. Patient Absorption Strategies

1. Overspill wait areas (escalation beds): When pressure on accident and emergency departments in hospitals is high there is little choice but to accommodate patients as best as possible, which means using temporary admission wards, corridors and ambulances.
2. Transfer of unscheduled patients to scheduled beds (boarders or outliers): Another way of making room for unscheduled (emergency) patients is to transfer them to scheduled (elective) beds.

2.2. Patient Expulsion and Exclusion Strategies

1. Early/premature hospital discharge: The early discharge of patients is a means of freeing up beds on an individual basis.

2. Hospital demand management: Demand management is defined here to mean reductions in GPs referrals from primary to secondary health care, which is now often carried out with commissioning group approval.
3. Spot purchase of social care beds: The purchase of Social Care beds directly by hospitals to facilitate patient discharge is a way of freeing up beds on a group basis, with some hospitals actually buying Care Homes for this purpose.

The unintended consequences of these coping strategies are complex and will be described in the cascaded archetypes presented later in the paper.

3. A Review of Generic Systems Archetypes

Causal loop diagrams (CLDs) have long been part of the system dynamics approach as a way of extracting the underlying feedback loops in organisations and models, responsible for their behaviour over time. However, CLDs can themselves be complex.

System archetypes simplify understanding of feedback structure by capturing and categorising common groups of feedback loops [21,22] responsible for generic patterns of behaviour over time and numerous archetypes have been reported [23–26].

Since there are only two types of feedback loop (reinforcing and balancing), it was suggested by this author that archetypes could be simplified even more. That is by condensing them down to 4 core types, representing the four ways of ordering the two loop types [17] and defining them in two forms; problem and solution archetypes. This core group were shown to be capable of subsuming a wide range of existing archetypes [17].

The 4 core, generic archetypes representing the four ways of ordering a pair of reinforcing and balancing feedback loops, were defined as:

1. Underachievement: where intended reinforcing action is diminished by balancing unintended consequences,
2. Out of Control: where intended balancing control is diminished by reinforcing unintended consequences,
3. Relative achievement: where intended reinforcing action is diminished by reinforcing unintended consequences,
4. Relative control: where intended balancing control is diminished by balancing unintended consequences.

This paper will focus on under-achievement and out-of-control archetypes since they are the ones used in the later hospital analysis. Figures 1–4 show these two archetypes in problem and solution forms.

In contrast to earlier writing by this author [17], the intended outcome for a reinforcing feedback loop will be defined as the realisation of an opportunity and the intended outcome for a balancing feedback loop will be defined as containment of a threat.

Notation: Actions and intended consequences will be shown in thick causal links and bold text. Unintended consequences will be shown in thin causal links and italics. A positive sign will be used to depict a causal link between variables in the same direction. A negative sign will be used to depict a causal link between variables in the opposite directions. A balancing feedback loop is defined as one which contains an odd number of negative causal links which gives rise to its control behaviour over time towards a target. A reinforcing feedback loop is defined as one which contains none or an even number of negative causal links which gives rise to its exponential behaviour over time (virtuous or vicious).

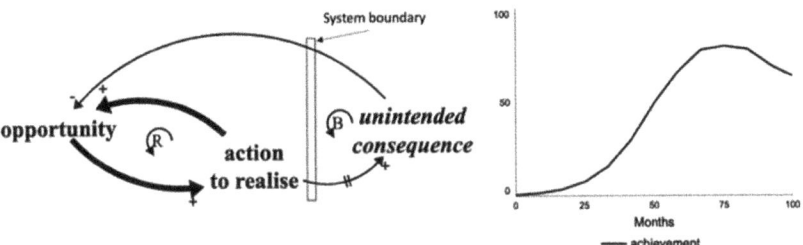

Figure 1. The generic underachievement problem archetype and an example of its behaviour over time.

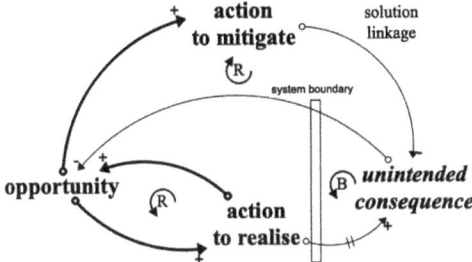

Figure 2. The generic under-achievement solution archetype.

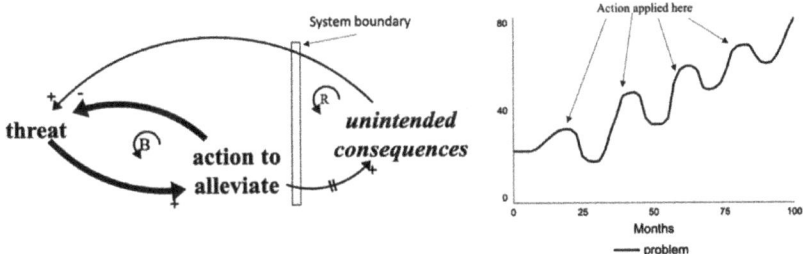

Figure 3. The generic out-of-control problem archetype and an example of its behaviour over time.

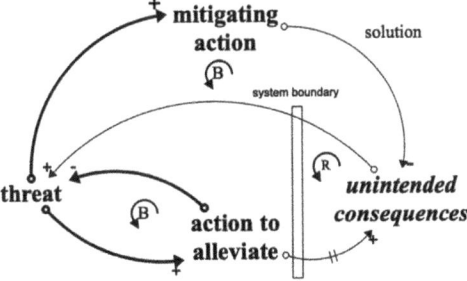

Figure 4. The generic out-of-control solution archetype.

3.1. Underachievement Archetype

The problem version of this archetype (Figure 1) consists of a reinforcing loop intended to generate growth in an opportunity over time, but this is countered by a balancing unintended consequence loop which inhibits the growth, occurring across a boundary (physical or mental barrier) and after a delay, both of which can mask the unintended consequence. Although shown as two loops, in practice the unintended consequence loop of the archetype may subsume a number of detrimental balancing effects giving rise to a variety of behaviours over time. Figure 1 shows an example of one such behaviour.

When the underachievement happens it is only too easy to blame external factors, rather than accept it as being seeded by the earlier action—a realisation of the systems message that today's problems are often yesterday's solutions.

The solution version of the archetype is shown in Figure 2. This suggests that if the unintended consequence can be pre-empted, a possible solution exit by introducing a second action in parallel with the first to reduce the impact of the unintended consequence and hence compliment the intended reinforcing loop.

A health-related example of this archetype would be investment in hospital capacity to increase the number of interventions, but this might result in more delayed discharges and actually reduce the effective capacity. A solution might be to make a corresponding investment in Social Care capacity.

3.2. Out-of-Control Archetype (Figures 3 and 4)

In this case, the problem archetype consists of a balancing feedback loop intended to reduce an exogenous rising threat (Figure 3), perhaps to a target level, but this is undermined by a reinforcing unintended consequence loop, again occurring across a boundary and after a delay, which mask the unintended consequences. Again, in practice, the unintended consequence loop may subsume a number of (this time) detrimental reinforcing effects giving rise to a variety of behaviours over time. Figure 3 shows one of these where each time the action is applied control is re-established, but only for limited periods.

As before, if the unintended consequence can be pre-empted, a possible solution exit by introducing a second action in parallel with the first to reduce the impact of the unintended consequence and hence compliment the intended balancing loop (Figure 4).

A health-related example would be the introduction of additional beds to control (reduce) patient waiting times, but these might stimulate demand and quickly fill up with waiting times increasing again. A solution might be to combine this action with measures to inhibit demand.

4. An Introduction to Cascaded and Interlocking Systems Archetypes

The generic archetypes in the last section were originally perceived as being useful in an individual context. However, it is suggested here that they can have a wider role collectively in tandem to capture actions and reactions in complex feedback situations. This is particularly true where solution links in individual archetypes have been identified, but proved difficult, if not impossible, to implement.

Rather than deploy solution links, it is far more common for new reactive strategies to be employed by groups of stakeholders to deal with unintended consequences. Such reactions can spawn a new archetype to address the unintended consequence of the first archetype. The key to drawing this situation is to understand that the unintended consequence variable of the first archetype becomes the driving variable of the second archetype. It is then possible to consider that the action of the second archetype (in addition to countering the unintended consequence of the first archetype), may have its own unintended consequence(s) which could be depicted with in a third archetype.

This sequence can happen repeatedly and give rise to chains of archetypes, defined here as a set of cascaded archetypes.

Each archetype in a chain may well be linked to the same system and these links would all be shown in a full causal loop diagram. Such causal maps can be self-defeating as a means of communication due to the number of interconnections contained and cascaded archetypes strive to reduce the links. In order to achieve this simplifying role, each archetype can be introduced separately in turn within a story telling context, before the composite picture of the full cascade is presented.

Some interesting choices must be made between keeping each archetype free-standing for simplicity, whilst showing important interlocking between them. The term interlocking archetypes applies to those cascaded archetypes whose unintended consequences link directly to an opportunity or threat variable of earlier ones. They may in fact be the same variables.

Within the overall picture, the pattern of each archetype (opportunity/threat-action-unintended consequence) provides familiar structure and simplicity. It is suggested that this approach has an intermediate role in communication between the more conventional use of individual system archetypes and the use of full causal loop diagrams.

It is of interest to note that reactions in each cascaded archetype may be carried out by different stakeholders reacting in their own interests or by the same group as in the first archetype, perhaps trying multiple attempts to solve the original problem.

Figure 5 shows an example of a generic representation of cascaded and interlocking archetypes. This is a cascade of 4 archetypes starting with an underachievement archetype (top) and 3 out-of-control archetypes. The last of which feeds back on the first. This is a similar sequence to the one used later to describe hospital congestion. The choice of the number of archetypes to use is subjective and should be made on the basis of clarity, ease of grouping of coping actions and their dynamic phasing.

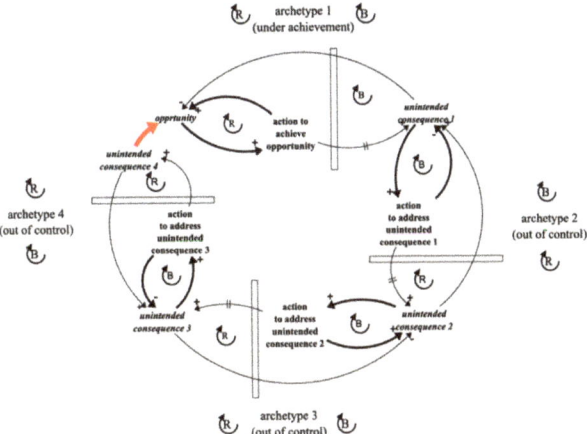

Figure 5. A cascade of 4 archetypes with the last one interlocking with the first.

Starting at the top of Figure 5:
1. archetype 1, underachievement: a reinforcing action to exploit an opportunity is undermined by balancing unintended consequence 1.
2. archetype 2, out-of-control: in the absence of a solution link, a balancing action to address the threat of unintended consequence 1 is undermined by reinforcing unintended consequence 2.
3. archetype 3, out-of-control: again, in the absence of a solution link, a balancing action to address the threat of unintended consequence 2 is undermined by a reinforcing unintended consequence 3.
4. archetype 4, out-of-control: again, in the absence of a solution link, a balancing action to address the threat of unintended consequence 3 is undermined by a reinforcing unintended consequence 4. This unintended consequence has strong links to the

variables in the opportunity loop of archetype 1 (or may be the same variables), hence it is referred to as interlocking with archetype 1.

The important point is that the original actions in the first (prime) archetype in the chain are not only undermined by their own unintended consequences, but also by the unintended consequences arising from subsequent actions to counter them.

Cascaded archetypes raise an interesting question not encountered in using individual archetypes. The convention with individual archetypes is to either start with a reinforcing feedback loop (opportunity) or a balancing loop (threat) as described earlier. However, if an archetype is started with a balancing feedback loop, cascaded thinking begs the question as to whether this threat is already an unintended consequence of a preceding archetype? It may have a linear source, but it is always worth exploring whether there is some reinforcing driver of the threat. It there is, it leads to the further question as to whether all cascaded archetypes should begin with a reinforcing feedback loop? This is certainly true in the hospital congestion example to follow.

5. Using Cascaded and Interlocking Archetypes to Trace the Links between Delayed Hospital Discharges, Hospital Congestion and Integrated Care Systems—A Case of 3 Interlocking Archetypes

5.1. Archetype 1

Health service underachievement (an underachievement archetype): investment in successful hospital interventions increases demand and is limited by delayed discharges, Figure 6.

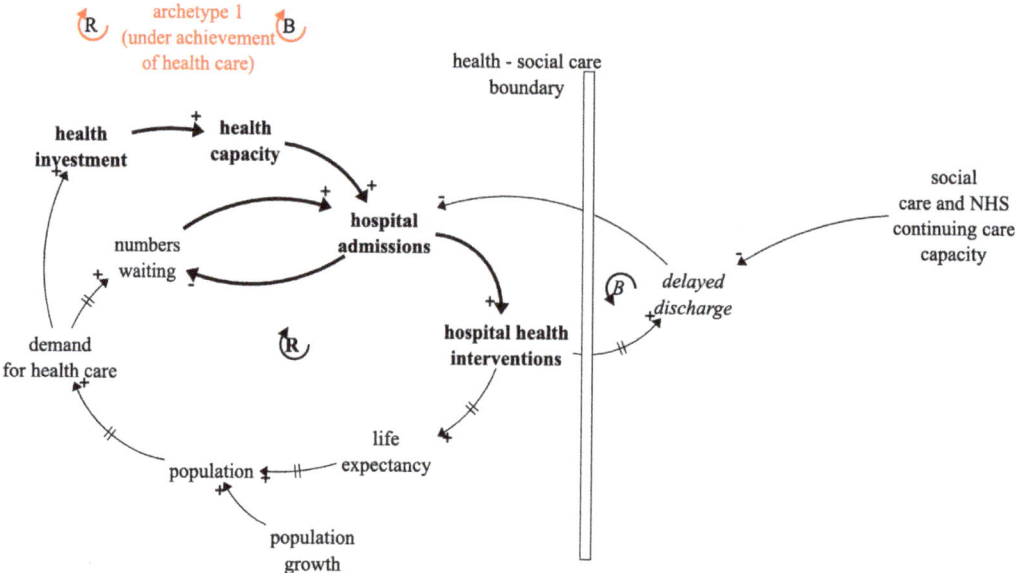

Figure 6. Archetype 1: The underachievement problem archetype involving health and social care.

This archetype is a classic example of underachievement and captures the way in which the demand for health services is driven by both population growth and aging, but also by health services being a victim of their own success by increasing longevity [27]. The supply response is investment in all types of hospital capacity with the intention of facilitating admissions and interventions. However, even if this is forthcoming, it results in problems with delayed discharges resulting from inadequate social care capacity, which feedback to reduce admissions and to cause underachievement in the number of hospital interventions.

The good news is that solutions do exist for this archetype which are shown in Figure 7.

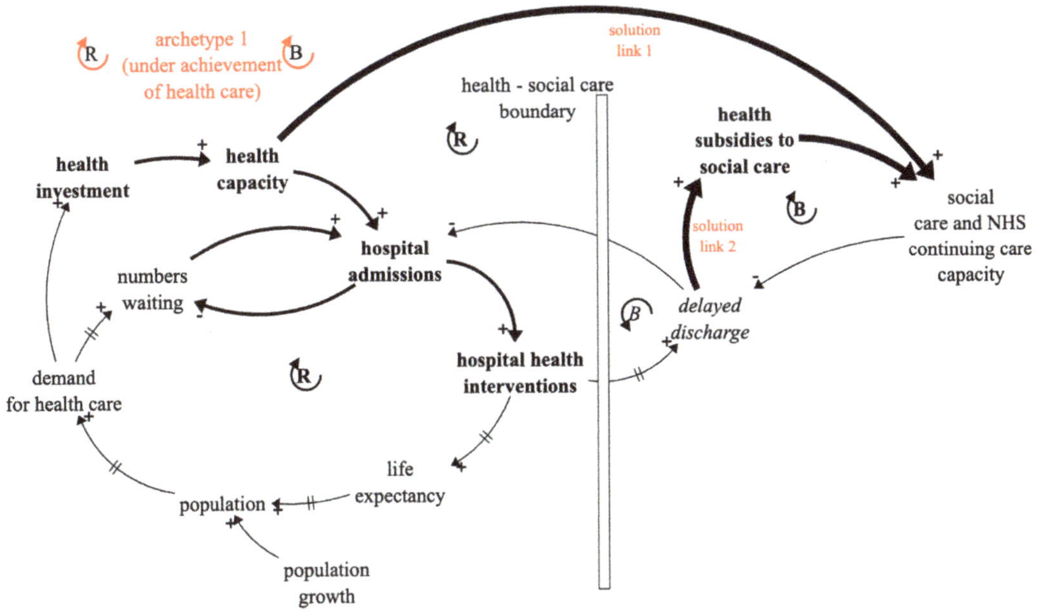

Figure 7. Archetype 1: The underachievement solution archetype involving health and social care.

First, solution link 1 is to expand Social Care capacity in line with Heath capacity and much previous has work has been aimed at demonstrating the merits of this link. The assumption has been that being that the government would provide this spending. However, the reality of implementing this solution has remained elusive since Health is funded from central government and Social Care is funded from local government. The new approach, motivating the thinking in this paper, is that an alternative solution might be pursued. That is for Health to subsidise Social Care to the benefit of both. Figure 7 shows this as solution link 2 and it is the purpose of this paper is to provide more justification for it by showing the congestion that arises from not doing so.

In the absence of solutions, hospitals have had to resort to numerous coping strategies, which can disguise the plight of their predicament.

5.2. Archetype 2

Patient absorption (an out-of-control archetype): using boarders and overspill waiting areas to counter delayed discharges leads to deteriorating services and rising costs, Figure 8.

The idea of using cascaded archetypes for improved communication is that they can be introduced one at a time. So, at this point archetype 1 is put to one side and archetype 2 starts with the threat from the unintended consequence of archetype 1—delayed discharges (highlighted).

However, rather than tackle delayed discharges head on, attention in hospitals is usually focussed on the consequential problem of delayed admissions at the 'front end' of the patient pathways. In fact, delayed admissions have often not been linked to delayed discharges, but more to lack of emergency room capacity. A clear case of looking for obvious solutions close to the symptoms of problems, when the best levers might be quite remote from the symptoms. This situation is changing, and hospitals now have sophisticated bed management systems and see freeing up discharges as a key to improving admissions.

These 'front end' issues are addressed by 'patient absorption' strategies comprising 'boarders' and 'overspill waiting areas.

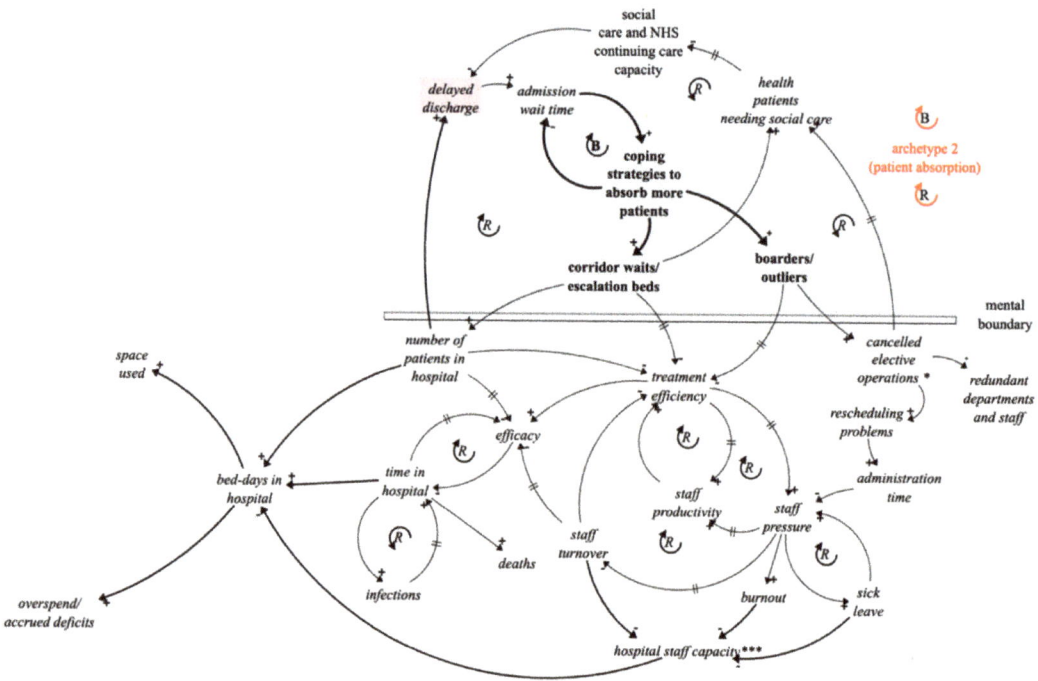

Figure 8. Archetype 2: The out-of-control archetype arising from patient absorption coping strategies.

Archetype 2 shows how these 2 coping strategies, are applied in response to admission problems. Both strategies lead to multiple and reinforcing unintended consequences.

The use of corridor and ambulance waits can lead to treatment inefficiencies and complications for patients. The use of temporary admissions wards restricts space for other conditions, and regular out-patient clinics, particularly long-term conditions clinics, have to be suspended. The use of boarders leads to the cancellation of elective procedures, redundant surgical teams, unused theatres and increases in the hospital elective waiting list. The resulting prioritising and rescheduling of elective procedures, places a massive demand on management and clinical time. Additionally, patients awaiting suspended clinics and elective operations may need social care, taking valuable capacity away from hospital discharges.

Both of these coping measures, like any form of bed capacity expansion, can quickly fill up without solving the flow problem. It is somewhat ironic that, whilst acknowledging the need for long term bed reductions, hospitals are forced into short term bed expansion. The coping measures are intended to provide a temporary solution to congestion, but periods of high demand and suspension of regular treatments are becoming more frequent and of longer duration. In recent years, there have been times when UK hospitals have formally cancelled elective operations during periods of high emergency demand.

Boarders and temporary admissions accommodation can also result in patients having longer stays in hospital, increased mortality rates [28] and reductions in treatment efficiency and efficacy [29,30]. Treatment efficiency is vital to care and recovery and when diminished has implications for both patients and staff. The longer patients are in hospital the greater the chance of infection and increased risk of fatalities. There are significant external issues in recruiting and retaining Health staff, but these are compounded by internal coping strategies. As patient to staff ratios increase staff disillusionment quickly shows up in staff productivity decline, increases in sick leave, burnout and higher staff turnover, with its associated loss of knowledge. Space becomes at a premium and budget deficits rise, perhaps to a point where new investment funds have to go to pay off accrued deficits rather than to enhance the supply of services [31].

It becomes more and more difficult for hospital management to address these vicious spirals of declining services and the net effect of the coping strategies is more patient bed-days in hospital and rising costs with delayed discharges increasing, rather than reducing.

An interesting question is whether there is a solution link for this second archetype on its own. It is easy to see in hindsight how absorbing more patients might inevitably lead to congestion and impact staff and patients. However, essential firefighting gives little time to think ahead to mitigate against these eventualities.

5.3. Archetype 3

Patient expulsion and exclusion (an out-of-control archetype): using early discharge, demand management and spot purchase of social care to counter deteriorating services and rising costs leads to reduced investment and increases in unmet need and latent demand Figure 9.

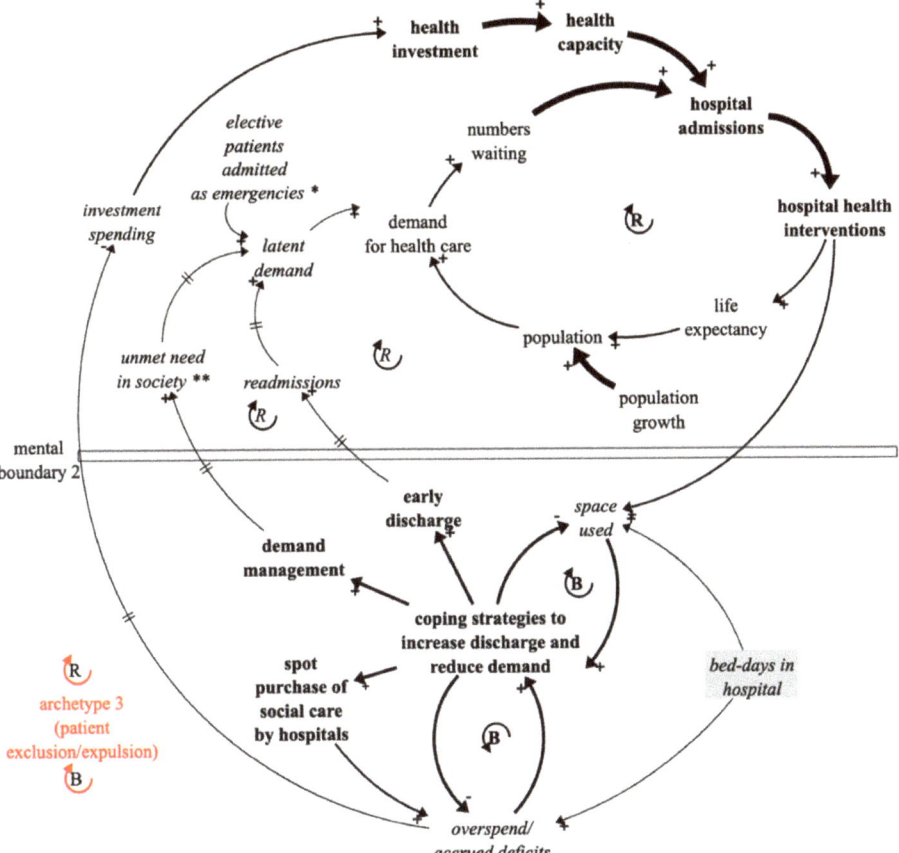

Figure 9. Archetype 3: The out-of-control archetype arising from patient exclusion/expulsion coping strategies. (The links between variables with asterisks exist but are not shown explicitly).

As overspending and provision of extra space become more and more difficult to address, attention of hospital managers and clinicians are inclined towards more radical coping strategies to relieve congestion pressures. In control engineering terms, from which System Dynamics emerged, there is a need to find a safety valve. The actions taken tend to have a 'rear end' focus with the intention of directly accelerating hospital discharge, but they also include stemming demand and hence admissions. They consist of early discharge of patients, the 'spot' purchase by health of social care capacity and demand management. This second group of coping strategies, in contrast to 'patient absorption', are referred to here as 'patient expulsion/exclusion' strategies.

In methodological terms Archetypes 1 and 2 are now put to one side and archetype 3 starts with how to address bed days in hospital (highlighted), space limitation and accrued deficits.

Early discharge can have serious unintended consequences by compromising patient safety. It can lead to readmissions and despite many guidelines poor hospital discharge is a recurring problem [32–36].

Demand management results in pushing demand further back upstream and ultimately this has to be absorbed by primary health care and society [37]. Demand can get pushed back on to families, charities and communities to create a cumulative unmet need which can result in further demands on Social Care.

The latent demand associated with early discharge and demand management eventually adds to demand on hospital services and interventions which add to the need for more coping strategies and space rather than to relieve them. Interestingly, due to delays, when extra demand impacts it can be puzzling as why it has happened, rather than seen as an inevitable consequence of earlier actions.

Purchasing Social Care beds by hospitals can be much more expensive than beds bought from social care under block contracts [38–40] and can also result in more variable quality of care. The cost of spot purchases also adds further to budget deficits.

The important point about archetype 3 is that it impacts directly on (interlocks with) variables which were the fundamental drivers of archetype 1. There is a double impact on achievement with investment reducing and demand increasing.

Again, the question might be raised as to whether there is a solution loop for this archetype, perhaps associated with providing help in the community to support early discharges and unmet need. Ironically, this would require more Social Care, the shortage of which caused the problems in the first place.

5.4. The Composite Picture

Figure 10 shows a composite picture of the 3 cascaded and interlocking archetypes, all on one page and without any crossed lines.

Whilst still complex, the structure of each individual generic archetype can be recognised in Figure 10, comprising opportunities/threats, actions and unintended consequences. The picture captures the phases of the coping strategies (patient absorption and patient expulsion/exclusion) and conveys the barriers and time delays conspiring to mask the unintended consequences in the early stages of action. In the composite picture it is also perhaps easier to see some of the feedback effects through the whole picture, rather than just within each archetype.

The key point, and a core point about interlocking archetypes, is that not only is archetype 1 inhibited by its own unintended consequence (delayed discharges), but this leads to a series of cascaded reactions which have implications for patients, staff and costs that undermine its achievement even more.

Figure 10 also includes the solution links and the message hopefully communicated is that investment in social care by government of Health in the form of Integrated Care Systems has the potential to both reduce delayed hospital discharges (direct cost saving), but to greatly reduce the use of coping strategies and congestion (indirect cost saving).

The financial costs of coping strategies are yet to be assessed but are underway and indications are that these could be much greater than a modest social care investment increase in the first place. However, financial costs pale into insignificance compared with the loss of efficacy and increased risk of patient illness and death arising from congestion. Additionally, eliminating the need for coping strategies would bring much-needed stress relief to both clinical and nursing staff.

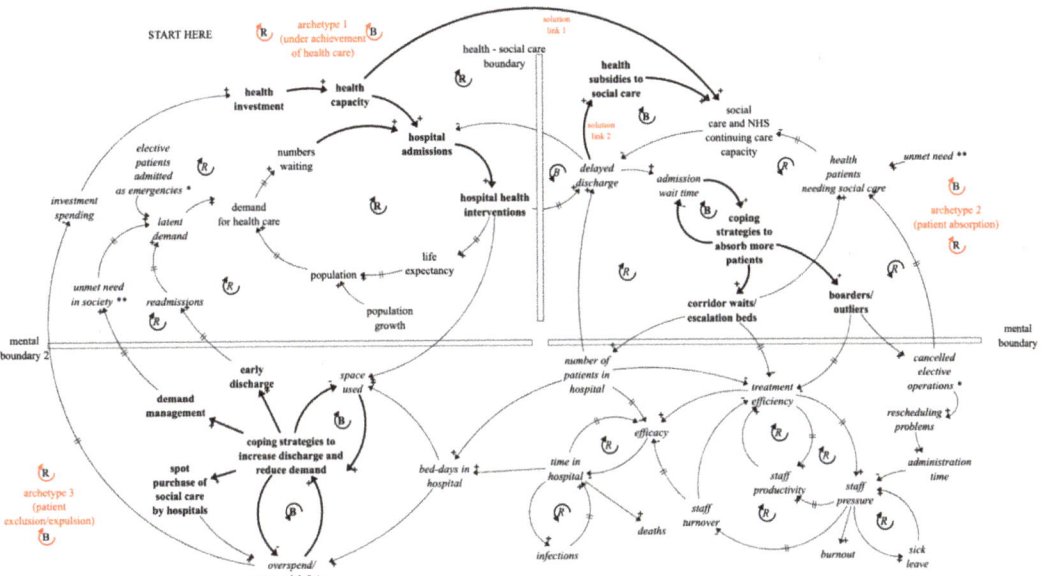

Figure 10. A composite picture of the 3 interlocking archetypes linking health and social care though delayed discharges and hospital congestion coping strategies. (The links between variables with asterisks exist but are not shown explicitly).

6. Benefits and Limitations of the Cascaded Archetype Approach

Whilst feedback loops do not in themselves provide definitive quantitative solutions to problems, they are very important at each stage of system dynamics modelling. They are useful both for conceptualising models and to extract insights from them. The idea of alternating between these two modes to develop models and thinking makes maximum use of both attributes. The work here has extrapolated early quantitative modelling results into a broad and succinct hypothesis, capable of drawing attention for further testing, which is already starting. Qualitative thinking is particularly important when some consequences in the situation described, such as mortality are intangible.

Cascaded archetypes enable complex feedback structures to be easily understood at a high level of aggregation and are proving useful to explain interconnections between Health and Social Care. Whether this is true in other domains is yet to be seen, but they have the potential to be helpful wherever obvious solutions prove elusive and informal strategies dominate system performance.

7. Conclusions

This paper has created a hypothesis that indicates that additional spending on Social Care, either by the government or Health (NHS) to reduce hospital-delayed discharges could bring very significant benefits to hospital management, staff and patients. It suggests that health spending on social care though Integrated Care Systems can be justified not only in the direct cost savings of expensive hospital beds, but by the indirect and wide-ranging benefits and savings associated with reducing hospital congestion. Whilst no specific integrated care initiatives are defined, it is recommended that linking Integrated Care Systems generally to relieving coping strategies and communicating the wider savings in a compelling manner could boost the case for and number and shape of the initiatives.

Methodologically, the paper has suggested that individual generic two-loop system archetypes can be usefully deployed collectively to improve the clarity of communication and storytelling of complex issues and to explain why unintended consequences occur. This is achieved by decomposing complex causal loop maps into recognisable and understandable structures. The process is particularly apposite to situations where the solution links of individual archetypes can be very difficult to implement and reactive actions by multiple stakeholders dominate.

It is suggested that further research is necessary to explore the full potential and limitations of the approaches described in other contexts and involving other types and combinations of generic archetypes. The generic nature of the method could have wide application in other systems where capacity constraints inhibit achievement and informal strategies need to be surfaced.

Funding: This research received no external funding.

Institutional Review Board Statement: Not applicable.

Informed Consent Statement: Not applicable.

Data Availability Statement: Not applicable.

Acknowledgments: The author would like to thank ISEE Systems, the creator of the Stella Architect software used to draw the figures in this paper, for their continuing support of his research.

Conflicts of Interest: The author declares no conflict of interest.

References

1. Bate, A. Delayed Transfers of Care in the NHS—House of Commons Library. 2017. Available online: https://commonslibrary.parliament.uk/research-briefings/cbp-7415 (accessed on 2 June 2022).
2. National Audit Office. *Annual Report: Discharging Older Patients from Hospital*; National Audit Office: London, UK, 2016.
3. Age UK, 1.4 million Older People Aren't Getting the Care and Support They Need—A Staggering Increase of Almost 20% in Just Two Years'. 2022. Available online: https://www.ageuk.org.uk/latest-news/articles/2018/july/1.4-million-older-people-arent-getting-the-care-and-support-they-need--a-staggering-increase-of-almost-20-in-just-two-years (accessed on 3 July 2018).
4. Nuffield Trust, The Health Foundation and The King's Fund. The Autumn Budget: Joint Statement on Health and Social Care. 2017. Available online: https://www.nuffieldtrust.org.uk/research/autumn-budget-2017 (accessed on 20 November 2017).
5. Kings Fund Newsletter. The NHS Budget and How It Has Changed. *Part of the NHS in a Nutshell*. 2022. Available online: https://www.google.com/search?client=safari&rls=en&q=%5B%5D+Kings+Fund%2C+Newsletter+(2022)+The+NHS+Budget+and+how+it+has+changed.+Part+of+the+NHS+in+a+nutshell.&ie=UTF-8&oe=UTF-8 (accessed on 14 July 2022).
6. NHS England. Better Care Operating Guide; 2016. Available online: https://www.england.nhs.uk/ourwork/part-rel/transformation-fund/better-care-fund/ (accessed on 2 August 2019).
7. Thorstensen, C. Integrated Care, The King's Fund. 2022. Available online: https://www.kingsfund.org.uk/topics/integrated-care?gclid=Cj0KCQjw1tGUBhDXARIsAIJx01ln_mqVn2FZpj8A-zFip89t9MwoXcoimhbqTXiSMYLf1wIzCPp-kUEaAujyEALw_wcB (accessed on 4 August 2022).
8. Ham, C. Making Sense of Integrated Care Systems, Integrated Care Partnerships and Accountable Care Organisations in the NHS in England, The King's Fund. 2018. Available online: https://www.kingsfund.org.uk/publications/making-sense-integrated-care-systems (accessed on 4 June 2019).
9. NHS England. Integrating Care: Next Steps to Building Strong and Effective Integrated Care Systems across England. 2022. Available online: https://www.england.nhs.uk/publication/integrating-care-next-steps-to-building-strong-and-effective-integrated-care-systems-across-england (accessed on 4 August 2022).
10. Home Care Investment Plan to Help Residents Through Winter. 2022. Available online: https://www.northstaffsccg.nhs.uk/news-events/1758-home-care-investment-plan-to-help-residents-through-winter (accessed on 4 August 2022).
11. The NHS Strategy Unit. Securing the Future of Domiciliary Care. 2022. Available online: https://www.strategyunitwm.nhs.uk/news/securing-future-domiciliary-care (accessed on 4 August 2022).
12. Wolstenholme, E.F.; McKelvie, D. Integrated Care. In *The Dynamics of Care*; Springer: Cham, Switzerland, 2019. [CrossRef]
13. Wolstenholme, E.F. A Case Study in Community Care using Systems Thinking. *J. Oper. Res. Soc.* **1993**, *44*, 925–934. [CrossRef]
14. Wolstenholme, E.F. A Patient Flow Perspective of UK Health Services. *Syst. Dyn. Rev.* **1999**, *15*, 253–273. [CrossRef]

15. Wolstenholme, E.F.; McKelvie, D. Hospital Delayed Transfer of Care (Delayed Discharges). In *The Dynamics of Care*; Springer: Cham, Switzerland, 2019. [CrossRef]
16. Wolstenholme, E.F.; Monk, D.; McKelvie, D.; Smith, G. Influencing and Interpreting Health and Social Care Policy in the UK. In *Complex Decision Making: Theory and Practice*; Qudrat-Ullah, H., Spector, M., Davidsen, P., Eds.; New England Complex Systems Institute Book Series on Complexity; Springer: Berlin/Heidelberg, Germany, 2007.
17. Wolstenholme, E.F. Towards the definition and use of a core set of archetypal structures in system dynamics. *Syst. Dyn. Rev.* **2003**, *19*, 7–26. [CrossRef]
18. Wolstenholme, E.F. Using generic system archetypes to support thinking and learning. *Syst. Dyn. Rev.* **2004**, *20*, 341–356. [CrossRef]
19. Wolstenholme, E.F.; McKelvie, D. Towards a Dynamic Theory of How Hospitals Cope in Times of High Demand. In *The Dynamics of Care*; Springer: Cham, Switzerland, 2019. [CrossRef]
20. Wolstenholme, E.F.; Monk, D.; McKelvie, D.; Arnold, S. Coping but not Coping in Health and Social Care—masking the reality, of running organisations well beyond safe design capacity. *Syst. Dyn. Rev.* **2008**, *23*, 371–389. [CrossRef]
21. Sterman, J.D. *Business Dynamics: Systems Thinking and Modelling for a Complex World*; Irwin McGraw-Hill: Boston, MA, USA, 2000.
22. Richardson, G.P. *Feedback Thought in Social Science and Systems Theory*; University of Pennsylvania Press: Philadelphia, PA, USA; Pegasus Communications: Waltham, MA, USA, 1999.
23. Senge, P.M. *The Fifth Discipline: The Art and Practice of the Learning Organization*; Doubleday/Currency: New York, NY, USA, 1990.
24. Wolstenholme, E.F. *System Enquiry: A System Dynamics Approach*; John and Wiley and Sons: Chichester, UK, 1990.
25. Stroth, P.L. *Systems Thinking for Social Change*; Chelsea Green Publishing: White River Junction, VT, USA, 2015.
26. Sherwood, D. *Seeing the Forest for the Trees: A Manager's Guide to Applying Systems Thinking*; Nicholas Brearley: London, UK, 2002.
27. Nolte, E. *NHS 70 Series—70 Years on, How Is the NHS Performing on Life Expectancy and Mortality?* London School of Hygiene and Tropical Medicine: London, UK, 2018.
28. Stylianou, N.; Fackrell, R.; Vasilakis, C. Are medical outliers associated with worse patient outcomes? *BMJ Open* **2017**, *7*, e015676. [CrossRef] [PubMed]
29. Santamaria, J.D.; Tobin, A.E.; Anstey, M.H.; Smith, R.J.; Reid, D.A. Do outlier inpatients experience more emergency calls in hospital? An observational cohort study. *Med. J. Aust.* **2014**, *200*, 45–48. [CrossRef]
30. Portsmouth Hospitals NHS Trust. *Adult Outlier Policy*, 5th ed.; Portsmouth Hospitals NHS Trust: Portsmouth, UK, 2018.
31. Ewbank, L.; Thompson, J.; Mckenna, H. *NHS Hospital Bed Numbers: Past, Present, Future*; THE Kings Fund: London, UK, 2017.
32. Nguyen, O.K.; Makam, A.N.; Clark, C. Vital Signs Are Still Vital: Instability on Discharge and the Risk of Post-Discharge Adverse Outcomes. *J. Gen. Intern. Med.* **2017**, *32*, 42–48. [CrossRef]
33. Buie, V.C.; Owings, M.F.; DeFrances, C.J.; Golosinskiy, A. National Hospital Discharge Survey: Summary. *Vital Health Stat.* **2010**, *13*, 168.
34. Smith, K.O.; Jackson, S. *It's Not All about Reducing Length of Stay*; Carlike: Atlanta, GA, USA, 2017. Available online: https://stage.carelike.com/providers/resources/its-not-all-about-reducing-length-of-stay (accessed on 4 December 2018).
35. Healthwatch News Report. *NHS Needs to Do More to Understand Why People Are Returning to Hospital after Discharge*; Healthwatch England: London, UK, 2017.
36. Oxtoby, K. Preventing unsafe discharge from hospital. *Nurs. Times* **2018**, *112*, 14–15.
37. Campbell, D. GPs Offered Cash to Refer Fewer People to Hospital. *Health Policy Guardian*, 28 February 2018.
38. Triggle, N. Care Homes Could Solve NHS Bed-Blocking. *BBC Health News*, 1 March 2016.
39. Smyth, C. NHS Hospitals Open Own Care Homes to Tackle Beds Crisis. *Times Newspaper*, 15 October 2016. Available online: https://www.thetimes.co.uk/article/nhs-hospitals-open-own-care-homes-to-tackle-beds-crisis-w8pvsztch (accessed on 10 June 2018).
40. Adam. Moving on from Spot Purchasing in Domiciliary Care Commissioning. 2018. Available online: http://www.useadam.co.uk/news/moving-on-from-spot-purchasing-in-domiciliary-care-commissioning (accessed on 2 September 2019).

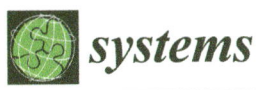

Article

How Can a Community Pursue Equitable Health and Well-Being after a Severe Shock? Ideas from an Exploratory Simulation Model

Bobby Milstein [1,2,*], Jack Homer [2,3] and Chris Soderquist [4,5]

1. ReThink Health and Rippel Foundation, Morristown, NJ 07960, USA
2. MIT Sloan School of Management, Cambridge, MA 02142, USA
3. Homer Consulting, Barrytown, NY 12507, USA
4. Pontifex Consulting, Atlanta, GA 30341, USA
5. Darden School of Business, University of Virginia, Charlottesville, VA 22903, USA
* Correspondence: bmilstein@rippel.org

Abstract: Local communities sometimes face severe shocks, such as the COVID-19 pandemic or economic recession, which inflict widespread harm, intensify injustice and test the ties that bind people together. A recent "Springboard" theory proposes a way to spring forward toward an equitable, thriving future by altering priorities among four structural drivers of population well-being: the extent of vital conditions, equity, urgent services capacity, and belonging and civic muscle. To explore the strategic implications of the Springboard theory, we developed the Thriving Together Model, a system dynamics simulation model that lets users play out alternative investment priorities and track changes over a decade as they try to maximize the number of people thriving and minimize suffering. The prototype model is exploratory, subject to further refinement and empirical support, but it has already sparked creative conversations among hundreds of changemakers who have interacted with it through an interactive theater. This paper presents the model's structure, illustrative results, and tentative insights. The Thriving Together Model extends Ostrom's Nobel Prize-winning work on shared stewardship by offering a general explanation about how stewards of a divided community can heal through a traumatic shock and spring forward toward a future with greater well-being and justice.

Keywords: population health and well-being; equity; stewardship; resilience; simulation modeling

1. Introduction

All communities must contend with persistent gaps in health and well-being as well as sudden crises that may make things even worse and test a community's resilience. Shocks (such as economic recessions, fires, floods, heat waves, mass violence, pandemics, etc.) typically unfold quickly, intensify pre-existing injustice, and lead to greater morbidity and mortality. When faced with such a shock, how can community changemakers establish conditions for everyone to heal and enhance life satisfaction, without leaving anyone behind?

A large body of evidence connects the health and well-being of individuals to features in the communities they inhabit [1,2]. Two sets of community-level contributors are especially crucial [3]: (1) adequacy of urgent services, which anyone may need temporarily in a crisis (e.g., acute care for injury or physical/mental illness; addiction treatment; crime response; environmental clean-up; homeless services; unemployment and food assistance); and (2) the presence of vital conditions, which everyone needs consistently to reach their full potential. Seven vital conditions are widely recognized: a thriving natural world; basic needs for health and safety; humane housing; meaningful work and wealth; lifelong learning; reliable transportation; and a sense of belonging and civic muscle (which is both a

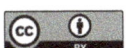

vital condition as well as practical capacity necessary for equitable progress in every other area) [4].

When a shock occurs, it tests community resilience and usually hits the most disadvantaged members hardest, widening pre-existing inequities. Much is known about the details of disaster recovery [5,6], but few studies explore what it takes to spring forward with greater levels of justice and equitable well-being.

At the start of the COVID-19 pandemic, more than 100 contributors came together to develop a general theory of how a shock that inflicts widespread loss might be converted into equitable renewal. The result was *"Thriving Together: A Springboard for Equitable Recovery and Resilience in Communities Across America"* [7]. The Springboard theory emphasizes four key elements for thriving together through periods of intense adversity:

1. Affirm racial justice and full inclusion for all people;
2. Strengthen belonging and civic muscle by working across differences, which, in turn, unlocks new assets for concerted action;
3. Expand all vital conditions with local stewards in the lead;
4. Renew civic life; economic life; and social, emotional, and spiritual life.

In conjunction with the Springboard, our system dynamics modeling team at ReThink Health (an initiative of the nonprofit Rippel Foundation) developed a model-based simulation to help changemakers understand the strategic challenges they would inevitably face when trying to spring forward toward an equitable, thriving future. The resulting Thriving Together Model (TTM), though still exploratory, enables community stewards to play out the dynamics of renewal over a 10-year time horizon, while they experiment with various ways to balance investment priorities among vital conditions, equity, belonging and civic muscle, and the adequacy of urgent services. This paper describes the structure, empirical foundation, illustrative results, and strategic insights from the prototype Thriving Together Model, as well as how it might be further refined.

2. Materials and Methods

2.1. Extending an Earlier Line of Research

The current TTM continues our inquiry into the dynamics of population well-being, which initially explored how to set investment priorities in communities that are contending with multiple interrelated or "tangled" threats [8]. That study compared the relative value of investing in one or more vital conditions. For that analysis, each of the seven vital conditions (other than reliable transportation) was operationalized using metrics available from the US County Health Rankings [9].

The TTM is broader than the earlier tangled threats analysis. It portrays a decade-long strategic challenge to equitably renew well-being after a severe shock using four interconnected investment priorities. However, it is also admittedly still exploratory, not yet as well grounded in data and community experiences as it could be. In the Discussion, we describe directions for further development to assure that this tool becomes more accurate and useful. Nonetheless, the current TTM has provoked strong interest from several hundred changemakers who have experienced it, making its preliminary findings worth documenting.

2.2. Representing Well-Being and Its Drivers

The TTM takes a broad view of population outcomes, looking not only at conventional measures of health status but more generally at population well-being using the Cantril Ladder categories of thriving, struggling, and suffering [10]. These self-reported life evaluation metrics are measured regularly in the US and around the world by Gallup.

Users of the TTM must find a way to allocate community assets over a period of 10 years so that more people are thriving and fewer are struggling and suffering. This involves generating greater equity, more secure vital conditions, adequate urgent services, and a stronger sense of belonging and civic muscle. Time starts at Year 0; shocks occur in Year 1; and the overall path toward renewal is tracked from Year 2 to Year 12.

2.3. Model Structure

Figure 1 presents an overview of the causal logic of the TTM (see Supplementary File S1 for a complete list of equations).

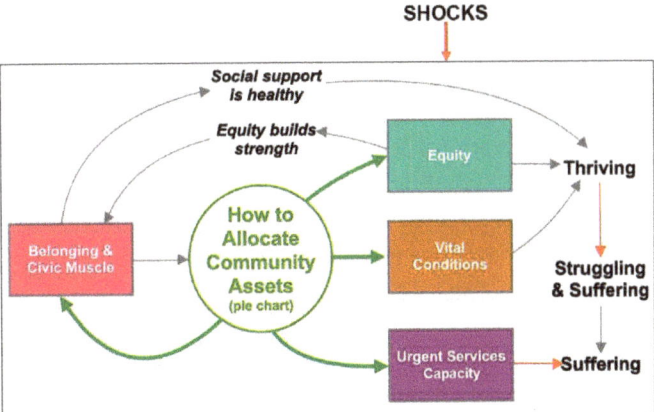

Figure 1. Structural logic of the Thriving Together Model (TTM).

On the right are sub-groups of people thriving, struggling, and suffering. There are three ways to increase the thriving percent: (a) expand vital conditions, (b) increase equity; and (c) strengthen social support (via higher levels of belonging and civic muscle). Those who are not thriving are struggling or suffering. Thus, one way to reduce suffering is to increase thriving. The other way is to increase urgent services capacity.

Vital conditions, equity, and belonging and civic muscle are all represented in the model as stock variables (rectangular boxes in Figure 1) measured as 0–1 indices. Vital conditions here refers to all of the vital conditions mentioned previously other than belonging and civic muscle, which is represented separately because of its distinct dynamic effects. The vital conditions index is initialized at Year 0 in the simulation as a weighted average of multiple indicators of household income, housing, education, physical activity, non-smoking, and health insurance across all US counties.

Belonging and civic muscle here describes the extent to which people feel they belong and have the power—as well as the practical capacity—to shape their common world. It is a shared community asset used to build all others. Additionally, as indicated in Figure 1, greater belonging and civic muscle not only increases community assets, but also drives peoples' sense of social support, which, in turn, helps boost the percent of people thriving. In lieu of an established multivariate measure, the belonging and civic muscle index is initialized based on social associations per capita across all US counties (again from the US County Health Rankings (CHR) [9]).

Equity here refers to whether there is just and fair inclusion for everyone as opposed to systemic exclusion rooted in institutional policies, practices, programs, and priorities. In lieu of an established multivariate measure, the equity index is based on the Gini Index for the US, which measures how fairly income is distributed [11]. As indicated in Figure 1, greater equity not only improves the percent of people thriving, but also tends to boost belonging and civic muscle through wider inclusion of people in civic life.

Urgent services capacity is expressed as a percent of the population. If the capacity to deliver urgent services is less than the current urgent need percent (a portion, e.g., 20%, of non-thriving people), then its adequacy will be something less than 100%, and people will suffer accordingly for lack of urgent services. For example, if the urgent need percent is 9% (20% of 45% non-thriving) and urgent services capacity is 5.4%, then its adequacy will be 60% (=5.4/9%), and the suffering percent will be 3.6% (=9−5.4%).

2.4. Gathering Assets

It can be difficult for a community to spring forward from a severe shock using only its usual resources and funding. However, shocks often unleash the potential to acquire special resources and dedicated funding for some number of years after the shock. The extent to which these assets for renewal can be gathered depends on the community's state of belonging and civic muscle: with greater belonging and civic muscle, community stewards can gather even more assets (e.g., through fundraising, grants, and in-kind support). Seeking assets beyond a certain point (or threshold) may impose obligations that begin to erode civic muscle. If that erosion is strong enough, it can counteract the benefit of the additional assets (creating a dysfunctional trap of depending on assets that also undermine their own capabilities). For the simulation analysis here, none of the scenarios exceed that threshold. Instead, this study explores what can happen with assets that can be gathered and managed relatively easily, without encumbering the community with onerous outside obligations or dependencies.

2.5. Allocating Assets

In the model, there are four distinct ways to allocate community assets. They can be used in various combinations to expand any of the four drivers of well-being (depicted as boxes in Figure 1): (1) vital conditions; (2) equity; (3) urgent services capacity; and/or (4) belonging and civic muscle. Any allocation scheme may be depicted as a pie chart dividing 100% of community assets among the four drivers. At any moment, available assets are finite, therefore a decision to prioritize one area of work necessarily means paying somewhat less attention to the others. Investments in belonging and civic muscle, however, can enable the community to gather even more assets over time, as shown in Figure 1. The overall resilience of a community after a shock depends on how effectively local stewards negotiate these four investment priorities over time.

How community assets are allocated among the four drivers of well-being is determined by the model's initial assumptions at Year 0 and then, starting in Year 2, by the model user. The initial allocations in the model may be suboptimal and leave room for improvement. Model users can adjust this allocation every two years starting at Year 2 (immediately after the shock) and for the last time at Year 10 before the simulation ends at Year 12.

Each of the four stock variables is subject to gradual erosion if they are not continuously maintained, as well as the possibility of a sudden, unexpected, adverse shock. The shocks may reflect rapid external occurrences, such as a pandemic, or internal ones, such as the loss of organizational leaders.

2.6. Parametric Assumptions

The model is configured with several parametric assumptions we have set based on data for the US overall (see Supplementary File S2 for a complete list with sources). Some of the most prominent parameters include initial values for the population well-being and its four drivers. Those include the initial thriving percent (55%; Gallup 2019), suffering percent (3.5%; Gallup 2019), vital conditions index (0.80; CHR 2006–2012), equity index (0.52; Gini 2011–2017), belonging and civic muscle index (0.50; CHR social associations per capita 2014–2017), and social support index (0.80; BRFSS "have social/emotional support" 2006–2012).

Other parameter values were estimated more impressionistically with the help of ReThink Health collaborators across the country who evaluated the model as it was being developed. These include estimates of the initial adequacy of urgent services; the strengths of causal links in Figure 1; the natural erosion rates of the four stock variables in Figure 1; and the initial allocation of community assets to those same four stocks.

To enhance clarity when interpreting simulated results, all variables in the model start in a dynamic equilibrium, unchanging over time absent any shock. This means that initially (prior to any shock) the normal erosion outflow for each of the four stock variables is exactly offset by a corresponding inflow which replenishes the stock.

Together, the model's parameters determine not only how well the community is doing initially, but also how close to optimal its starting priorities are, in terms of its ability to spring forward after a shock. A community that begins with suboptimal starting priorities will have to shift its priorities more dramatically to spring forward. Because of the model's complexity and nonlinearity, the optimal set of investment priorities is not directly calculable but can only be determined by testing the simulator under different conditions.

Any of the four allocation areas may be shocked; these shocks occur during Year 1 and take one year to have their full effect. For all tests described below, we used the same set of relative shock values: vital conditions (−12.5%), equity (−11.5%), urgent services capacity (−5.8%), belonging and civic muscle (0%). We configured these parameters to approximate what occurred in the US during March to April 2020, as COVID-19 swept through the country, a time when Gallup reported that the percent of Thriving adults in the US dropped sharply [12]. The decision not to alter the level of belonging and civic muscle was informed by observations that people and organizations were simultaneously separating and coming together.

2.7. Summary Measures

The model calculates several summary measures of cumulative performance. First is the change in average life expectancy, measured relative to Year 0. In line with national data, we assume that struggling (relative to thriving) reduces life expectancy by three years, while suffering reduces life expectancy by 20 years [13].

We also calculate a "renewal score" determined by cumulative changes in thriving and suffering over a decade relative to where those well-being metrics were at Year 2, immediately after the shock. If either metric moves in the wrong direction, a double penalty is applied. This renewal score starts at zero, with a minimum value of −100 and a maximum value of +100.

2.8. Illustrative Model Tests

We have performed hundreds of model tests, varying uncertain parameters as well as allocation decisions. Here, we present six tests that illustrate noteworthy dynamics of renewal. Each scenario is based on a particular allocation of community assets to the model's four drivers of well-being (i.e., vital conditions, equity, urgent services capacity, belonging and civic muscle).

1. *Status Quo*: continue the historical, pre-shock allocation, which gives greatest priority to urgent services capacity (40%) and vital conditions (30%), and far less to equity (15%) and belonging and civic muscle (15%).
2. *Vital Conditions 40%*: switch at Year 2 to a new stable allocation emphasizing vital conditions (40%), with the other three at 20%.
3. *Equity 40%*: switch at Year 2 to a new stable allocation emphasizing equity (40%), with the other three at 20%.
4. *Belonging and Civic Muscle 40%*: switch at Year 2 to a new stable allocation emphasizing belonging and civic muscle (40%), with the other three at 20%.
5. *Even Balance 25%*: switch at Year 2 to a new stable allocation with all four at 25%.
6. *Best Pivot*: switch at Year 2 to emphasize equity first (65%) and belonging and civic muscle (25%), with the other two at 5% each; then, from Years 4–6, pivot back toward urgent services and vital conditions, for an eventual stable allocation at Year 6 of urgent services (45%), vital conditions (35%), belonging and civic muscle (15%), and equity (5%).

2.9. Tests in a More Disorganized Community

In addition to tests using community settings based on US national averages, we also conducted the same battery of simulated scenarios using settings that portray a more disorganized community. Relative to the baseline assumptions above, we used an alternative setup to explore the potential for renewal in a community that begins with twice as many people suffering, as well as half as much equity, social support, and belonging and civic muscle. See Supplementary File S3 for parameter assumptions and results of those alternative tests.

3. Results

The six illustrative renewal strategies result in different outcome trajectories for thriving and suffering and consequently average life expectancy. See Figures 2–4.

Vital conditions and equity are the strongest drivers of thriving (Figure 2). Throughout *Vital Conditions 40%* (red line) and *Equity 40%* (green line), the sum of the asset allocations to vital conditions and equity is a strong 60%; accordingly, thriving rises the farthest in these two runs. Thriving also rises strongly at first in *Best Pivot* (brown line), but slows after Year 6, as the sum of the allocations to vital conditions and equity declines from 70% in Year 2, to 60% in Year 4, and finally to 40% in Years 6 and beyond. Both *Even Balance 25%* (black line) and *Belonging and Civic Muscle 40%* (grey line) initially have modest effects, but by Year 12, both produce slightly better results for Thriving than *Best Pivot*.

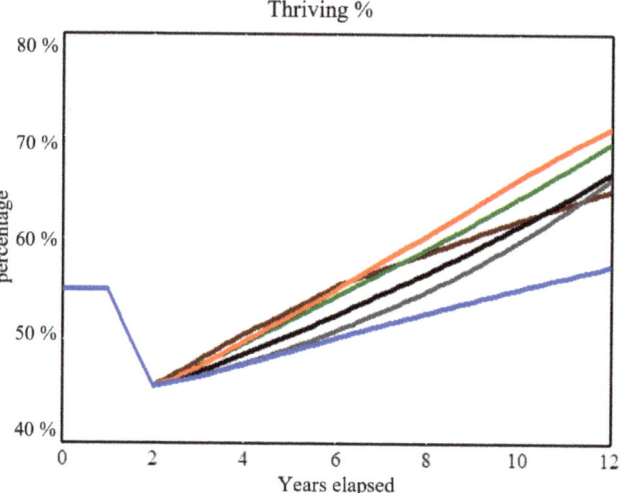

Figure 2. Thriving percent under six allocation scenarios. Blue = *Status Quo*, Red = *Vital Conditions 40%*, Green = *Equity 40%*, Grey = *Belonging and Civic Muscle 40%*, Black = *Even Balance 25%*, Brown = *Best Pivot*.

When attempting to reduce the suffering percent (Figure 3), the two most influential forces are the size of the thriving percent and urgent services capacity. Because *Status Quo* devotes a large 40% allocation to urgent services capacity, suffering declines consistently throughout. In all other runs, suffering rises at first (even with the increases in thriving seen in Figure 2) because there is less allocation to urgent services capacity. However, the trajectory is very different in *Best Pivot*, where suffering falls rapidly after Year 6—declining below *Status Quo* by Year 9. This turnaround occurs for two reasons. First, the allocation to urgent services capacity in *Best Pivot* starts at only 5% in Year 2 but rises to 45% in Years 6 and beyond. Second, thriving is much greater in *Best Pivot* than it is in *Status Quo*.

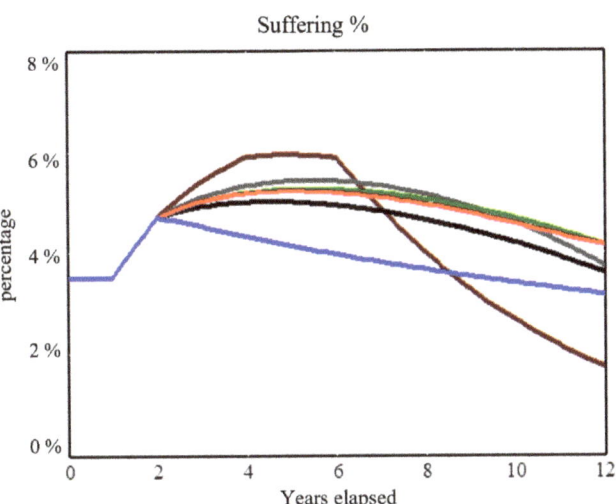

Figure 3. Suffering percent under six allocation scenarios. Blue = *Status Quo*, Red = *Vital Conditions 40%*, Green = *Equity 40%*, Grey = *Belonging and Civic Muscle 40%*, Black = *Even Balance 25%*, Brown = *Best Pivot*.

The trajectories for the change in life expectancy (Figure 4) (measured relative to Year 0) all show rebound after the shock, but with significant differences in magnitude and timing.

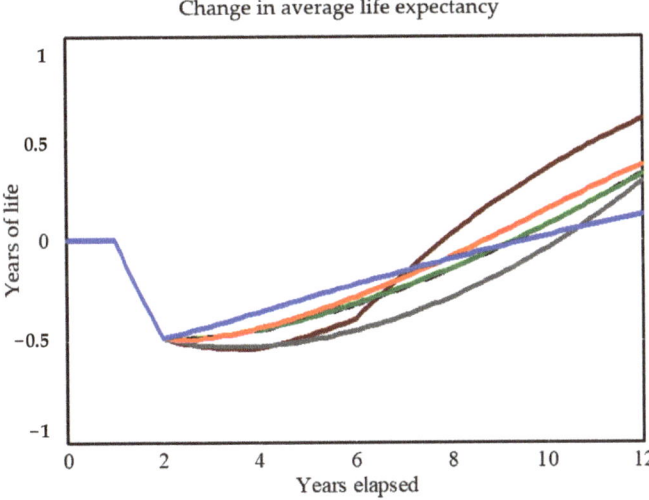

Figure 4. Change in average life expectancy under six allocation scenarios. Blue = *Status Quo*, Red = *Vital Conditions 40%*, Green = *Equity 40%*, Grey = *Belonging and Civic Muscle 40%*, Black = *Even Balance 25%*, Brown = *Best Pivot*. Note the black line is nearly indistinguishable from the green line here.

Status Quo looks best for the first several years. With its heavy emphasis on urgent services capacity, it is the only strategy that avoids a further rise in suffering after the shock. However, *Status Quo* is also the worst strategy for increasing the thriving percent; as a result, it is the worst of the six investment scenarios on life expectancy by Year 12. Runs with a fixed emphasis on drivers other than urgent services capacity (*Vital Conditions 40%*, *Equity 40%*, *Belonging and Civic Muscle 40%*, *Even Balance 25%*) all do better on thriving but not as well on suffering, ultimately producing modest net gains in life expectancy.

The clear winner on this metric, from Year 7 onward, is *Best Pivot*. This strategy allocates 65% of assets to equity in Year 2, and then pivots decisively to urgent services capacity and vital conditions. The early emphasis on equity works because it activates a virtuous reinforcing feedback loop (designated in Figure 1 as "equity builds strength"): equity helps build belonging and civic muscle, which builds more community assets, which, in turn, help expand equity even more—as well as all other drivers of well-being.

Although *Best Pivot* does worse on life expectancy than most of the other strategies immediately after the shock, it establishes equity as an immediate priority and builds a reservoir of belonging and civic muscle, both of which continue to yield benefits for years even after attention pivots back to expanding urgent services capacity and vital conditions– both of which become stronger and more equitable than under the other strategies. By concentrating first on equity and belonging and civic muscle, *Best Pivot* prepares the ground for building adequate urgent services but without sacrificing vital conditions and thriving (as occurs in *Status Quo* and *Belonging and Civic Muscle 40%*).

Furthermore, tests using alternative initial conditions (described in Supplementary File S3) show that (1) a more disorganized community would have a harder time recovering; but (2) even a community with twice as many suffering people and half the amount of equity, social support, and belonging and civic muscle can still recover fully and reach greater levels of equitable well-being within a decade if they commit to the *Best Pivot* strategy.

4. Discussion

4.1. Tentative Strategic Implications

The results above illustrate dynamics that we have seen consistently from the Thriving Together Model. Although the model is still exploratory, we hypothesize that the basic logic of the Springboard (e.g., the idea that belonging and civic muscle is a critical, yet constrained and contested resource) may lead to the following conclusions:

1. The best resilience strategy may require decisive shifts from historical priorities.
2. The best strategy requires investing early in both equity and belonging and civic muscle so that one may build on those assets later: a kind of self-reinforcing, asset-building maneuver. The value of those early investments is not only because they support thriving by helping people connect and heal through collective trauma. It is also because they support the infrastructure needed for shared stewardship. In a diverse and divided community, it takes dedicated resources to establish greater interdependence and enable stewards to work across differences, devise shared plans, gather and manage assets, and adapt to challenges over time.
3. Efforts to transition toward an equitable, thriving future may involve some inevitable sacrifice of greater suffering in the shorter term; a "worse before better" dynamic. This dynamic has been described previously with respect to downstream and upstream health investments [14], as well as business process improvements and the concept of the "capability trap" [15].
4. A risk-averse approach (changing priorities little from the status quo and leaving them fixed over time) may avoid the worse-before-better pattern, but the lack of a decisive pivot will result in a mediocre trajectory over time. Safe, static allocation avoids sacrifice, but it does not build the reservoirs of equity or belonging and civic muscle needed to both boost thriving and drive down suffering.
5. A community that can pivot strongly toward building equity and belonging and civic muscle after a severe shock may be best positioned to spring forward and maximize well-being over time. Although that maneuver is superior in principle (under the conditions of this analysis), it may be perceived as infeasible in practice– especially if it entails somewhat greater suffering immediately after a shock. Actual

feasibility, however, depends on how effectively community stewards make the case for equitable system change [16]. For instance, savvy casemakers could portray long-overdue investments in equity and belonging and civic muscle as a decisive break from a status quo that for generations has caused far greater unjust suffering and would otherwise continue to leave the entire community weaker and more vulnerable.

4.2. Contributions

The Thriving Together Springboard [7] lays out clear goals and principles but does not provide a detailed strategy for allocating assets over time. To help community stewards play out investment scenarios, we developed the *Thriving Together Model* as an exploratory tool that puts the Springboard concepts into motion. As far as we know, this is the first formal simulation model to represent dynamic connections among equity, belonging and civic muscle, vital conditions, and urgent services capacity as drivers of population levels of thriving, struggling, and suffering over a multiyear time horizon. This project also builds on Elinor Ostrom's Nobel Prize-winning work on shared stewardship [17] by developing a general explanation about how a divided community can heal through a traumatic shock and spring forward toward a future with greater well-being and justice. The practical contributions of the TTM include:

1. A focus on summary measures of population-level health and well-being, as opposed to focusing only on a particular subset of health or social outcomes. The model's main outcome measures (i.e., the Cantril categories of people thriving, struggling, and suffering) are routinely tracked across the US and around the world, allowing standardized comparisons over time and geography.
2. Representation of equity as a structural driver affecting the entire system, as opposed to only accounting for differences among certain subpopulations (e.g., by race, gender, or income).
3. Broad analytic boundary, encompassing concepts of well-being, vital conditions, urgent services, equity, and belonging and civic muscle and portraying their dynamic interactions.
4. Ability to explore alternative paths toward equitable renewal over a decade. The model does not tell leaders what to do, but rather strengthens their ability to interpret local data and negotiate local priorities, spot opportunities, weigh tradeoffs, and think creatively about navigating a multiyear path from crisis to renewal.
5. Ability to explain the dynamics of shock and renewal by tracking a suite of interacting variables and outcome metrics over time.

ReThink Health also used the TTM to create the Thriving Together Theater [18]. Guided by input from several hundred contributors, this interactive experience combines dynamic simulation, powered by the TTM, with dramatic role-play to explore how a group of community stewards can spring forward through an unjust shock. It is an immersive experience in shared stewardship that asks, "How will you and your fellow stewards exercise civic muscle while looking for an equitable path from crisis to renewal?" As in real life, the story depends on who shows up. The experience helps stewards rehearse high-stakes negotiations and play out potential consequences of their own investment priorities. Participants learn for themselves how to weigh tradeoffs and navigate the dynamics of equitable well-being in a community experiencing unjust adversity. The Thriving Together Theater has provoked creative conversations with hundreds of changemakers across the country, including community-led multisector partnerships, government agencies, and graduate schools. It is a reliable way to surface participants' mental models about equitable long-term resilience, while also emphasizing the importance of adaptive, shared stewardship.

4.3. Limitations and Extensions

The TTM incorporates multiple sources of available evidence, but it requires further development and validation in line with system dynamics modeling best practice [19,20] to generate more definitive insights. This would likely entail working closely with colleagues in several communities that have experienced shock and attempts at renewal. Data collection and group model building with community leaders would inform a new iteration of the TTM that is more historically grounded and usefully detailed. This enhanced model would likely have more precise and operational measures for concepts such as equity as well as belonging and civic muscle. Ideally, it would also have a straightforward data-driven method for calibration to represent characteristics of any given community as they explore their own path toward an equitable, thriving future.

Supplementary Materials: The following supporting information can be downloaded at: https://www.mdpi.com/article/10.3390/systems10050158/s1, Supplementary File S1: Equation List; Supplementary File S2: Parameter Assumptions; Supplementary File S3: Tests in a more disorganized community.

Author Contributions: Conceptualization and design, J.H., B.M., and C.S.; data acquisition and analysis, J.H.; data visualization, J.H., B.M., and C.S.; writing—original draft preparation, J.H. and B.M.; writing—review and editing, J.H., B.M., and C.S. All authors have read and agreed to the published version of the manuscript.

Funding: The Rippel Foundation supported this work through the ReThink Health initiative.

Data Availability Statement: All data are publicly available. Simulated scenarios can be explored with our free online interface at: http://tiny.cc/thriving-dynamics (accessed on 13 September 2022).

Acknowledgments: This study was inspired by 100+ fellow contributors to the *Thriving Together Springboard*. We are grateful for early guidance from colleagues at ReThink Health (Laura Landy, Anna Creegan, Ella Auchincloss), Community Initiatives Network (Monte Roulier, Elizabeth Hartig, Stacy Wegley); as well as the Well Being in the Nation (WIN) Network (Somava Saha and the WIN Measurement and Research Collaborative).

Conflicts of Interest: The author declares no conflict of interest.

References

1. Botchwey, N.; Dannenberg, A.; Frumkin, H. *Making Healthy Places: Designing and Building for Well-Being, Equity, and Sustainability*, 2nd ed.; Island Press: Washington, DC, USA, 2022.
2. Braveman, P.; Cubbin, C.; Egerter, S.; Pedregon, V. *Neighborhoods and Health*; Robert Wood Johnson Foundation: Princeton, NJ, USA, 2011; Available online: https://www.rwjf.org/en/library/research/2011/05/neighborhoods-and-health-.html (accessed on 5 August 2022).
3. Milstein, B. Thriving Together through Shared Stewardship. ReThink Health. 2021. Available online: http://tiny.cc/SharedStewardshipVideo (accessed on 5 August 2022).
4. Rethink Health. Vital Conditions for Well-Being and Justice. 2022. Available online: http://www.rethinkhealth/about/#1 (accessed on 5 August 2022).
5. Institute of Medicine. *Healthy, Resilient, and Sustainable Communities after Disasters: Strategies, Opportunities, and Planning for Recovery*; National Academies Press: Washington, DC, USA, 2015; Available online: https://nap.nationalacademies.org/catalog/18996/healthy-resilient-and-sustainable-communities-after-disasters-strategies-opportunities-and (accessed on 5 August 2022).
6. Walpole, E.H.; Loerzel, J.; Dillard, M. *A Review of Community Resilience Frameworks and Assessment Tools: An Annotated Bibliography*; National Institute for Standards and Technology: Washington, DC, USA, 2021. Available online: https://nvlpubs.nist.gov/nistpubs/TechnicalNotes/NIST.TN.2172.pdf (accessed on 5 August 2022).
7. Milstein, B.; Roulier, M.; Hartig, E.; Kelleher, C.; Wegley, S. (Eds.) *Thriving Together: A Springboard for Equitable Recovery and Resilience in Communities across America*; Well Being Trust: Oakland, CA, USA, 2020; Available online: http://www.thriving.us (accessed on 5 August 2022).
8. Milstein, B.; Homer, J. Which Priorities for Health and Well-Being Stand out after Accounting for Tangled Threats and Costs? Simulating Potential Intervention Portfolios in Large Urban Counties. *Milbank Q.* **2020**, *98*, 372–398. [CrossRef] [PubMed]
9. University of Wisconsin Population Health Institute. *County Health Rankings & Roadmaps*; University of Wisconsin Population Health Institute: Madison, WI, USA, 2022; Available online: http://www.countyhealthrankings.org (accessed on 5 August 2022).
10. Gallup. Understanding How Gallup Uses the Cantril Scale: Development of the "Thriving, Struggling, Suffering" Categories. 2020. Available online: https://news.gallup.com/poll/122453/understanding-gallup-uses-cantril-scale.aspx (accessed on 5 August 2022).
11. World Bank. Gini Index for the United States. Available online: https://fred.stlouisfed.org/series/SIPOVGINIUSA (accessed on 5 August 2022).

12. Witters, D.; Harter, J. In U.S., Life Ratings Plummet to 12-Year Low. Gallup. 2020. Available online: https://news.gallup.com/poll/308276/life-ratings-plummet-year-low.aspx (accessed on 5 August 2022).
13. Arora, A.; Spatz, E.; Herrin, J.; Riley, C.; Roy, B.; Kell, K.; Coberley, C.; Rula, E.; Krumholz, H.M. Population Well-Being Measures Help Explain Geographic Disparities in Life Expectancy at the County Level. *Health Aff.* **2016**, *35*, 2075–2082. Available online: http://content.healthaffairs.org/content/35/11/2075.abstract (accessed on 5 August 2022). [CrossRef] [PubMed]
14. Homer, J.B.; Hirsch, G.B. System Dynamics Modeling for Public Health: Background and Opportunities. *Am. J. Public Health* **2006**, *96*, 452–458. [CrossRef] [PubMed]
15. Repenning, N.P.; Sterman, J.D. Nobody Ever Gets Credit for Fixing Problems That Never Happened: Creating and Sustaining Process Improvement. *Calif. Manag. Rev.* **2001**, *43*, 64–88. [CrossRef]
16. Manuel, T.; Milstein, B. To Catalyze System Change, Become a Better Casemaker. ReThink Health, 10 March 2020. Available online: https://rethinkhealth.org/blog/Resource/to-catalyze-system-change-become-a-better-casemaker/ (accessed on 5 September 2022).
17. Ostrom, E. Beyond Markets and States: Polycentric Governance of Complex Economic Systems. Stockholm, Sweden: Nobel Prize Lecture, 2009. Available online: http://www.nobelprize.org/nobel_prizes/economic-sciences/laureates/2009/ostrom-lecture.html (accessed on 5 August 2022).
18. Milstein, B.; Homer, J.; Soderquist, C.; Belsky, M. Playbill for the Thriving Together Theater. ReThink Health. Available online: http://tiny.cc/thriving-playbill (accessed on 5 August 2022).
19. Sterman, J.D. *Business Dynamics: Systems Thinking and Modeling for a Complex World*; Irwin McGraw-Hill: Boston, MA, USA, 2000.
20. Homer, J. Best Practices in System Dynamics Modeling, Revisited: A Practitioner's View. *Syst. Dyn. Rev.* **2019**, *35*, 177–181. [CrossRef]

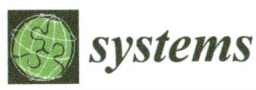

Article

Resilience Development in Multiple Shocks: Lessons in Mental Health and Well-Being Deterioration during COVID-19

Ke Zhou [1,*] and Mengru Zhang [2]

1 UCL Institute for Environmental Design and Engineering, The Bartlett Faculty of The Built Environment, University College London, London WC1H 0NN, UK
2 The Wright Institute, Berkeley, CA 94704, USA
* Correspondence: ke.zhou@ucl.ac.uk

Abstract: Resilience describes individuals' and organizations' recovery from crises and adaptation to disturbances and adversities. Emerging research shows the deterioration of the population's mental health and well-being during the multiple waves of the COVID-19 pandemic, suggesting that the resilience developed is insufficient to address the system's persistent shocks. Drawing on the findings on mental health and well-being during the COVID-19 pandemic and the psychological and organizational resilience theories, we developed a system dynamics theory model exploring how the presence of multiple shocks to the system challenges the population's health and well-being. We initiated the model with three shocks with the same intensities and durations, and then experimented with scenarios in which the strength of multiple shocks (duration and intensity) was attenuated and amplified. The model showed that temporary environmental adjustments with limited long-term stabilized solutions and a lack of health service provision can increase the accumulative risks of health and well-being deterioration. We highlight the role of essential health service sectors' resilience and individuals' and organizations' tolerance of adversities and disturbances in providing sustainable resilience. We conclude by discussing critical factors in organizational and psychological resilience development in crises with multiple shocks to the system.

Keywords: COVID-19; resilience; system dynamics

1. Introduction

As of August 2022, COVID-19 has caused over six million deaths and approximately 600 million confirmed cases worldwide [1]. While many of us hoped that COVID-19 would be over before the summer of 2020 after the first wave, the pandemic continued with multiple ongoing waves of increasing diseases and cases. Despite the attempts and responses to the pandemic from multiple levels, the system has not developed enough resilience to address the ongoing shocks and waves of the crisis. In the U.K., multiple studies have shown the population's deterioration in mental health and overall well-being between March and May 2020 [2]. Followed by a period of improvement in the summer of 2020, there was a second deterioration in population mental health and well-being between October 2020 and February 2021. Studies have shown that inequality in population mental health and psychological distress was significantly higher in the second wave [3]. The threat of persistent stress on health is also lasting. Trajectory analysis of psychological well-being in the COVID-19 waves showed that nearly two-fifths of the population experienced elevated distress risk [4]. The risk of persistent deterioration shows that the experience of distress in the first wave was not transformed into resilience to respond to following shocks in the second and third waves.

Resilience describes how the system recovers and adapts to the disturbances in crises. At the individual level, resilience refers to how individuals retrieve stability in healthy functioning and develop insights and learnings to positively adapt to future disturbances [5,6].

Crises bring multiple shocks to a complex system in which individual resilience interconnects with social and physical ecology factors at the group and organizational levels [7–9]. Pandemics require integrated systems to provide prevention and treatment services [10], as well as require organizations and their members to provide and adjust to new norms of collaboration and communication. However, mitigation measures might upend people's economic and social lives, leading to increases in psychological distress [4]. The mental health and well-being deterioration during the COVID-19 pandemic indicates that resilience development has not been activated or is insufficient for handling persistent stress, strains, and adversity.

While the resilience literature views adversity, strain, and significant barriers as bringing opportunities for adaptation and development [11,12], it is unclear how human–environment resilience is interconnected and provides the population and system with sustainable recovery during the multiple waves of crises.

System dynamics modeling offers opportunities to explore and theorize resilience development by exploring the causal and feedback mechanisms of the risk of accumulative interruptions and resilience development [13,14]. System dynamics focus on the feedback structures that underlie complex behaviors [15]. Through computer-aided simulation models, we can explore the underlying mechanisms to advance theory development [16,17]. By drawing on the findings of mental health and well-being during the COVID-19 pandemic and psychological and organizational resilience theories, we developed a small system dynamics theory model exploring how the presence of multiple shocks to the system challenges the population's health and well-being.

Our contributions are two-fold: First, drawing on the psychosocial (individual) and organizational resilience literature, we contribute to the theorizing of multisystemic approaches in resilience development, especially when the system is exposed to risks of multiple shocks. Second, we explore the accumulative risk of the population's health and well-being deterioration and propose interventions that can help mitigate and protect population well-being in long-crisis events such as COVID-19.

2. COVID-19 and Multisystemic Perspectives in Resilience Development

This section summarizes the resilience perspectives in relation to COVID-19 and provides an overview of psychological resilience and organizational resilience theories.

2.1. Resilience Development during COVID-19

The systematic review revealed that the deterioration of health and well-being, especially the negative impact on mental well-being, including high rates of anxiety, depression, posttraumatic stress disorder, and psychological and emotional distress, is widespread worldwide [18]. In the U.K., the COVID-19 mental health and well-being surveillance report [2] published by Public Health England showed that mental health and well-being during the pandemic has demonstrated an "up-and-down" pattern, in that there have been continuous deteriorations in health and well-being throughout the multiple waves. The report synthesized insights from multiple data sources, such as the University College London's COVID-19 Social Study and national data from the Office for National Statistics. The report highlighted a general increase in psychological stress during the pandemic, particularly for young people aged between 18 to 34 years. Analysis from the U.K. Householder Longitudinal Study further suggested that the second wave of COVID-19 was associated with a significant increase in psychological distress [19]. As Figure 1 shows, the proportion of people with clinically significant levels of psychological distress rose from 20.7% to 29.8% compared to the pre-pandemic levels. Between October 2020 and February 2021, a second deterioration in the population's mental health and well-being was observed [19]. By March 2021, the distress levels increased to 27.1%, significantly higher than the pre-pandemic level [19]. Even though the majority of the population are resilient or recovered quickly, two-fifths of the population experienced significant and severe distress repeatedly and continuously [4].

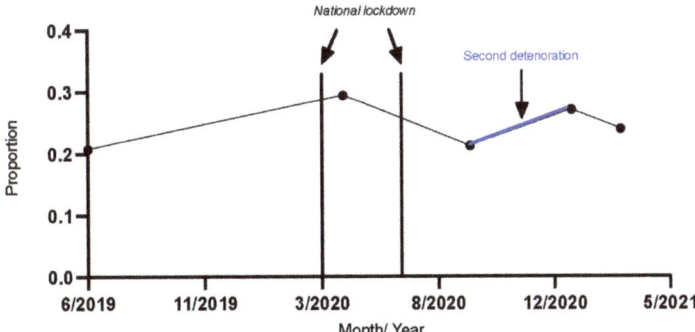

Figure 1. Changes in population mental health and well-being. Adapted from Daly and Robinson [19]. Copyright (2022), with permission from Elsevier.

Long-term distress exposure increases mortality risk and results in poor health outcomes [20]. Due to the nature of the long-lasting and prolonged effect of COVID-19, researchers pay increasing attention to trajectory changes in the multiple waves of crises [3,4,21,22]. Health systems' resilience in governance, health workforce, provision of medical products, and health service delivery has been stressed [23]. Aside from vaccination and hospital capacity, health workers' well-being also influences service capacity. Greenberg et al. [24] suggested that the National Health Service (NHS), as an organization, needs to provide post-trauma social support to healthcare workers during the COVID-19 pandemic facing increasing numbers of working hours.

Emerging research presents a resilience perspective that the unprecedented and prolonged pandemic brings shocks to individuals' health and well-being [22], and the health service system [25], and significant disturbances at all societal levels [26]. However, despite the attention to resilience development in relation to COVID-19, there is limited knowledge and theory of resilience development in crises with multiple shocks.

2.2. Clinical and Multisystemic Perspectives in Psychological Resilience

Psychological resilience at the clinical level promotes personal assets and protects them from the adverse effects of stressors [6]. Psychological resilience indicates less appraisal of negative emotions, higher capacity of meta-cognition in response to felt emotions [5,6], more insights and self-reflection [27], positivity [28], psychological flexibility [29], and adaptive coping strategies. A multisystemic perspective in psychological resilience theory concerns a process where various systems (biological, psychological, social, and ecological) interact in ways that help individuals to regain, sustain, or improve their mental well-being in contexts of adversity and distress [9]. Psychological resilience can vary among different populations and cultural communities. It reinforces positive and protective/preventive aspects at different stages of the stress process.

The multisystemic perspective has broadened the understanding and facilitation of psychological resilience. At the individual level, the study of children with abuse experience recognizes cognitive appraisal, high rumination, high distress tolerance, low suppression of emotion, low expression of aggression, and a secure attachment relating to high psychology resilience [30]. Family- and community-level factors such as family cohesion, parental involvement, social support, and household income contribute to psychological and behavioral changes in resilience [30]. Recent findings have recognized that biological genes, confounded by factors such as the environment, population, and demographic features, are associated with the complexity of individual resilience [31]. Furthermore, cultural dynamics and contexts and environmental safety and security also impact how individuals adjust to adversity [8]. Compared to narrow perspectives on individual dynamics, the multisystemic perspective stresses that psychological resilience is a complex phenomenon of intersectionality, which dynamically varies and shifts alongside individuals, communities, and societal systems.

Clinical facilitation of psychological resilience may relate to interventions on the individual psyche to achieve protective psychological features and personal development, as mentioned above, to prevent individuals from being overwhelmed by emotional distress and adversity. By strengthening one's tolerance of distress, individuals are equipped with a range of coping skills and strategies for adjusting and coping with adversity. Clinical contact, as a kind of interpersonal contact with its frame, provide relational social support, companionship, and a process where the individual has the space to explore and experience their own resilience and personal assets. Relevant psychoeducation, taking into account intersectionality, can include contextual factors, such as cultural identity, community environment, and external systems, in interventions. Lastly, community clinical settings can identify and bridge an individual with needed social welfare support, resources, and social advocacy, so that one may regain homeostasis in their social and ecological systems.

2.3. Organizational Resilience and Impact

Exploring interconnections between individual and organizational resilience is crucial from the multisystemic perspective as organizations underly the complex system and generate mitigation and actions [32]. Discontinuity and disruption not only cause adversity for individuals to respond to [7], but also raise a question regarding to what extent the environment is stable for people in acute distress. Crisis events such as climate change, energy (gas) crises, and extreme weather events leave high-level complexities and uncertainties for organizations to adapt to [33]. Thus, the idea of organizational resilience and how organizations adapt to exogenous changes are becoming increasingly relevant and essential. For example, Bryce et al. [25] argued that the U.K. government and NHS need to "readjust" to the new environment by operating through national emergency preparedness, aside from coping with the challenge of inadequate resource provision in terms of virus tests, ventilators, and personal protective equipment.

Organizational resilience describes the environment attempting to adjust to disturbances in the environment. While turbulence and adverse events are often viewed negatively, resilience studies have the underlying aim of shifting from the tendency to focus on "failures, decline, and maladaptive or pathological cycles" to "how organizations continually achieve desirable outcomes amid diversity" [11]. Meyer [34] framed sudden and unprecedented events as "environmental jolts" that create transient perturbations and force organizations to adapt to the environment. The process of averting maladaptive outcomes involves the organizations, their units, and members developing and mobilizing cognitive, emotional, relational, and structured resources to cope with adverse events. When organizations face sudden and unprecedented events, according to Meyer [34], resilience occurs if the organization absorbs the environmental jolt's impacts and decreases deviation from the previous order. Specifically, the process of adapting to environmental stimuli includes three phases: Anticipating changes and risks of failure, responding to and providing changes, and then readjusting the strategies and resources after the shocks.

The psychodynamic perspective in organizational research has shed light on some of the unintended consequences of organizational defenses against disturbances derived from external threats, internal conflicts, or the nature of work [35]. Understanding the interplays of individual and organizational narratives in organizational changes is essential, as collective learning can develop "critical self-reflexivity and an identify-focused dialogue" to mitigate maladaptive defenses such as denial, rationalization, and idealization [36].

In facing threats and potential risks in functioning and performance, learnings and insights can inform strategy-making to be resilient to future disturbances [34]. Organizational adaptations and learnings are "dynamic" and require "multi-institutional working" in broader systems [37]. Williams et al. [38] described that organizational members' and organizations' responses to disturbance can change over time and shape future interpretations and responses to adverse events. The responses depend on individuals' cognitive, behavioral, emotional, and relational capabilities and their interactions with organizational efforts in risk reduction and reliability, forming "feedback causal mechanisms" between individuals and organizations [38].

Although the connection between individual and organizational psychosocial resilience has been recognized—for example, individual employees' response to and coping with adverse or significant traumatic events may influence their capacity to perform their roles [33]—mainstream research on organizational resilience uses business performance as one of the key indicators. According to Ilseven et al. [39], the critical components in measuring resilience are the magnitude and rate of the both drop and recovery in organizations' performance. The operational or engineering frame of organizational resilience is helpful in that the functioning of organizations is essential. However, the frame misses the multisystemic perspective that individuals and members of organizations face psychosocial risk or challenges, which influences how individuals collaborate and perform. As Kahn et al. [40] suggested, if the relational systems that underlie organizations remain disturbed, even when operational performance interruptions have been resolved, organizations can still face dysfunctional patterns of behavior and longer-term performance issues.

3. Methods

System dynamics modeling is a methodology that explores the complexity of circular causality or feedback loops and how interactions between factors can result in non-linear behaviors in the systems [15]. It can be applied to generate robust policies in specific real-world issues such as public health (e.g., [41–43]), climate and environmental (e.g., [44,45]), and operational and managerial issues (e.g., [46,47]). It is also widely used to inform theory building and testing [48], especially in organizational and management theories (e.g., [49–52]). The significant difference between theoretical and applied system dynamics modeling regards the steps in the modeling process (if specifics of policy arrangements need to be provided), data (if the collection of primary data is needed), and model boundaries (if the omission of specific variables and relationships is acceptable) [17]. While applied modeling is about developing a model to develop specific policy suggestions for the phenomenon under investigation, theory-based modeling focuses on generalizability and providing incremental knowledge to explain and theorize a phenomenon without the absolute need to collect empirical data on a specific instance [16,17,48,53]. Through model-based theory building, more profound insights can be gained and tested to inform the development of "minor and middle-range theories" that attempt to build generic and overall explanations of a problem but have not yet been formed as a unified theory [53].

A theory-based modeling approach was chosen to contribute to the theorizing of resilience development in multiple shocks and to provide some generic learnings regarding health and well-being deterioration during the COVID-19 pandemic. A resilience model was developed via the following steps: First, health and well-being deterioration phenomena are defined through reports and data. The COVID-19 mental health and well-being surveillance report [2] was chosen mainly to aid in forming a definition of the problem, as it is one of the earliest publications synthesizing evidence in health and well-being deterioration during the COVID-19 pandemic. Second, a dynamic hypothesis was formed through reviewing the broader theories of psychological and organizational resilience. Third, the conceptualized model was developed iteratively by revising the initial structures and conceptualization [54]. Lastly, the model was tested and provided equilibrium runs and different combinations of shock duration and intensity, providing directions for policy testing and insight.

4. Model Conceptualization

This section describes the causal mechanisms and main feedback loops in the model conceptualization.

4.1. Resilience and Disturbance

The model starts with a stock of *Disturbance Events* (see Figure 2. Resilience and disturbance interconnections), representing the accumulation of disturbance events in the system. Disturbance events cause a departure from a standard or desired state [55]. We followed the definition of disturbance by White and Pickett [56] (p.7), that "a disturbance is any relatively discrete event in time that disrupts ecosystem, community, or population structure and changes resources, substrate availability, or the physical environment." In the model, the stock of *Disturbance Events* increases with an inflow of *average disturbance events per month*, assuming that there is a constant exogenous inflow of disturbance events for individuals to address. The stock decreases after the disturbances are processed by individuals, which depends on the *time needed to resolve events, effect of environmental resilience*, and *effect of individual resilience* on *decreasing disturbance events*.

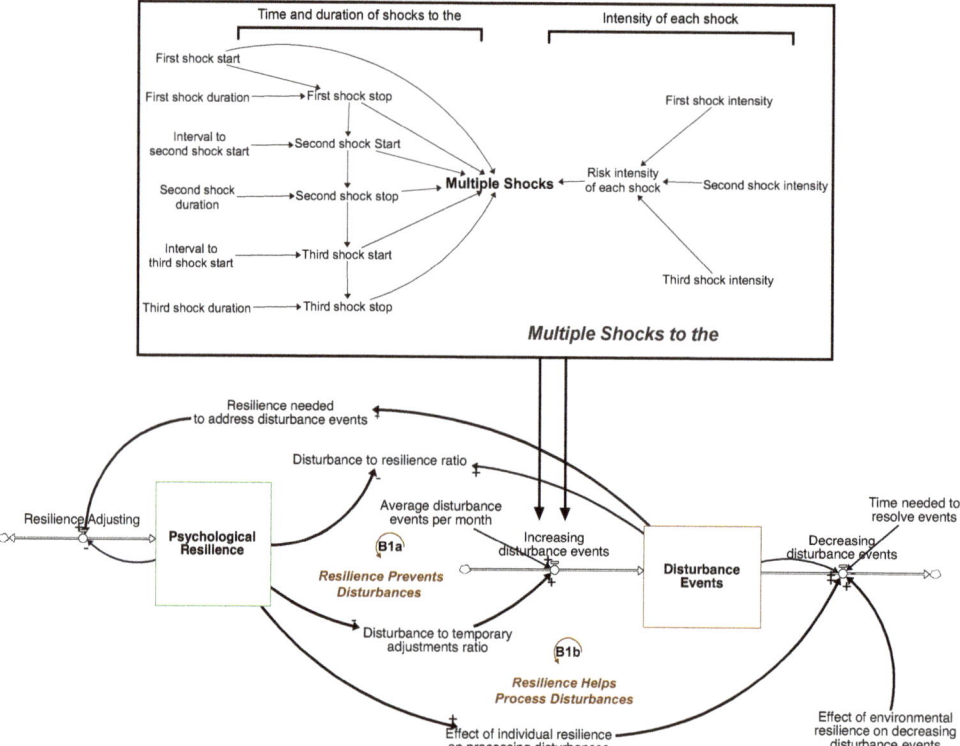

Figure 2. Resilience and disturbance interconnections. The top box describes the conceptualization of multiple shocks to the system. The bottom part of the figure shows the causal links between resilience and disturbance. *Note*: A positive (+) sign implies positive arrow polarity, meaning that an increase (decrease) in the cause variable will result in an increase (decrease) in the effect variable, compared to what would have been otherwise and if everything else stays the same. A negative (−) sign implies positive causality, meaning that an increase (decrease) in the cause variable will result in a decrease (increase) in the effect variable, compared to a what would have been otherwise and if everything else stays the same. 'B' represents 'balancing loops, meaning that an increase (decrease) of one variable would trigger a decrease (increase) of this variable after travelling the full loop.

Another stock in Figure 2 is *Psychological Resilience*, which represents the accumulation of resilience that individuals retain to address disturbances in the system. Resilience describes how individuals recover from shock, acquire stability in healthy functioning, and adapt to disturbances. *Increasing disturbance events* increases the *resilience needed to address disturbance events*, demanding individuals to develop resilience and decreasing the disturbance events perceived, which forms the first balancing loop—B1a: Resilience Prevents Disturbances. As individuals resolving disturbance events, the stock of *Disturbance Events* decreases, decreasing the demand for resilience, which forms another balancing loop—B1b: Resilience Helps Process Disturbances.

As shown in Figure 2, multiple shocks can create waves of disturbances in the system, increasing the inflow of the stock of *Disturbance Events*. To understand the impact of the multiple waves of crises on the system, we added three waves to the system, with the intensity and duration of each crisis that can be specified and changed.

4.2. Psychological Resilience at the Population Level

"Stress" describes people's general experience of psychosocial distress, including anxiety, depressive symptoms, sleep problems, self-reported mental health, loneliness, and general stress. We used three stocks in the population structure to describe changes in distress levels at the population level: *Low/mild Stress People, Highly Stressed People without Health and Well-being (HW) Services,* and *Highly Stressed People with HW Services* (see Figure 3). When low/mild stress people are exposed to crises or disturbance events, they move to the *Highly Stressed People without HW Services* through the flow *Stressing up*. The speed of moving to high-stress stock depends on two variables: (1) The *disturbance to resilience ratio*, which measures individuals' experience of disturbance level relative to their resilience level; (2) *time to change the stress level*. Although crises with multiple waves can hit all three population stocks, in the model, we assumed that the shocks do not bring additional adversities for the people who are already in the two high-stress stocks.

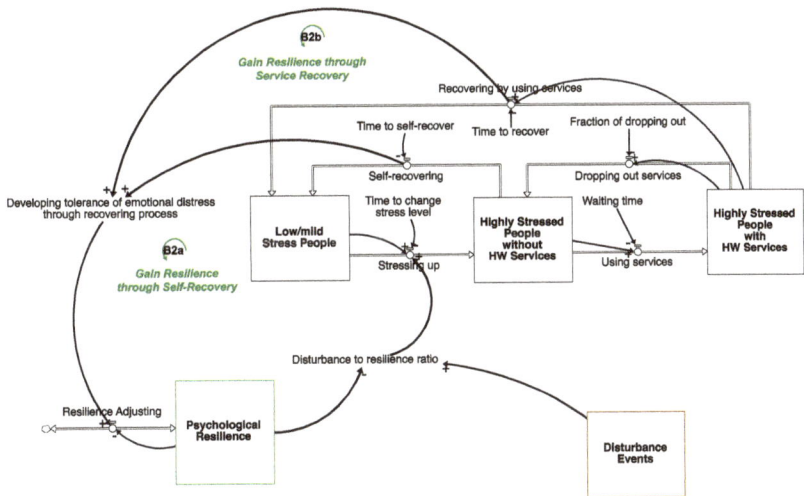

Figure 3. Population structure linking with resilience and disturbance.

Short-term deterioration in health and well-being does not directly indicate an increase in mental illness or a need for HW service support. As this model aims to understand the connections between individual and organizational resilience and potential policies, we assumed that a fraction of highly stressed people will use HW services and move to the third stock: *Highly Stressed People with HW Services*. A fraction of people from the service-using population might drop out and move to the *Highly Stressed People without HW Services* stock. People from the two high-stress stocks can recover after a specific time (2.5–3 months in the model) and move back to the *Low/mild Stress People* stock. The flow *recovering by using services* describes the process for people to gain higher tolerance of emotional distress and disturbance. The recovering process increases *Psychological Resilience*, which decreases the *Stressing up* process, decreasing highly stressed people with or without HW services, forming two balancing loops—B2a: Gain Resilience through Self-recovery and B2b: Gain Resilience through Service Recovery.

4.3. Health and Well-Being Service Sector Resilience

At the organizational level, the health service sector is critical in supporting and helping highly stressed people recover and gain emotional tolerance to adversity and distress. HW services include a range of therapies, case management, and community-based support. For example, brief treatments provide clinical intervention to decrease emotional distress, identify and reinforce strength and protective factors, introduce coping skills, increase relative insights, and provide social support and relational connection. HW services include triage systems that refer people to the appropriate level of care services. The process includes assessing the severity of psychological distress and can provide case management services with needed resources.

We used the stock of *HW Service Staff* to measure the health and well-being service sector capacity (see Figure 4). We measured how many health and well-being support sessions can be provided monthly. In this model, *Highly Stressed People without HW Services* increase the *total sessions demand*, requiring HW organizations to hire more staff to increase the service capacity, forming the third balancing loop—B3: Reduce Out of Services. Here, we also considered the demand of the existing clients in the system. Highly stressed people using HW services are also part of the session's demand. Providing services to the people already in the HW system indicates a further increase in the *total sessions demand*, which increases *HW Service Staff* as the capacity increase, forming the first reinforcing loop—R1: Adjust HW Service Capacity. Prioritizing services to people indicates a decrease in the remaining capacity, creating the fourth balancing loop—B4: Prioritize Existing Clients.

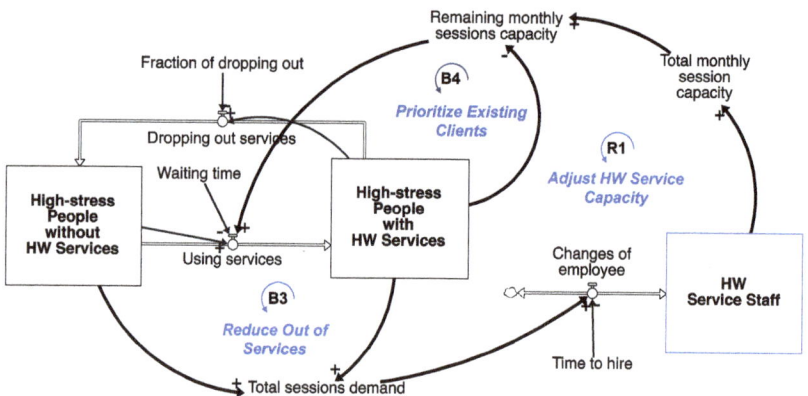

Figure 4. Health and well-being service provision. *Note:* 'R' represents 'reinforcing' loops, meaning that an increase (decrease) of one variable would trigger an increase (decrease) of this variable after travelling the full loop.

4.4. Organizational Resilience in the Environment

Aside from the health service sector mentioned above, another critical factor that connects individuals' and organizations' resilience is how the surrounding environment and organizations can mitigate the adversities and disturbances that individuals face. Multiple crisis events are "environmental jolts" that potentially bring opportunities for organizational transformation, which might also create disturbances for individuals. With "crisis shocks" in the system, the average number of disturbance events increases, increasing the number of people experiencing increased stressing.

In this model, we used the stock of *Environment Temporary Adjustments* to describe the organization's attempts to provide solutions (see Figure 5). Increasing disturbance events requires organizations such as workplaces to accommodate the events and increase temporary adjustments, which increases the disturbance events that individuals need to adjust to, forming the second reinforcing loop—R2: Temporary Environmental Disturbance. *Environment Temporary Adjustments* are settled and moved to the stock of *Stabilized Adjustments*, forming the fifth balancing loop—B5: Long-term Stabilization. For example, vaccination programs, work-from-home guidelines, and traveling notices formed some of the stabilized adjustments during the COVID-19 pandemic. *Environment Stabilized Adjustments* could be revisited after a specific time in multiple shocks, being moved to *Temporary Adjustments*.

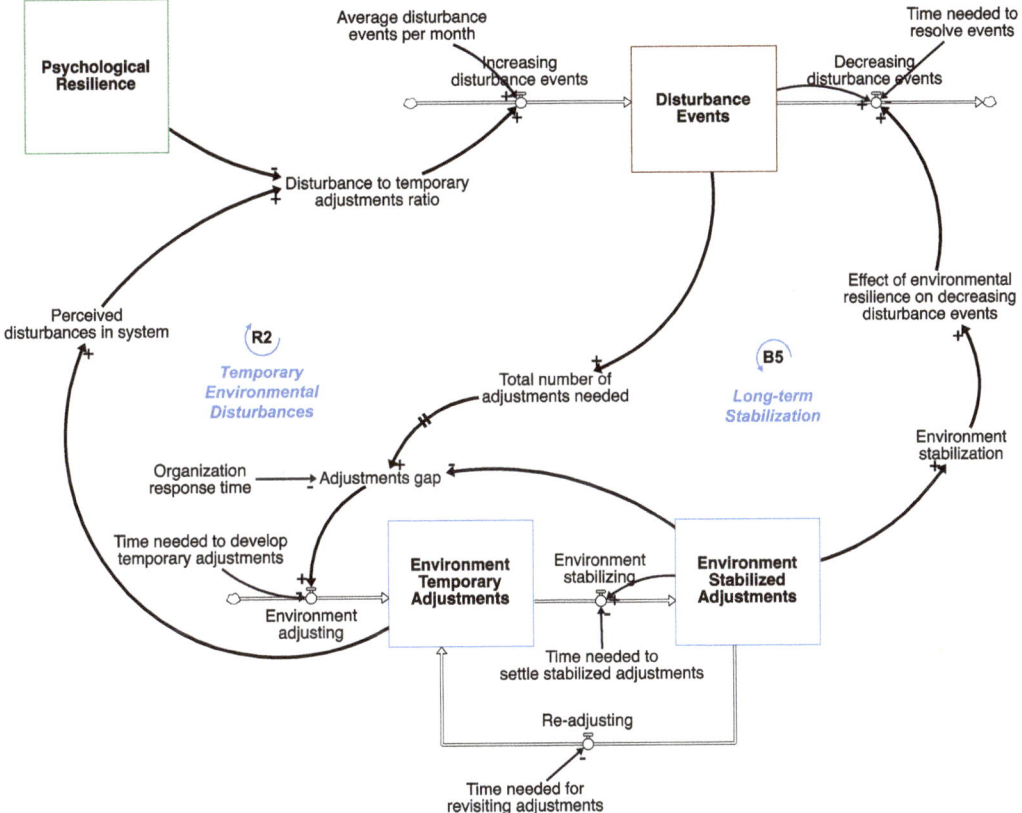

Figure 5. Organizational resilience in the environment.

In Figure 6, we present an overview of the main causal mechanisms and the interconnections between four sectors that we described.

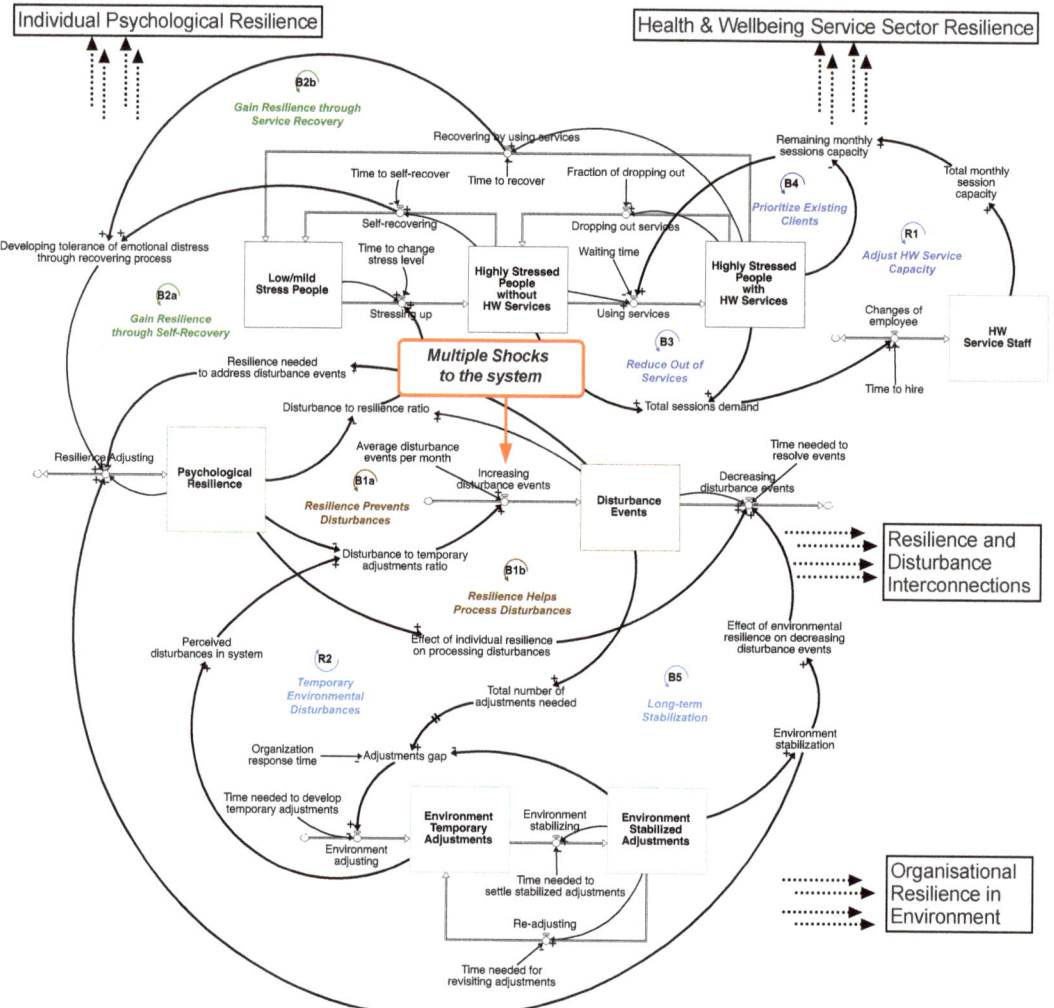

Figure 6. Stock and flow structure of the resilience model. The red box highlights the impact of multiple shocks to the system.

5. Model Results

The simulation model had a 200-month time horizon. In this section, we describe the model equilibrium conditions and how the model responds to different scenarios of multiple shocks.

5.1. Model Equilibrium

We initialized the model in equilibrium without any shocks to the system. The model equations are included in Appendix A. With an average of 2.5 disturbance events happening every month, the psychological resilience remained 0.6 throughout the model's running time of 200 months. The number of temporary adjustments remained the same as the adjustments demanded by the disturbance events, leaving the disturbance to temporary adjustments ratio at 1. The environmental stabilization ratio remained 0.23, indicating that the environment was stable in providing support. The model was initialized with

12,300 people, with 10,000 people having low/mild stress, 1.74k people not using HW services, and 543 highly stressed people using HW services. The mental health services had 57 staff throughout the model running time, providing 5700 sessions monthly to support the population's health and well-being.

5.2. Multiple Shocks in the Base Run

For the base run, we simulated the model with three consecutive shocks with equal intensities and durations. The model's time horizon was 200 months, while the shocks only presented in the initial 60 months, which is less than one-third of the running time. The reason is that a long time horizon can show the long-term impact and the process for the system to regain steady status. Each shock lasted five months, with an interval of six months and an equal intensity of three. The three shocks from month 20 to month 47 indicate that there were approximately two years of elevated disturbance, ensuring the investigation of the long-term impacts. A shock intensity of three increased the number of disturbances of events to 10 events per month. The first shock started by month 20. Figure 7 shows that the number of highly stressed people without HW services rose to 4200 by month 26.5, which shows that the peak of the first wave shocks had a 6.5-month delay. The maximum number of highly stressed people was a third of the total population. The next two waves displayed the same delays as the first wave. The peak of highly stressed people without HW services remained the same as in the first wave in the second wave, and then decreased to 3240 in the third wave. The psychological resilience ratio increased over the three consecutive shocks from 0.63 to 0.66, indicating that people recovering from using HW services or self-recovery gained tolerance toward the same intensity and duration of shock, increasing the population's resilience to future shocks. The psychological resilience ratio describes the general trend and changes in psychological resilience. The impact of the multiple shocks on the system lasted for the remaining simulation time, with a relatively stable increase in highly stressed people without HW services. Overall, the number of highly stressed people without HW services remained lower compared to pre-multiple shocks, due to the overall improvement in psychological resilience gained from the multiple shocks. The base run showed two interesting results:

- Resilience developed in multiple shocks can lower the number of highly stressed people without HW services compared to pre-shock conditions.
- Under the scenario of three consecutive shocks with the same durations and intensities, the psychological resilience at the population level increased over time, but was not sufficiently high enough to decrease the overall risk of deterioration of health and well-being.

5.3. Attenuation of Multiple Shocks

In the real world, the level of disturbances and adversities from crises varies. To explore the system's response to different crisis scenarios, we changed the durations, intervals, and intensities of the three consecutive shocks. The first scenario that we were interested in was the "attenuation of multiple shocks," in which the duration and intensity of the three shocks decreased over time. The first shock lasted 12 months with an intensity of six, the second shock lasted five months with an intensity of three, and the third shock lasted two months with an intensity of two. As Figure 8 shows, the number of highly stressed people without HW services increased immediately after the starting point of the first crisis in month 20 and kept increasing during the first wave for 10 months, reaching 6720 in month 30. Afterward, the number of highly stressed people without HW services started to decline before the end of the first wave, which occurred by month 32. Toward the end of the subsequent two waves of crises, the number of highly stressed people without HW services reached 3090 and 1670 per month.

The number of highly stressed people without HW services showed a stable decreasing-over-time pattern after the first wave, and the overall increase in psychological resilience was enormous compared to the base run throughout the 200 months. One of the reasons is that the duration and intensity of the shocks to the system decreased. Another reason is that the amplified first wave increased the total number of environmental adjustments needed for stabilizing the environment in comparison to the base run. While it brought more short-term disturbances to individuals to adjust (see R2: Temporary Environmental Disturbance in Figure 6), in the long run, the temporary solutions were transformed to stabilized adjustments that were relatively more sufficient to address the second and third waves as the shocks to the systems were also attenuated (see B5: Long-term Stabilization in Figure 6). Moreover, as more people experienced disturbances and adversities in the first wave, the recovering process increased the population's psychological resilience by increasing the emotional tolerance of distress and prevented individuals from becoming more stressed when the second and third shocks happened (see B2a and B2b: Gain Resilience through Self-recovery and Service Recovery, respectively in Figure 6). The health service system tried to increase the number of staff in the first significant wave, reaching approximately 139 staff by month 36.5 (after 4.5 months of the end of the first crisis), which was approximately 40 more staff in the same month in comparison to the base run. Consequently, the maximum number of flows of people becoming more stressed was significantly lower in the second and third waves. The environment became stable, providing more transformational adjustments throughout the crisis. The attenuation run showed another significant result:

- When the intensity and duration of the shocks decreased over time, the system's rapid responses in providing health services and environmental stabilization in the first significant shock were critical in improving the population's resilience in addressing the risk of health and well-being deterioration in later shocks.

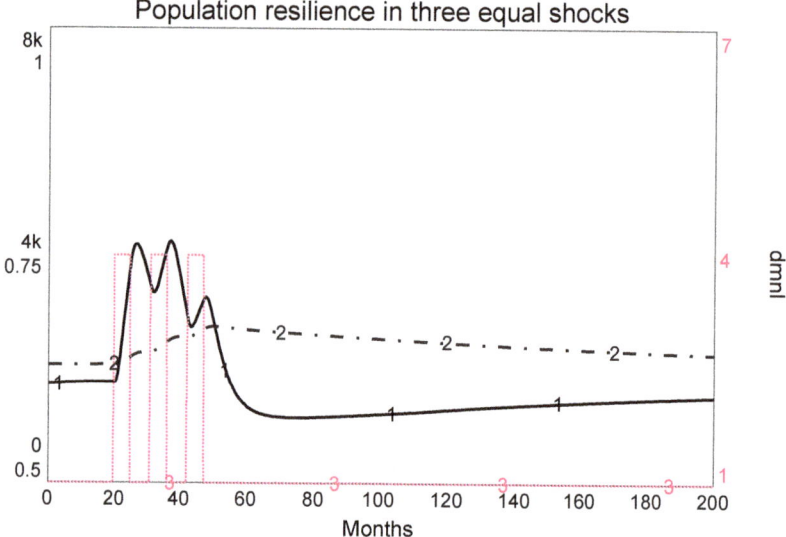

Figure 7. Population resilience with input of three shocks. Each shock lasted five months, with an interval of six months (dashed dot pink, right axis). Two indicators of population resilience were included: The number of highly stressed people without HW services (solid black, left axis, scale: 0~8000 people) and the psychological resilience ratio (dashed dot black, left axis, scale: 0.5~1).

5.4. Amplification of Multiple Shocks

The second scenario we were interested in was the "amplification of multiple shocks." The duration and intensity of the three shocks increased over time. In this scenario, we reversed the setting conditions of the "attenuation of multiple shocks" scenario. Here, the first shock lasted two months with an intensity of two, the second shock lasted five months with an intensity of three, and the third shock lasted 12 months with an intensity of six. Figure 9 shows that the number of highly stressed people without HW services kept increasing during the first and second waves for 10 months, reaching 4350 by month 34, which is higher than the base run. Afterward, until month 48, the number of highly stressed people without HW services rose exponentially to 5620 as the third shock hit the system by month 39 for another 12 months. The number of people without HW services started to decline from month 48, three months before the third shock ended, indicating that the stabilized solutions and HW services provided by the HW sector were effective before the third wave ended.

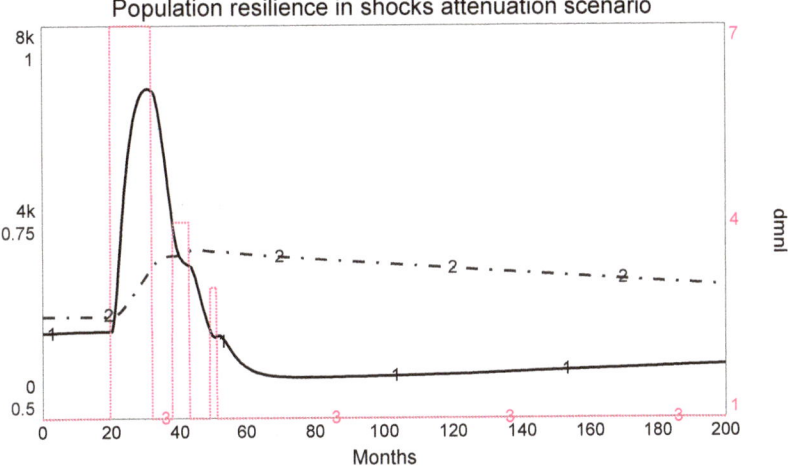

- 1 Attenuation shocks Highly Stressed People without HW Services (people)
- 2 Attenuation shocks Psychological resilience ratio (dmnl)
- 3 Attenuation shocks Multiple shocks to the system (dmnl)

Figure 8. Population resilience with an input of three attenuated shocks. The shocks (right axis) are shown in dashed dot lines in pink. The first shock lasted 12 months with an intensity of six, the second shock lasted five months with an intensity of three, and the third shock lasted two months with an intensity of two. The intervals between shocks remained six months.

Changes in the sequence of primary, mild, and minor shocks resulted in changes in the number of people who were stressed. Figure 10 shows comparisons of the accumulation of people became increasingly stressed and highly stressed people without HW services in four runs: Equilibrium, base run, shocks attenuation, and amplification. Before month 50, the accumulative number of people who became increasingly stressed in the attenuation scenario was the highest among the four runs, as the first wave was primary, leaving 6700 people without HW services (Figure 10b). However, from month 48 onward, the accumulative number of people stressed in the amplification scenario was higher than in the attenuation scenario throughout the simulation time. The outbreak of the third wave in the amplification scenario between months 39 and 51 left 5600 people without HW services (Figure 10b), which is lower than the peak in the attenuation stage. However, in the case of shock amplification, the psychological resilience and environmental stabilization solutions developed in the last two waves were not sufficient to prevent deterioration in the third wave (see B1a and B1b: Resilience Prevents Disturbances and Resilience Helps Process Disturbances, respectively in Figure 6), the accumulative number of people without HW services remaining in the amplification scenario was higher in comparison to that in the attenuation stage. After the disturbances were processed and resilience development caught up (see B2a and B2b: Gain Resilience through Self-recovery and Service Recovery, respectively, in Figure 6), the number of people who became increasingly stressed was lower than that in the equilibrium and base run. The amplification run and comparisons leave us with a final point that:

- When the intensity and duration of the shocks increased over time, while the direct consequences of the first minor and mild shocks can be relatively smaller, a higher risk of health and well-being deterioration can present in the following major shock if the resilience development process does not sufficiently prepare the system.

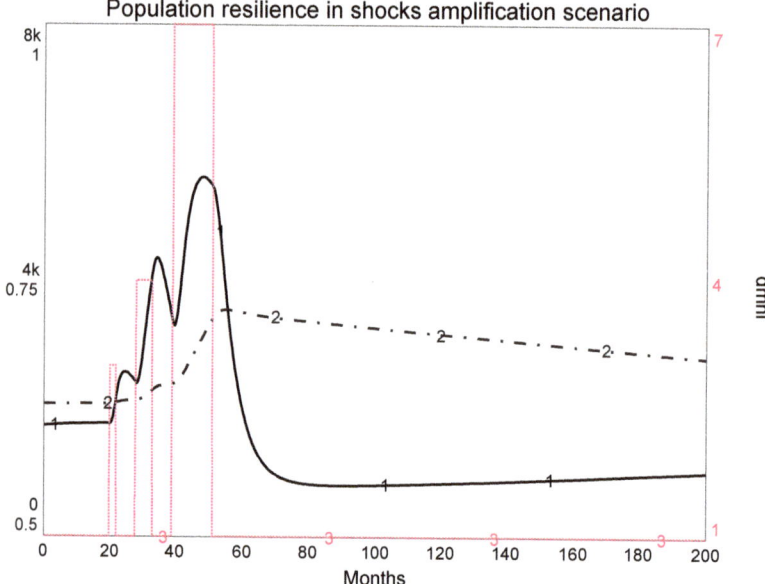

- 1- Amplification shocks Highly Stressed People without HW Services (people)
- 2 Amplification shocks Psychological resilience ratio (dmnl)
- 3 Amplification shocks Multiple shocks to the system (dmnl)

Figure 9. Population resilience with input of three amplified shocks. The shocks (right axis) are shown in dashed dot line in pink. The first shock lasted two months with an intensity of two, the second shock lasts five months with an intensity of three, and the third shock lasted 12 months with an intensity of six. The intervals between shocks remained six months.

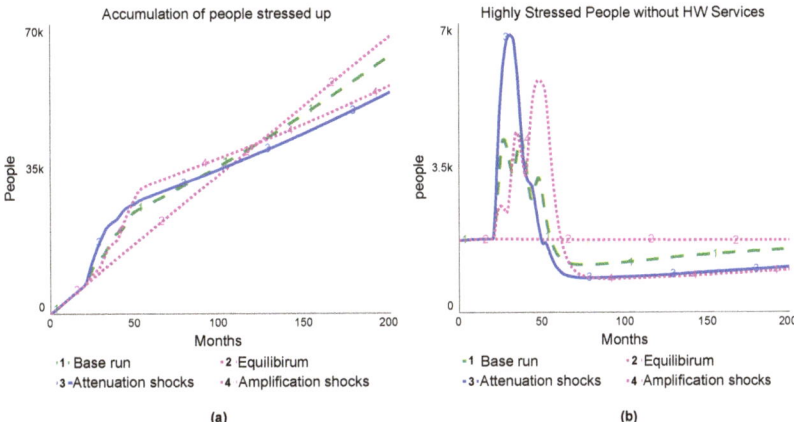

Figure 10. Comparisons of four runs: (**a**) Accumulation of people becoming increasingly stressed; (**b**) highly stressed people without HW services.

6. Policy Testing

The four runs suggest the importance of policies that develop resilience pre- and during multiple shocks of crises to decrease the risk of health and well-being deterioration. In this section, we describe how different policies can potentially reduce the number of highly stressed people without HW services in crises and increase the system's resilience to withhold future shocks.

Table 1 shows three policies and their dynamic principles and target loops. The first policy (P1) focuses on organizational adjustments—specifically, how organizations respond to crises and help individuals adjust to crises early when the shock hits the system. The second policy (P2) focuses on the health service sector's response to health service demand. The third policy (P3) focuses on individual and organizational learning during crises, which can help individuals develop a higher tolerance of distress and adversities. Moreover, organizations require stabilized adjustment when there are multiple and consecutive shocks as waves of crises.

Table 1. Policies for enhancing individual and organizational resilience when facing multiple crises.

Policy	Policy Description	Dynamic Principle	Targeted Loops
P1: Environment-based fast adjustments	Speeding up the environment's adjustments in providing temporary solutions. Organizations monitor changes, quickly respond to crises, and attempt to develop temporary plans and revisit them quickly once the shock hits the system.	The organizational response time is one month (base run is three months), the time needed for temporary plans equals two months (base run is four months), and every six months (base run is 12 months), the organization revisits the plan.	B2, B1a, B1b
P2: Health service sector-based fast responses	Providing health services to support health and well-being throughout crises. The health service sector responds to the demands of health services quickly and provides programs to encourage the use of health services.	The fraction of people reaching out to health and well-being services is 0.8 (base run is 0.5). The waiting time to access these services equals two months (base run is four months), and the time to hire new staff is now three months (base run is 12 months).	R1, B3, B4, B2b, B1a, B1b
P3: Collective growth	Facilitating organizations' and individuals' evolution and adjustment for long-term stabilization in crises. Specifically, individuals develop more resilience in tolerating distress and adversities through self-recovery and using health services. Moreover, organizations can provide stabilized adjustments (such as guidelines, arrangements, long-term strategies, and solutions) more quickly in crises.	The emotional tolerance acquired from the recovery process is four times that of the original baseline, which is now 4 (base run is 1), and the time for organizations to settle their stabilization adjustment is now three months (base run is 12 months).	B2a, B2b, B5, B1a, B1b

Figure 11a shows the accumulation of people becoming increasingly stressed, which is the sum of the flow "becoming increasingly stressed" over the 200 months. The accumulation shows the long-term impact of disturbance and resilience development. For the scenario of attenuation shocks (see runs 2~5 in Figure 11) and the scenario of amplification shocks (see runs 6~9 in Figure 11), while the first policy P1 managed to lower the number of highly stressed people with no HW services in the long run, it unexpectedly increased the maximum number of highly stressed people with no HW services in the major waves (runs 3 and 7 in Figure 11b), which suggests that the recovery from services cannot be placed to support the population's psychological resilience development, leaving more people at risk of becoming increasingly stressed. The unintended consequence of increasing the number of highly stressed people with no HW services is that the adjustment in P1 only considered the increase in short-time adjustments rather than stabilization of the long-term adjustment, which increased the disturbance level significantly in a short time, resulting in an increase in the number of highly stressed people with no HW services. As a result, the increased psychological resilience was not sufficient to address the increased level of disturbances in the environment.

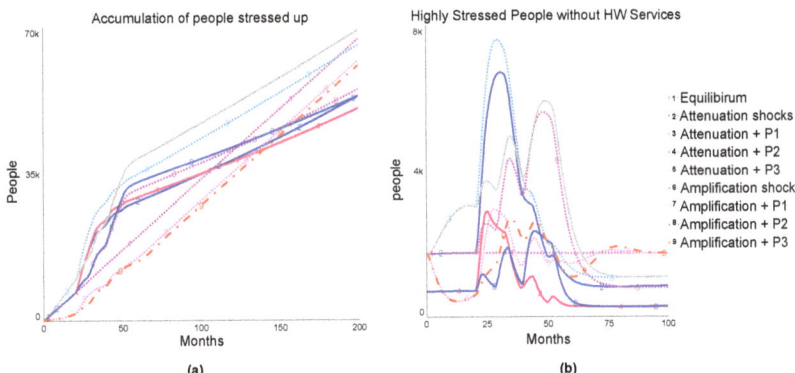

Figure 11. Policy tests. Comparisons of the three policies P1, P2, and P3 for the scenario of attenuation and amplification shocks, in comparison to the equilibrium conditions: (**a**) Accumulation of people becoming increasingly stressed in 200 months; (**b**) highly stressed people without HW services in the initial 100 months.

P2 (see runs 4 and 8 in Figure 11) showed the best outcome in reducing the number of highly stressed people with no HW services, compared to all other runs. Under P2, more than 200 health service staff, four times the initial number of health service staff in the system, were hired to provide services and help individuals gain resilience through the recovery process in both the attenuation and amplification scenarios. P2 significantly reduced the accumulation of stressed people over the long run after month 150. However, between months 50 and 125, a significant number of people still experienced adversity and distress, which shows that the reliance on service capacity changes is not the best policy.

Policy P3, collective growth (see runs 5 and 9 in Figure 11), significantly reduced the maximum number of stressed people with no HW services. As Figure 11b shows, the number of highly stressed people without HW services started to decline before the onset of the first shock in both the attenuation and amplification shocks scenarios, and the peaks were reduced by approximately 50%, suggesting that the prevention and pre-crises responses were activated before the crises. Consequently, disturbances and adversities can be addressed without being stressed. As Figure 11a shows, the accumulation of people becoming increasingly was significantly reduced throughout the simulation time. However, the impact of the shocks did not reach equilibrium until month 60 in Figure 11b, showing the accumulative risk of multiple shocks in the system again.

In summation, the policy test showed the critical role of health services in hiring staff to meet the service demand. However, it did not solve the fundamental problem of how multiple crisis shocks increase disturbance and stress for individuals, thus not sufficiently addressing the challenges of multiple shocks. Moreover, without long-term stabilization adjustments, rapid temporary adjustments can create unintended consequences in terms of increasing the number of disturbances over a short time, challenging the resilience of the system. Furthermore, providing individuals' and organizations' learnings and reflections on tolerating adversities and disturbances seems vital to improving resilience and preventing a significant level of distress at the population level.

7. Discussion, Limitations, and Implications

This paper adopted a feedback view of resilience development and drew theories of psychological and organizational resilience to determine how resilience is developed during multiple shocks in crises. The multisystemic perspective in connecting psychological and organizational resilience was used to develop a simulation model based on the learnings from mental health and well-being deterioration during the COVID-19 pandemic, which extends resilience theories. Model analysis illuminated that multiple shocks in crises, the rise of temporary adjustments, and limited service provision resources can increase the accumulative risk of the deterioration of health and well-being. Simulations and multiple combinations of intensities and durations of shocks demonstrated that the learnings developed during the first few shocks could potentially provide the system with a significant level of prevention that decreases the chances of continuous deterioration. In Figure 12, we show the how psychological resilience, environmental resilience, and the HW service provision form this "resilience," which can grow and buffer shocks in the multiple waves of a crisis. The simulation model contributed a few critical implications in theorizing the dynamics of resilience development in multiple shocks.

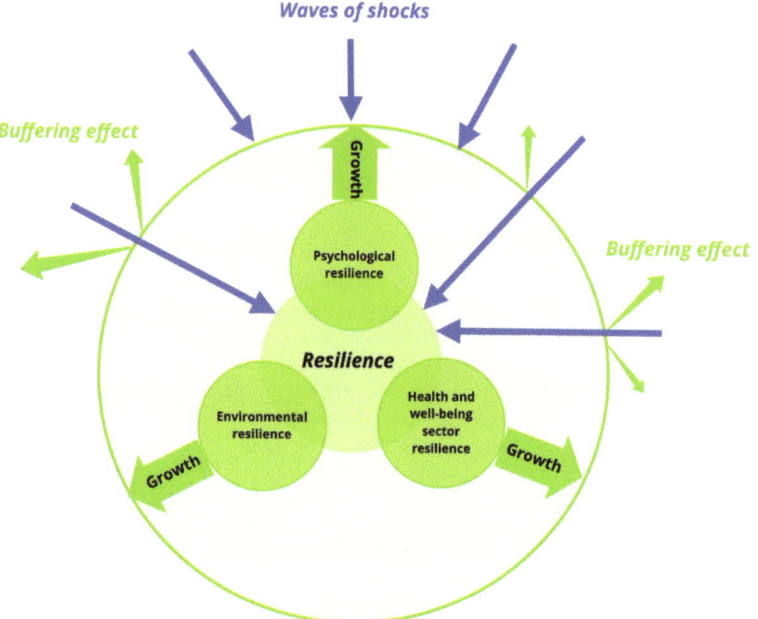

Figure 12. Resilience development in multiple shocks.

The first implication is extending the multisystemic perspectives in resilience development by seeing resilience as a complex adjustment process involving multiple systems and contexts. The risk of crises accumulates as the number of disturbance events rises beyond the resilience level. Abrupt, significant, temporary, and frequent changes in surrounding organizations may cause unintended difficulties for individuals, primarily when changes concern essential resources or support for one's immediate stabilization and grounding. For people who struggle with acute abruptions and disturbances, these changes may become another burdensome object that people need to become acquainted with quickly, which is likely to contribute to emotional disturbance in the sense of experiencing the unknown, uncertainty, and feelings of powerlessness, helplessness, and hopelessness.

The second implication relates to strengthening and reinforcing protective factors in producing systemic efforts of strategy development and policy design in population resilience. At an individual level, resilience developed through recovering from previous shocks of the exact nature is critical as it provides higher tolerance of distress and adversity. The recovery process requires individuals to constantly build on personal assets such as self-esteem and emotional positivity. It is also critical to develop adequate insights into one's external reality, nuanced emotions, and intrapsychic experiences. Individuals can present with psychological flexibility, reflect, and wonder about goals and visions of oneself and life, as well as present with adaptive coping skills and strategies, which support individuals' counter against appraisal of negative emotions and destructive responses. Involving multi-sector organizations such as the education, workplace, and public service sectors across systems is essential, as resilience development is a process of experiencing human relationships, connections, rapport, and trust across the boundaries of multiple systems. Resilience of multiple systems serves not only certain designed functions, but also forms stable systems to protect individuals, families, and even groups from being shattered by crises and forceful interruptions. As the model suggested, systemic efforts such as equipping parents with skills and knowledge about crises and providing supportive resources, strategic guidelines, and financial and employment security are needed to facilitate the growth of resilience.

The third implication is conceptualizing organizational resilience from individual resilience development perspectives. Persistent crises require organizations to respond with mitigations, but short-term adjustments that only focus on securing organizational performance and functioning without considering individual resilience can increase the accumulative disturbances individuals face within the short term, which hinders the development of psychological resilience during crises. Organizational and individual learnings are critical to help the growth of resilience and decrease the number of people becoming increasingly stressed during a crisis. When crises and shocks to the system regard health and well-being, such as COVID-19, measurements of organizational resilience should expand from organizational functionality and performance. An individual–environment view of organizational resilience should incorporate indicators such as to what extent the organization provides insights and learnings from the adverse events for individuals, and to what extent the organization's capacity to adapt to disturbances and mobilize resources to sustain changes and provide transformational adjustments.

The last implication regards COVID-19 lessons. Significant changes have been observed in conducting and receiving health and well-being services. As all parties strive to adjust to the long-pandemic, we wonder how we may learn and reflect from our experiences of the pandemic and continuously support people in need. When the population faces constant and enduring waves of a pandemic, policies and multiple sectors should facilitate the development of psychological assets such as self-esteem, psychological flexibility, adaptive self-care or coping strategies, and supportive social welfare. The present reality is that the pandemic has a high level of uncertainty, and the unknown may not be eliminated, which requires us to live with these disturbing and uncomfortable dynamics. A resilience perspective can cultivate tolerance of disturbances and distress, reinforcing the population's growth to strive for a happy life.

In terms of limitations, while we used the COVID-19 pandemic as an example to explore the interconnections between individual and organizational resilience, the model is not calibrated with empirical data and does not consider variations across subpopulations. Emerging longitudinal research shows that young generations aged 19–30 years and females had a higher risk of distress during the pandemic and its lockdowns [57]. Additionally, younger age (<40 years), female gender, psychological illness, student status, exposure to social media/news, and unemployment are common risk factors that have been shown to be associated with mental distress caused by the pandemic [18]. The model was not calibrated with empirical data, as the focus of this model is to provide theoretical exploration. Empirical evidence decides the realism and reliability of the model's validity, which requires both structural and behavior-over-time data [58]. While we believe theory-based modeling was useful and proper for the purpose of this paper, the model was not calibrated with behavior-over-time data; thus, the model should be considered exploratory with tentative and uncertain conclusions. To improve the evidence level of the model, future studies can calibrate the model using data on the population's health and well-being, service provision, and environmental changes. Future research can further include the impact of accumulative risk on different socioeconomic or age groups to show the different levels of vulnerability.

The model provided theoretical insights but was overall simplified at quite a high level. A more systematic review of theoretical orientations or models in clinical psychology can be used to improve the structural conceptualization. For example, resilience can be closely linked to psychological development, insights, judgments, resourcefulness, behavioral regulation, distress tolerance, etc. For organizational resilience, we simplified the conceptualization of organization resilience by using the number of staff in the health and well-being service sector. In practice, different agencies have broader approaches to health services, such as crisis intervention and community-based health services. Agencies that provide community health services and care might have more significant challenges in responding to crisis interventions during multiple pandemic waves. Future research can integrate broader service provision challenges by different agencies. Meanwhile, it could be meaningful to include resilience in different cultures, communities, and groups, so this concept and thinking can be further nuanced to different cultural norms and identities.

Author Contributions: Conceptualization, K.Z.; methodology, K.Z.; modeling, K.Z.; writing—original draft preparation, K.Z. and M.Z.; writing—review and editing, K.Z. and M.Z.; visualization, K.Z. All authors have read and agreed to the published version of the manuscript.

Funding: K.Z. was funded by the National Institute for Health and Care Research (NIHR) School for Public Health Research (SPHR), grant reference number PD-SPH-2015. The views expressed are those of the authors and not necessarily those of the NIHR or the Department of Health and Social Care.

Institutional Review Board Statement: Not applicable.

Informed Consent Statement: Not applicable.

Data Availability Statement: Not applicable.

Acknowledgments: The authors appreciate Christina Gkini, Jefferson Rajah, and Birgit Kopainsky for their valuable feedback on the model. They are also grateful for feedback received at the 2022 System Dynamics Conference in Frankfurt, Germany.

Conflicts of Interest: The authors declare no conflict of interest.

Appendix A Model Equations

****

Crises_multiple_shocks:

****

First_shock_duration = 5
    UNITS: month
First_shock_intensity = 3
    UNITS: dmnl
First_shock_start = 20
    UNITS: month
First_shock_stop = First_shock_start+First_shock_duration
    UNITS: month
Interval_to_second_shock_start = 6
    UNITS: month
Interval_to_third_shock_start = 6
    UNITS: month
Multiple_Shocks[First_wave] = STEP(Risk_intensity_of_each_shock[First_wave], First_shock_start)-STEP(Risk_intensity_of_each_shock[First_wave], First_shock_stop)
    UNITS: dmnl
Multiple_Shocks[Second_wave] = STEP(Risk_intensity_of_each_shock[Second_wave], Second_shock_Start)-STEP(Risk_intensity_of_each_shock[Second_wave], Second_shock_stop)
    UNITS: dmnl
Multiple_Shocks[Third_wave] = STEP(Risk_intensity_of_each_shock[Third_wave], Third_shock_start)-STEP(Risk_intensity_of_each_shock[Third_wave], Third_shock_stop)

UNITS: dmnl
"MULTIPLE_SHOCKS_Switch_1=_crisis_on" = 1
UNITS: dmnl
Risk_intensity_of_each_shock[First_wave] = First_shock_intensity
UNITS: dmnl
Risk_intensity_of_each_shock[Second_wave] = Second_shock_intensity
UNITS: dmnl
Risk_intensity_of_each_shock[Third_wave] = Third_shock_intensity
UNITS: dmnl
Second_shock_duration = 5
UNITS: month
Second_shock_intensity = 3
UNITS: dmnl
Second_shock_Start = Interval_to_second_shock_start+First_shock_stop
UNITS: month
Second_shock_stop = Second_shock_duration+Second_shock_Start
UNITS: month
Third_shock_duration = 5
UNITS: month
Third_shock_intensity = 3
UNITS: dmnl
Third_shock_start = Second_shock_stop+Interval_to_third_shock_start
UNITS: month
Third_shock_stop = Third_shock_start+Third_shock_duration
UNITS: month

****
Disturbance_and_Psychological_resilience:
****

Disturbance_events_that_can_be_dealt_with_resiliency = Psychological_Resilience//Resilience_needed_per_disturbance_event
UNITS: event
Fractional_emotional_tolerance_acquired_from_recovering = IF P3_Collective_growth =1 THEN Normal_fractional_emotional_tolerance_acquired_from_recovering*Intensity_of_P3_on_distress_tolerance ELSE Normal_fractional_emotional_tolerance_acquired_from_recovering
UNITS: dmnl
Goal_of_resilience = Resilience_needed_per_disturbance_event*Disturbance_events
UNITS: resilience
Initial_individual_resilience = INIT(Goal_of_resilience)
UNITS: resilience
Normal_fractional_emotional_tolerance_acquired_from_recovering = 1
UNITS: dmnl
Psychological_Resilience(t) = Psychological_Resilience(t - dt) + (Resilience_adjusting_by_Recovering_from_shocks) * dt
INIT Psychological_Resilience = Initial_individual_resilience
UNITS: resilience
Psychological_resilience_ratio = EXP(Psychological_Resilience)/(1+EXP(Psychological_Resilience))
UNITS: dmnl
Resilience_adjusting_by_Recovering_from_shocks = (Goal_of_resilience-Psychological_Resilience)*(Fractional_effect_of_tolerating_emotional_distress_through_recovering_process_per_month)*Environment_stabilization_ratio
UNITS: resilience/month
Resilience_needed_per_disturbance_event = 0.053

UNITS: resilience/event
****
Environment_adjustments:
****
Adjustments_Gap = MAX(0, SMTH3(Total_adjustments_needed-Environment_Stabilized_Adjustments, Organization_response_time))
   UNITS: adjustment
Environment_adjusting = MAX(0, (Adjustments_Gap)//Time_needed_to_develop_temporary_adjustments)
   UNITS: adjustment/month
Environment_Stabilized_Adjustments(t) = Environment_Stabilized_Adjustments(t - dt) + (Environment_stabilizing - "Re-adjusting") * dt
   INIT Environment_Stabilized_Adjustments = Initial_stabilised_adjustments
   UNITS: adjustment
Environment_stabilizing = Fractional_adjustments_that_move_to_stabilized_adjustments*Environment_Temporary_Adjustments//Time_needed_to_settle_permanent_solutions
   UNITS: adjustment/month
Environment_Temporary_Adjustments(t) = Environment_Temporary_Adjustments(t - dt) + (Environment_adjusting + "Re-adjusting" - Environment_stabilizing) * dt
   INIT Environment_Temporary_Adjustments = Initial_temporary_adjustments
   UNITS: adjustment
Fractional_adjustments_that_move_to_stabilized_adjustments = 0.3
   UNITS: dmnl
Initial_stabilised_adjustments = Total_adjustments_needed
   UNITS: adjustment
Initial_temporary_adjustments = Total_adjustments_needed*Time_needed_to_settle_permanent_solutions/(Time_needed_for_revisiting_adjustments*Fractional_adjustments_that_move_to_stabilized_adjustments)
   UNITS: adjustment
Normal_organizational_response_time = 3
   UNITS: month
Normal_time_needed_to_develop_temporary_adjustments = 4
   UNITS: month
Normal_time_needed_to_revisit_adjustments = 12
   UNITS: month
Normal_time_needed_to_settle_permanent_adjustments = 12
   UNITS: month
Organization_response_time = IF P1:_Environment_Fast_Adaptation=1 THEN Normal_organizational_response_time/Intensity_of_P1_on_organizational_response_time ELSE Normal_organizational_response_time
   UNITS: month
"Re-adjusting" = Environment_Stabilized_Adjustments//Time_needed_for_revisiting_adjustments
   UNITS: adjustment/month
Time_needed_for_revisiting_adjustments = IF P1:_Environment_Fast_Adaptation=1 THEN Normal_time_needed_to_revisit_adjustments/Intensity_of_P1_on_revisiting_adjustments ELSE Normal_time_needed_to_revisit_adjust ments
   UNITS: month
Time_needed_to_develop_temporary_adjustments = IF P1:_Environment_Fast_Adaptation=1 THEN Normal_time_needed_to_develop_temporary_adjustments/Intensity_of_P1_on_temporary_adjustment_time ELSE Normal_time_needed_to_develop_temporary_adjustments
   UNITS: month

Time_needed_to_settle_permanent_solutions = IF P3_Collective_growth=1 THEN Normal_time_needed_to_settle_permanent_adjustments/Intensity_of_P3_on_stabilised-_adjustment ELSE Normal_time_needed_to_settle_permanent_adjustments
UNITS: month
****
Health and Well-being_service:
****
Changes_of_employee = CAPACITY_RESPOND_STWITCH* (Indicated_demanded-_number_of_MH_staff-HW_service_staff)//Time_to_hire
UNITS: people/month
HW_service_staff(t) = HW_service_staff(t - dt) + (changes_of_employee) * dt
INIT HW_service_staff = Initial_MH_service_staff
UNITS: people
Indicated_demanded_number_of_MH_staff = Total_sessions_demand/Number_of-_sessions_per_staff_per_month//Target_Waiting_Time
UNITS: people
Normal_target_waiting_time = 4
UNITS: month
Normal_time_to_hire = 12
UNITS: month
Number_of_sessions_per_staff_per_month = 100
UNITS: session/people/month
Remaining_monthly_sessions_capacity = MAX(0, Total_monthly_session_capacity-Total_monthly_sessions_occupied)
UNITS: session/month
Target_Waiting_Time = IF P2_Mental_Wellbeing_Service_Fast_Response=1 THEN Normal_target_waiting_time/Intensity_of_P2_on_waiting_time ELSE Normal_target_waiting_time
UNITS: month
Time_to_hire = IF P2_Mental_Wellbeing_Service_Fast_Response=1 THEN Normal_time_to_hire/Intensity_of_P2_on_time_to_hire ELSE Normal_time_to_hire
UNITS: month
Total_monthly_session_capacity = HW_service_staff*Number_of_sessions_per_staff_per_month
UNITS: session/month
Total_monthly_sessions_occupied = "Highly stressed_people_with_HW_services"*Frequency_of_sessions_attended_per_month_per_people
UNITS: session/month
Total_number_of_service_sessions_needed_per_person = 10
UNITS: session/people
Total_sessions_demand = ("Highly_stressed_people_without_HW_services"+"Highly_stressed_people_with_HW_services")*Total_number_of_service_sessions_needed_per_person
UNITS: session
****
Initial_numbers:
****
Fractional_recovering_by_own = Fraction_of_self_recover/"Time_to_self-recover"
UNITS: 1/month
Fractional_Stressing_up = Normal_fraction_of_highly_stressed_symptoms/Time_to_change_stress_level
UNITS: 1/month
Fractional_using_service = Fraction_of_service_using_among_highly_stressed_people/Target_Waiting_Time

UNITS: 1/month

INIT_highly_stressed_not_using_HW_services = INIT_low_stress_population*(fractional_Stressing_up)/(fractional_recovering_by_own+Fractional_using_service)

UNITS: people

INIT_highly_stressed_using_HW_services = INIT_highly_stressed_not_using_HW_services*Fractional_using_service*Time_to_recover/(1+Time_to_recover*Fraction_of_dropping_out_per_month)

UNITS: people

INIT_low_stress_population = 10000

UNITS: people

Initial_MH_service_staff = INIT(Indicated_demanded_number_of_MH_staff)

UNITS: people

Sum_of_population_stocks = "Low/mild_stress_people" + "Highly-stressed_people_with_HW_services" + "Highly-stressed_people_without_HW_services"

UNITS: people

****

Multiple_shocks_and_disturbance:

****

Decreasing_disturbance_events = (Effect_of_environmental_resilience_on_processing_disturbance_events*Effect_of_individual_resilience_on_processing_disturbances)*Disturbance_events/Time_needed_to_resolve_events

UNITS: event/month

Disturbance_events(t) = Disturbance_events(t - dt) + (Increasing_disturbance_events - Decreasing_disturbance_events) * dt

INIT Disturbance_events = Initial_disturbance_events

UNITS: event

Disturbance_to_temporary_adjustments_ratio = Environment_Temporary_Adjustments//Max_adjustment_depending_on_resiliency

UNITS: dmnl

Effect_of_environmental_resilience_on_processing_disturbance_events = GRAPH(Environment_stabilization_ratio)

Points: (0.000, 0.000), (0.100, 0.360), (0.200, 0.660), (0.330, 1.000), (0.400, 1.100), (0.500, 1.200), (0.600, 1.300), (0.700, 1.400), (0.800, 1.600), (0.900, 1.800), (1.000, 2.000)

UNITS: dmnl

Effect_of_individual_resilience_on_processing_disturbances = GRAPH(Psychological_Resilience)

Points: (0.000, 0.0133857018486), (0.100, 0.0359724199242), (0.200, 0.0948517463551), (0.300, 0.238405844044), (0.400, 0.53788284274), (0.423, 1.000), (0.600, 1.46211715726), (0.700, 1.76159415596), (0.800, 1.90514825364), (0.900, 1.96402758008), (1.000, 1.98661429815)

UNITS: dmnl

Effect_of_temporary_disturbance_on_increasing_disturbance_events = GRAPH(Disturbance_to_temporary_adjustments_ratio)

Points: (0.000, 0.0133857018486), (0.400, 0.0359724199242), (0.800, 0.0948517463551), (1.200, 0.238405844044), (1.600, 0.53788284274), (2.000, 1.000), (2.400, 1.46211715726), (2.800, 1.76159415596), (3.200, 1.90514825364), (3.600, 1.96402758008), (4.000, 1.98661429815)

UNITS: dmnl

Environment_stabilization_ratio = (Environment_Stabilized_Adjustments)//(Environment_Stabilized_Adjustments+Environment_Temporary_Adjustments)

UNITS: dmnl

Increasing_disturbance_events = Effect_of_temporary_disturbance_on_increasing_disturbance_events*Number_of_disturbance_events_per_month

UNITS: event/month

Initial_disturbance_events = Normal_disturbance_events_per_month*Time_needed_to_resolve_events*2

UNITS: event
Initial_Disturbance_ratio_input = INT(Environment_Temporary_Adjustments//Max_adjustment_depending_on_resiliency)
UNITS: dmnl
Max_adjustment_depending_on_resiliency = Disturbance_events_that_can_be_dealt_with_resiliency*Number_of_adjustments_needed_per_disturbance_events
UNITS: adjustment
Multiple_shocks_to_the_system = (1+"MULTIPLE_SHOCKS_Switch_1=_crisis_on"*SUM(Multiple_Shocks))
UNITS: dmnl
Normal_disturbance_events_per_month = 2.5
UNITS: event/month
Number_of_adjustments_needed_per_disturbance_events = 3
UNITS: adjustment/event
Number_of_disturbance_events_per_month = Normal_disturbance_events_per_month*Multiple_shocks_to_the_system
UNITS: event/month
Time_needed_to_resolve_events = 2
UNITS: month
Total_adjustments_needed = (Disturbance_events*Number_of_adjustments_needed_per_disturbance_events)
UNITS: adjustment

****

Policy_switches:

****

CAPACITY_RESPOND_STWITCH = 1
UNITS: dmnl
Intensity_of_P1_on_organizational_response_time = 3
UNITS: dmnl
Intensity_of_P1_on_revisiting_adjustments = 2
UNITS: dmnl
Intensity_of_P1_on_temporary_adjustment_time = 2
UNITS: dmnl
Intensity_of_P2_on_fraction_of_dropping_out = 2
UNITS: dmnl
Intensity_of_P2_on_fraction_of_using_services = 1.6
UNITS: dmnl
Intensity_of_P2_on_time_to_hire = 4
UNITS: dmnl
Intensity_of_P2_on_waiting_time = 2
UNITS: dmnl
Intensity_of_P3_on_distress_tolerance = 4
UNITS: dmnl
Intensity_of_P3_on_stabilised_adjustment = 4
UNITS: dmnl
P1:_Environment_Fast_Adaptation = 0
UNITS: dmnl
P2_Mental_Wellbeing_Service_Fast_Response = 0
UNITS: dmnl
P3_Collective_growth = 1
UNITS: dmnl

****

Psychological_resilience_structure:

****

Accumulative_people_stressed_up(t) = Accumulative_people_stressed_up(t - dt) + (stressing_up_flow) ∗ dt
  INIT Accumulative_people_stressed_up = 0
  UNITS: people
Disturbance_to_resilience_ratio = Disturbance_events//Disturbance_events_that_can_be_dealt_with_resiliency
  UNITS: dmnl
Dropping_out_services = IF P2_Mental_Wellbeing_Service_Fast_Response=1 THEN "Highly_stressed_people_with_HW_services"*Fraction_of_dropping_out_per_month/Intensity_of_P2_on_fraction_of_dropping_out ELSE Fraction_of_dropping_out_per_month*"Highly_stressed_people_with_HW_services"
  UNITS: people/month
Fraction_of_dropping_out_per_month = 0
  UNITS: 1/month
Fraction_of_self_recover = 0.2
  UNITS: dmnl
Fraction_of_service_using_among_highly_stressed_people = IF P2_Mental_Wellbeing_Service_Fast_Response=1 THEN Normal_fraction_of_service_using_among_highly_stressed_people*Intensity_of_P2_on_fraction_of_using_services ELSE Normal_fraction_of_service_using_among_highly_stressed_people
  UNITS: dmnl
Fractional_effect_of_tolerating_emotional_distress_through_recovering_process_per_month = ("Self-_recovering"+Recovering_by_using_services)*Fractional_emotional_tolerance_acquired_from_recovering//Sum_of_population_stocks
  UNITS: 1/month
Frequency_of_sessions_attended_per_month_per_people = 4
  UNITS: session/people/month
Highly_stressed_people_reaching_out_services = "Highly_Stressed_people_without_HW_services" *Fraction_of_service_using_among_highly_stressed_people
  UNITS: people
Highly_stressed_people_that_can_be_scheduled = Remaining_monthly_sessions_capacity//Frequency_of_sessions_attended_per_month_per_people
  UNITS: people
"Highly_Stressed_people_with_HW_services"(t) = "Highly_Stressed_people_with_HW_services"(t - dt) + (Using_services - Recovering_by_using_services - Dropping_out_services) ∗ dt
  INIT "Highly_Stressed_people_with_HW_services" = INIT_Highly_stressed_using_HW_services
  UNITS: people
"Highly_Stressed_people_without_HW_services"(t) = "Highly_Stressed_people_without_HW_services"(t - dt) + (Stressing_up + Dropping_out_services - "Self-_recovering" - Using_services) ∗ dt
  INIT "Highly_Stressed_people_without_HW_services" = INIT_highly_stressed_not_using_HW_services
  UNITS: people
"Low/mild_stress_people"(t) = "Low/mild_stress_people"(t - dt) + ("Self-_recovering" + Recovering_by_using_services - Stressing_up) ∗ dt
  INIT "Low/mild_stress_people" = INIT_low_stress_population
  UNITS: people
Normal_fraction_of_highly_stressed_symptoms = 0.2
  UNITS: dmnl
Normal_fraction_of_service_using_among_highly_stressed_people = 0.5
  UNITS: dmnl

Recovering_by_using_services = "Highly_Stressed_people_with_HW_services"//Time_to_recover
UNITS: people/month

"Self-_recovering" = "Highly_Stressed_people_without_HW_services"*Fraction_of_self_recover//"Time_to_self-recover"
UNITS: people/month

Stressing_up = "Low/mild_stress_people"*Disturbance_to_resilience_ratio*Normal_fraction_of_highly_stressed_symptoms//Time_to_change_stress_level
UNITS: people/month

Stressing_up_flow = Stressing_up
UNITS: people/month

Time_to_recover = Total_number_of_service_sessions_needed_per_person//Frequency_of_sessions_attended_per_month_per_people
UNITS: month

"Time_to_self-recover" = 3
UNITS: month

Time_to_change_stress_level = 6
UNITS: month

Using_services = MIN(Highly_stressed_people_that_can_be_scheduled, Highly_stressed_people_reaching_out_services)/Target_Waiting_Time
UNITS: people/month

References

1. World Health Organization WHO Coronavirus (COVID-19) Dashboard | WHO Coronavirus (COVID-19) Dashboard with Vaccination Data. Available online: https://covid19.who.int/info/ (accessed on 28 August 2022).
2. Office for Health Improvement & Disparities COVID-19 Mental Health and Wellbeing Surveillance: Report. Available online: https://www.gov.uk/government/publications/covid-19-mental-health-and-wellbeing-surveillance-report (accessed on 15 December 2021).
3. Gao, X.; Davillas, A.; Jones, A.M. *The COVID-19 Pandemic and Its Impact on Socioeconomic Inequality in Psychological Distress in the UK: An Update*; Institute of Labor Economics (IZA): Bonn, Germany, 2021.
4. Ellwardt, L.; Präg, P. Heterogeneous Mental Health Development during the COVID-19 Pandemic in the United Kingdom. *Sci. Rep.* **2021**, *11*, 15958. [CrossRef] [PubMed]
5. Fletcher, D.; Sarkar, M. Psychological Resilience: A Review and Critique of Definitions, Concepts, and Theory. *Eur. Psychol.* **2013**, *18*, 12–23. [CrossRef]
6. Schwarz, S. Resilience in Psychology: A Critical Analysis of the Concept. *Theory Psychol.* **2018**, *28*, 528–541. [CrossRef]
7. Burnard, K.; Bhamra, R. Organisational Resilience: Development of a Conceptual Framework for Organisational Responses. *Int. J. Prod. Res.* **2011**, *49*, 5581–5599. [CrossRef]
8. Ungar, M. The Social Ecology of Resilience: Addressing Contextual and Cultural Ambiguity of a Nascent Construct. *Am. J. Orthopsychiatry* **2011**, *81*, 1–17. [CrossRef]
9. Ungar, M.; Theron, L. Resilience and Mental Health: How Multisystemic Processes Contribute to Positive Outcomes. *Lancet Psychiatry* **2020**, *7*, 441–448. [CrossRef]
10. Rahmandad, H.; Lim, T.Y.; Sterman, J. *Estimating COVID-19 Under-Reporting Across 86 Nations: Implications for Projections and Control*; Social Science Research Network: Rochester, NY, USA, 2020.
11. Vogus, T.; Sutcliffe, K. Organizing for Resilience. In *Positive Organizational Scholarship: Foundations of a New Discipline*, Cameron, K., Dutton, J.E., Quinn, R.E., Eds.; Berrett-Koehler: Oakland, CA, USA, 2003; pp. 94–110.
12. Weick, K.E.; Sutcliffe, K.M. *Managing the Unexpected: Sustained Performance in a Complex World/Karl E. Weick, Kathleen M. Sutcliffe.*, 3rd ed.; Wiley: Hoboken, NJ, USA, 2015; ISBN 978-1-118-86241-4.
13. BlackDeer, A.A.; Hovmand, P.S.; Chew, K.; Zhou, K.; Fowler, P.J.; Auslander, W. Resiliency from a Feedback Perspective. Available online: https://exchange.iseesystems.com/public/psh/human-resiliency/index.html#page1 (accessed on 15 December 2021).
14. Rudolph, J.W.; Repenning, N.P. Disaster Dynamics: Understanding the Role of Quantity in Organizational Collapse. *Adm. Sci. Q.* **2002**, *47*, 1–30. [CrossRef]
15. Sterman, J.D. *Business Dynamics: Systems Thinking and Modeling for a Complex World /John D. Sterman*; Irwin/McGraw-Hill: Boston, MA, USA, 2000; ISBN 0-07-231135-5.
16. Lane, D.C.; Schwaninger, M. Theory Building with System Dynamics: Topic and Research Contributions. *Syst. Res. Behav. Sci.* **2008**, *25*, 439–445. [CrossRef]
17. de Gooyert, V.; Größler, A. On the Differences between Theoretical and Applied System Dynamics Modeling. *Syst. Dyn. Rev.* **2018**, *34*, 575–583. [CrossRef]

18. Xiong, J.; Lipsitz, O.; Nasri, F.; Lui, L.M.W.; Gill, H.; Phan, L.; Chen-Li, D.; Iacobucci, M.; Ho, R.; Majeed, A.; et al. Impact of COVID-19 Pandemic on Mental Health in the General Population: A Systematic Review. *J. Affect. Disord.* **2020**, *277*, 55–64. [CrossRef]
19. Daly, M.; Robinson, E. Psychological Distress Associated with the Second COVID-19 Wave: Prospective Evidence from the UK Household Longitudinal Study. *J. Affect. Disord.* **2022**, *310*, 274–278. [CrossRef]
20. Barry, V.; Stout, M.E.; Lynch, M.E.; Mattis, S.; Tran, D.Q.; Antun, A.; Ribeiro, M.J.; Stein, S.F.; Kempton, C.L. The Effect of Psychological Distress on Health Outcomes: A Systematic Review and Meta-Analysis of Prospective Studies. *J. Health Psychol.* **2020**, *25*, 227–239. [CrossRef] [PubMed]
21. Ahrens, K.F.; Neumann, R.J.; Kollmann, B.; Brokelmann, J.; von Werthern, N.M.; Malyshau, A.; Weichert, D.; Lutz, B.; Fiebach, C.J.; Wessa, M.; et al. Impact of COVID-19 Lockdown on Mental Health in Germany: Longitudinal Observation of Different Mental Health Trajectories and Protective Factors. *Transl. Psychiatry* **2021**, *11*, 392. [CrossRef] [PubMed]
22. Manchia, M.; Gathier, A.W.; Yapici-Eser, H.; Schmidt, M.V.; de Quervain, D.; van Amelsvoort, T.; Bisson, J.I.; Cryan, J.F.; Howes, O.D.; Pinto, L.; et al. The Impact of the Prolonged COVID-19 Pandemic on Stress Resilience and Mental Health: A Critical Review across Waves. *Eur. Neuropsychopharmacol.* **2022**, *55*, 22–83. [CrossRef] [PubMed]
23. Haldane, V.; De Foo, C.; Abdalla, S.M.; Jung, A.-S.; Tan, M.; Wu, S.; Chua, A.; Verma, M.; Shrestha, P.; Singh, S.; et al. Health Systems Resilience in Managing the COVID-19 Pandemic: Lessons from 28 Countries. *Nat. Med.* **2021**, *27*, 964–980. [CrossRef] [PubMed]
24. Greenberg, N.; Brooks, S.K.; Wessely, S.; Tracy, D.K. How Might the NHS Protect the Mental Health of Health-Care Workers after the COVID-19 Crisis? *Lancet Psychiatry* **2020**, *7*, 733–734. [CrossRef]
25. Bryce, C.; Ring, P.; Ashby, S.; Wardman, J.K. Resilience in the Face of Uncertainty: Early Lessons from the COVID-19 Pandemic. *J. Risk Res.* **2020**, *23*, 880–887. [CrossRef]
26. Sakurai, M.; Chughtai, H. Resilience against Crises: COVID-19 and Lessons from Natural Disasters. *Eur. J. Inf. Syst.* **2020**, *29*, 585–594. [CrossRef]
27. Sawyer, A.T.; Bailey, A.K.; Green, J.F.; Sun, J.; Robinson, P.S. Resilience, Insight, Self-Compassion, and Empowerment (RISE): A Randomized Controlled Trial of a Psychoeducational Group Program for Nurses. *J. Am. Psychiatr. Nurses Assoc.* **2021**. [CrossRef]
28. Milioni, M.; Alessandri, G.; Eisenberg, N.; Caprara, G.V. The Role of Positivity as Predictor of Ego-Resiliency from Adolescence to Young Adulthood. *Personal. Individ. Differ.* **2016**, *101*, 306–311. [CrossRef]
29. Gentili, C.; Rickardsson, J.; Zetterqvist, V.; Simons, L.E.; Lekander, M.; Wicksell, R.K. Psychological Flexibility as a Resilience Factor in Individuals with Chronic Pain. *Front. Psychol.* **2019**, *10*, 2016. [CrossRef] [PubMed]
30. Fritz, J.; de Graaff, A.M.; Caisley, H.; van Harmelen, A.-L.; Wilkinson, P.O. A Systematic Review of Amenable Resilience Factors That Moderate and/or Mediate the Relationship Between Childhood Adversity and Mental Health in Young People. *Front. Psychiatry* **2018**, *9*, 230. [CrossRef] [PubMed]
31. Niitsu, K.; Rice, M.J.; Houfek, J.F.; Stoltenberg, S.F.; Kupzyk, K.A.; Barron, C.R. A Systematic Review of Genetic Influence on Psychological Resilience. *Biol. Res. Nurs.* **2019**, *21*, 61–71. [CrossRef] [PubMed]
32. de Leon, H.J.H.; Kopainsky, B. Do You Bend or Break? System Dynamics in Resilience Planning for Food Security. *Syst. Dyn. Rev.* **2019**, *35*, 287–309. [CrossRef]
33. van der Vegt, G.S.; Essens, P.; Wahlström, M.; George, G. Managing Risk and Resilience. *Acad. Manag. J.* **2015**, *58*, 971–980. [CrossRef]
34. Meyer, A.D. Adapting to Environmental Jolts. *Adm. Sci. Q.* **1982**, *27*, 515–537. [CrossRef]
35. Petriglieri, G.; Petriglieri, J.L. The Return of the Oppressed: A Systems Psychodynamic Approach to Organization Studies. *Acad. Manag. Ann.* **2020**, *14*, 411–449. [CrossRef]
36. Brown, A.; Starkey, K. Organizational Identity and Learning: A Psychodynamic Perspective. *Acad. Manag. Rev.* **2000**, *25*, 102–120. [CrossRef]
37. Pring, E.T.; Malietzis, G.; Kendall, S.W.H.; Jenkins, J.T.; Athanasiou, T. Crisis Management for Surgical Teams and Their Leaders, Lessons from the COVID-19 Pandemic; A Structured Approach to Developing Resilience or Natural Organisational Responses. *Int. J. Surg.* **2021**, *91*, 105987. [CrossRef]
38. Williams, T.; Gruber, D.; Sutcliffe, K.; Shepherd, D.; Zhao, E.Y. Organizational Response to Adversity: Fusing Crisis Management and Resilience Research Streams. *Acad. Manag. Ann.* **2017**, *11*, 733–769. [CrossRef]
39. Ilseven, E.; Puranam, P. Measuring Organizational Resilience as a Performance Outcome. *J. Organ. Des.* **2021**, *10*, 127–137. [CrossRef]
40. Kahn, W.A.; Barton, M.A.; Fellows, S. Organizational Crises and the Disturbance of Relational Systems. *Acad. Manage. Rev.* **2013**, *38*, 377–396. [CrossRef]
41. Homer, J.B.; Hirsch, G.B. System Dynamics Modeling for Public Health: Background and Opportunities. *Am. J. Public Health* **2006**, *96*, 452–458. [CrossRef] [PubMed]
42. Homer, J.; Hirsch, G.; Milstein, B. Chronic Illness in a Complex Health Economy: The Perils and Promises of Downstream and Upstream Reforms. *Syst. Dyn. Rev.* **2007**, *23*, 313–343. [CrossRef]
43. Chichakly, K. Behavioral Implications in COVID-19 Spread and Vaccinations. *Systems* **2021**, *9*, 72. [CrossRef]
44. Rooney-Varga, J.N.; Kapmeier, F.; Sterman, J.D.; Jones, A.P.; Putko, M.; Rath, K. The Climate Action Simulation. *Simul. Gaming* **2020**, *51*, 114–140. [CrossRef]

45. Randers, J.; Rockström, J.; Stoknes, P.-E.; Goluke, U.; Collste, D.; Cornell, S.E.; Donges, J. Achieving the 17 Sustainable Development Goals within 9 Planetary Boundaries. *Glob. Sustain.* **2019**, *2*, e24. [CrossRef]
46. Rahmandad, H.; Ton, Z. If Higher Pay Is Profitable, Why Is It So Rare? Modeling Competing Strategies in Mass Market Services. *Organ. Sci.* **2020**, *31*, 1053–1071. [CrossRef]
47. Jalali, M.S.; Rahmandad, H.; Bullock, S.L.; Ammerman, A. Dynamics of Implementation and Maintenance of Organizational Health Interventions. *Int. J. Environ. Res. Public. Health* **2017**, *14*, 917. [CrossRef]
48. de Gooyert, V. Developing Dynamic Organizational Theories; Three System Dynamics Based Research Strategies. *Qual. Quant.* **2019**, *53*, 653–666. [CrossRef]
49. Zimmermann, N. *Dynamics of Drivers of Organizational Change*; Gabler Verlag: Wiesbaden, Germany, 2011; ISBN 978-3-8349-3051-4.
50. Sastry, M.A. Problems and Paradoxes in a Model of Punctuated Organizational Change. *Adm. Sci. Q.* **1997**, *42*, 237–275. [CrossRef]
51. Repenning, N.P. A Simulation-Based Approach to Understanding the Dynamics of Innovation Implementation. *Organ. Sci.* **2002**, *13*, 109–127. [CrossRef]
52. Hovmand, P.; Gillespie, D. Implementation of Evidence-Based Practice and Organizational Performance. *J. Behav. Health Serv. Res.* **2010**, *37*, 79–94. [CrossRef] [PubMed]
53. Schwaninger, M.; Grösser, S. System Dynamics as Model-Based Theory Building. *Syst. Res. Behav. Sci.* **2008**, *25*, 447–465. [CrossRef]
54. Homer, J.B. Why We Iterate: Scientific Modeling in Theory and Practice. *Syst. Dyn. Rev.* **1996**, *12*, 1–19. [CrossRef]
55. Newman, E.A. Disturbance Ecology in the Anthropocene. *Front. Ecol. Evol.* **2019**, *7*, 147. [CrossRef]
56. White, P.S.; Pickett, S.T.A. Chapter 1—Natural Disturbance and Patch Dynamics: An Introduction. In *The Ecology of Natural Disturbance and Patch Dynamics*; Pickett, S.T.A., White, P.S., Eds.; Academic Press: San Diego, CA, USA, 1985; pp. 3–13, ISBN 978-0-12-554520-4.
57. Henderson, M.; Fitzsimons, E.; Ploubidis, G.; Richards, M.; Patalay, P. Mental Health during Lockdown: Evidence from Four Generations. *Lond. UCL Cent. Longitud. Stud.* **2020**, *20*, 1–17.
58. Homer, J. Levels of Evidence in System Dynamics Modeling. *Syst. Dyn. Rev.* **2014**, *30*, 75–80. [CrossRef]

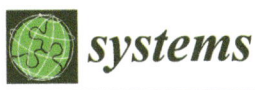

Article

Addressing Parameter Uncertainty in a Health Policy Simulation Model Using Monte Carlo Sensitivity Methods

Wayne Wakeland [1,*] and Jack Homer [2]

1 Systems Science Program, Portland State University, Portland, OR 97207, USA
2 Homer Consulting and MIT Research Affiliate, Barrytown, NY 12507, USA
* Correspondence: wakeland@pdx.edu

Abstract: We present a practical guide and step-by-step flowchart for establishing uncertainty intervals for key model outcomes in a simulation model in the face of uncertain parameters. The process starts with Powell optimization to find a set of uncertain parameters (the optimum parameter set or OPS) that minimizes the model fitness error relative to historical data. Optimization also helps in refinement of parameter uncertainty ranges. Next, traditional Monte Carlo (TMC) randomization or Markov Chain Monte Carlo (MCMC) is used to create a sample of parameter sets that fit the reference behavior data nearly as well as the OPS. Under the TMC method, the entire parameter space is explored broadly with a large number of runs, and the results are sorted for selection of qualifying parameter sets (QPS) to ensure good fit and parameter distributions that are centrally located within the uncertainty ranges. In addition, the QPS outputs are graphed as sensitivity graphs or box-and-whisker plots for comparison with the historical data. Finally, alternative policies and scenarios are run against the OPS and all QPS, and uncertainty intervals are found for projected model outcomes. We illustrate the full parameter uncertainty approach with a (previously published) system dynamics model of the U.S. opioid epidemic, and demonstrate how it can enrich policy modeling results.

Keywords: simulation model; uncertainty analysis; optimization; sensitivity testing; Monte Carlo randomization; opioid epidemic

Citation: Wakeland, W.; Homer, J. Addressing Parameter Uncertainty in a Health Policy Simulation Model Using Monte Carlo Sensitivity Methods. *Systems* **2022**, *10*, 225. https://doi.org/10.3390/systems10060225

Academic Editor: Peter Jones

Received: 17 September 2022
Accepted: 12 November 2022
Published: 18 November 2022

Publisher's Note: MDPI stays neutral with regard to jurisdictional claims in published maps and institutional affiliations.

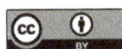

Copyright: © 2022 by the authors. Licensee MDPI, Basel, Switzerland. This article is an open access article distributed under the terms and conditions of the Creative Commons Attribution (CC BY) license (https://creativecommons.org/licenses/by/4.0/).

1. Introduction

1.1. Background and Approach

System dynamics (SD) models frequently employ parameters for which solid empirical data are not available. Modelers often use expert judgment to provide estimates of parameter values for which empirical data are not available. When several experts are available, and a formal process (such as Delphi) produces convergent estimates, modelers may have reasonable confidence in the parameter values despite the lack of data. Nevertheless, these parameter values remain uncertain to a degree—as is indeed true even for measured parameters, due to issues including small sample sizes and definitional variation.

To address parameter uncertainty, SD modelers test alternative parameter values in order to understand their degree of influence in the model. Formal sensitivity analyses can be run using features provided in popular SD software packages, and results can be displayed in a table or portrayed graphically as a "Tornado diagram" [1].

Once the modeler has identified influential parameters, additional effort is applied, as time and budget allow, to increase confidence that the values of these influential parameters are well supported. When reliable empirical data are available, ideally from multiple sources, the parameter value may be fixed and used with confidence. Usually, however, some, perhaps even many, parameter values typically remain uncertain.

This paper describes how the model analysis features available in the Vensim™ software package (as well as other popular packages including Stella®), can be used to represent and incorporate parameter uncertainty into the analysis of SD model results, including providing outcome uncertainty intervals.

In this paper, we present a flowchart describing a step-by-step process for incorporating parameter uncertainty in SD models. We then illustrate use of the method using a previously published model of the U.S. opioid epidemic [2]. We close with a discussion of how model results under uncertainty can be described for interested parties such as policy makers or other end users of the analyses.

1.2. Prior Work in This Area

Ford [3] and Sterman [4] discussed uncertainty analysis vis-à-vis dynamic models. Helton et al. [5] provided a general overview of sampling-based methods for sensitivity analysis, including traditional Monte Carlo (TMC). Dogan [6,7] discussed confidence interval estimation in SD models using bootstrapping and the likelihood ratio method. Cheung and Beck [8] explained Bayesian updating in Monte Carlo processes, and background material on the mathematics of Markov Chain Monte Carlo (MCMC) is readily available [9,10].

Background on sensitivity analysis methods for dynamic modeling, and SD in particular, including the TMC and MCMC methods being employed in this paper, may be found in Fiddaman and Yeager [11], Osgood [12], Osgood and Liu [13], and Andrade and Duggan [14]. Using TMC methods to search a parameter space is sometimes considered to be a brute force or totally random search, whereas the MCMC method uses a Bayesian update process to guide the search of parameter space. In at least some contexts, it has been shown that MCMC optimally creates statistically valid samples [9].

Although publications describing the application of these methods are plentiful in some scientific and engineering disciplines, publications featuring their use with SD models are scant. A search for "system dynamics" AND ("MCMC" or "monte carlo") returned only a handful of publications. Five relevant examples are Jeon and Chin [15], who described their use of TMC with an SD model of renewable energy; Sterman et al. [16], who applied MCMC in a model of bioenergy; Garfazadegan and Rahmandad [17] who used MCMC to estimate parameter values for a COVID-19 model, Lim et al. [18] who applied MCMC in a model of the U.S. opioid crisis; and Rahmandad et al. [19] who applied MCMC in another model of COVID-19.

2. Materials and Methods

2.1. The Process: Initial Steps

Figure 1 presents the initial steps of a process for incorporating uncertainty analysis into SD models, with further steps shown in Figures 2–4. The complete process is shown in a single flowchart in Supplement Part S1.

The process starts at **Create model & modify as needed**. This would be a model that employs uncertain parameters and includes dynamic outcome variables that strive to match the dynamics seen in real world reference behavior data. To use the methods described in Figure 1, one needs to **Define error metric variables** and **Add error metrics to model**. A useful example could be to compute the mean absolute error (MAE) between the model calculated time series and the reference behavior time series for each outcome variable. Care must be taken to consider how to compute MAE when reference data are incomplete so as not to distort results. When different outcomes have very different scales, it is useful to use MAEM, which stands for MAE over M, where M is the mean value of the metric. In addition, composite error statistics are added to the model, such as the average of the MAEMs over all the outcomes, and the maximum value of the individual MEAMs. These are used later in the process for identifying well-fitting parameter sets. There are statistical macros available for Vensim to help with this (Supplement Part S2).

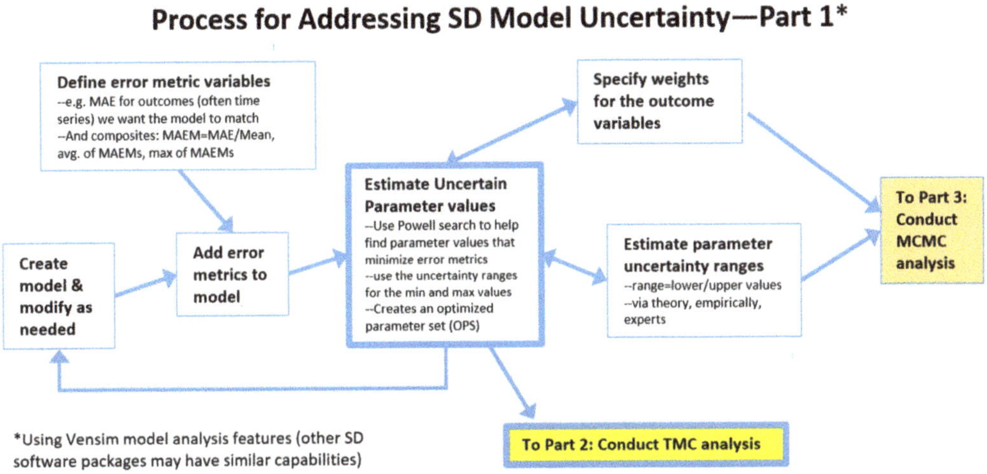

Process for Addressing SD Model Uncertainty—Part 1*

Define error metric variables
--e.g. MAE for outcomes (often time series) we want the model to match
--And composites: MAEM=MAE/Mean, avg. of MAEMs, max of MAEMs

Create model & modify as needed

Add error metrics to model

Estimate Uncertain Parameter values
--Use Powell search to help find parameter values that minimize error metrics
--use the uncertainty ranges for the min and max values
--Creates an optimized parameter set (OPS)

Specify weights for the outcome variables

Estimate parameter uncertainty ranges
--range=lower/upper values
--via theory, empirically, experts

To Part 3: Conduct MCMC analysis

To Part 2: Conduct TMC analysis

*Using Vensim model analysis features (other SD software packages may have similar capabilities)

Figure 1. Process for addressing simulation model uncertainty, initial steps.

Another initial step is to *Estimate parameter uncertainty ranges*, a lower and upper bound for each uncertain parameter, and to *Specify weights for the outcome variables*. These are needed for the algorithm used in a key part of the process: *Estimate uncertain parameter values*. This process employs a Powell optimization process that uses an objective function consisting of model outcomes vs. reference data. For more information, see Menzies et al. [20] for a tutorial on using Bayesian methods to calibrate health policy models. Each term of the objective function represents one of the outcome time series of interest. The algorithm strives to minimize the differences between model and reference data. Weights are needed because outcomes may have very different scales and variances. This tends to be an iterative process, so Figure 1 contains a feedback loop, and some of the connections are bidirectional. The end result of this step is a set of optimized parameter values for the uncertain parameters (OPS). Its average MAEM might be 0.1 and its maximum MAEM (worst MAEM for any one of the outcomes) might be 0.2.

2.2. The Process: Intermediate Steps for the Traditional Monte Carlo (TMC) Approach

At this point, the user may elect to use traditional Monte Carlo (TMC) or Markov Chain Monte Carlo (MCMC). TMC is discussed first; see Figure 2.

Make very large traditional Monte Carlo (TMC) run employs Vensim's sensitivity feature to perform a very large number of model runs, millions if there are many uncertain parameters. Using this feature requires the user to specify how many runs to perform, the seed to start with, the type of sampling (e.g., multivariate, Latin hypercube, etc.), and which parameters to vary and how. We used multi-variate, which is a totally random search process. Latin hypercube strives to cover a large parameter space more efficiently. Both may be valid choices. We experimented with Uniform but settled on Triangular with the mode specified as the value from the OPS. Since we were focused on overall error, we changed the output save period (SAVEPER) to be the length of the run. This kept the output file size manageable. We also specified some additional variables to be saved (all the parameters being varied are automatically saved). These additions were the average MAEM and maximum MAEM for the run.

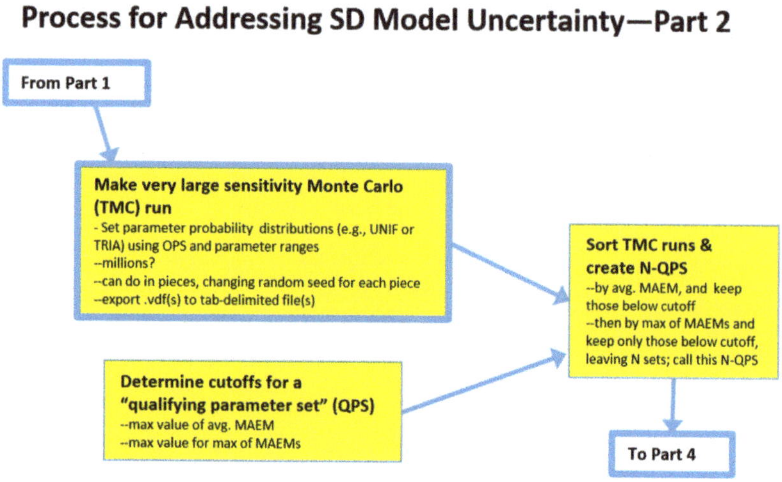

Process for Addressing SD Model Uncertainty—Part 2

Figure 2. Intermediate steps for the traditional Monte Carlo (TMC) approach.

Note that when more than one million runs are needed, we find it practical to perform one million at a time and to change the seed for each run. At the end of a sensitivity run, the data output file (.vdf in Vensim) is exported to a tab-delimited file for further analysis.

Next, the user needs to *Determine cutoffs for a qualified parameter set (QPS)* which involves determining how well-fitting a candidate parameter set must be to warrant its inclusion in the QPS. The vast majority of the TMC runs will not be well-fitting in the manner of the OPS. One rational approach would be to accept parameter sets that performed nearly as well as the OPS. For example, for a model in which the OPS has an average MAEM = 0.1 and the maximum MAEM = 0.2, the cutoffs for the inclusion of a candidate parameter set could be average MAEM < 0.12 and maximum MAEM < 0.25.

Sort TMC runs & create N-QPS employs Excel's data/import external data from file to read in the TMC results. The result will be M columns by N rows, where M is the number parameters being varied + K, and N is the number of runs. K is the number of saved variables times the number of saved times per variable, which could be one, two (start time and end time), or more. The results are then sorted by average MAEM and all rows > average MAEM cutoff are discarded. The remainder is sorted by maximum MAEM and all rows > maximum MAEM are discarded. This will likely leave a very tiny fraction of runs, perhaps a few hundred out of a million. These N runs are the qualified parameter sets (N-QPS).

2.3. The Process: Intermediate Steps for Markov Chain Monte Carlo (MCMC) Approach

A very different approach for creating a set of runs to be used to evaluate the impacts of parameter uncertainty is to use the MCMC approach; see Figure 3.

This begins with *Estimate Optimal Outcome Weights*. First, one adds to the model a weight variable for each outcome, instead of specifying the weights numerically as in the MC process. One also needs to specify the search range for outcome weight constants. The search ranges for the uncertain parameters can be the same as for the MC approach. Or, these ranges could be broader than those used with the prior approach. No sampling distribution such as Uniform or Triangular is specified because the search of parameter space is guided by a heuristic, not by random, sampling. Guidance regarding how broad to set the ranges for MCMC varies by expert. We have heard from some, the comment that very broad ranges will give the algorithm "room to work". Others have suggested that ranges should not include implausible values. Both comments are sensible, suggesting that a careful study of this question is needed. To proceed, first a Powell search is performed that optimizes the uncertain parameters and the weights simultaneously. In our experience, allowing larger ranges may allow the algorithm to find an optimum that achieves slightly lower average MAEM, but higher maximum MAEM. The reason is that some of the individual outcomes are sacrificed to achieve lower overall error. However, these results may be less realistic.

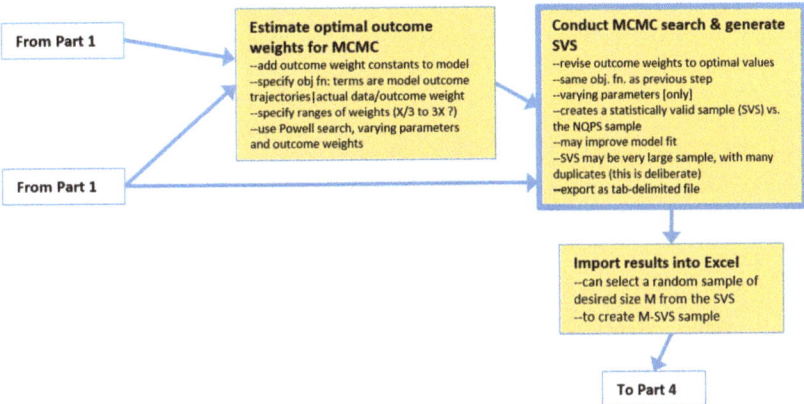

Figure 3. Intermediate steps for the Markov Chain Monte Carlo (MCMC) approach.

Next is to *Conduct MCMC search & generate SVS*. MCMC, in the manner of MC, varies the uncertain parameters over the specified ranges, but uses in the objective function the outcome weights that were found in previous step. The Markov Chain-driven search algorithm is designed to create a statistically valid sample (abbreviated here as SVS). It can be quite large and contain many duplicates (which apparently helps to assure a sample with the correct properties). Model fitness may be further improved, but be less plausible, as mentioned earlier. Results are then exported as a tab-delimited file.

One then must *Import results into Excel*, and, if the population of runs produced by the MCMC search is excessively large, one can select a random sample of desired size M from the SVS. This subsample of size M, which is still a statistically valid sample (M-SVS), is comparable to the N-QPS set of runs created by the conventional MC process described earlier. One can proceed to computing statistics by parameter using the M-SVS and/or use it to run file-driven sensitivity runs, analyze alternative scenarios, etc.

2.4. The Process: Final Steps for Both TMC and MCMC

The final steps of the process are shown in Figure 4.

Save sensitivity (TMC or MCMC) parameters as a tab-delimited txt file creates the file needed for file-driven sensitivity runs.

Within Excel, the user can proceed to ***Compute/graph statistics by parameter*** to see what the values in N-QPS (or M-SVS) file are for each parameter, for example, to see if the entire range of possible values for a given parameter is represented in N-QPS, if the mean of this sample is near the value of the parameter in the OPS. Additionally, it could be used to determine the confidence interval of the estimate for the mean of the parameter based on this sample and examine the distribution (shape) of the sample. Does this information raise any red flags with respect to the OPS or N-QPS? Or, does this information indicate that the N-QPS may be representative of the entire parameter space?

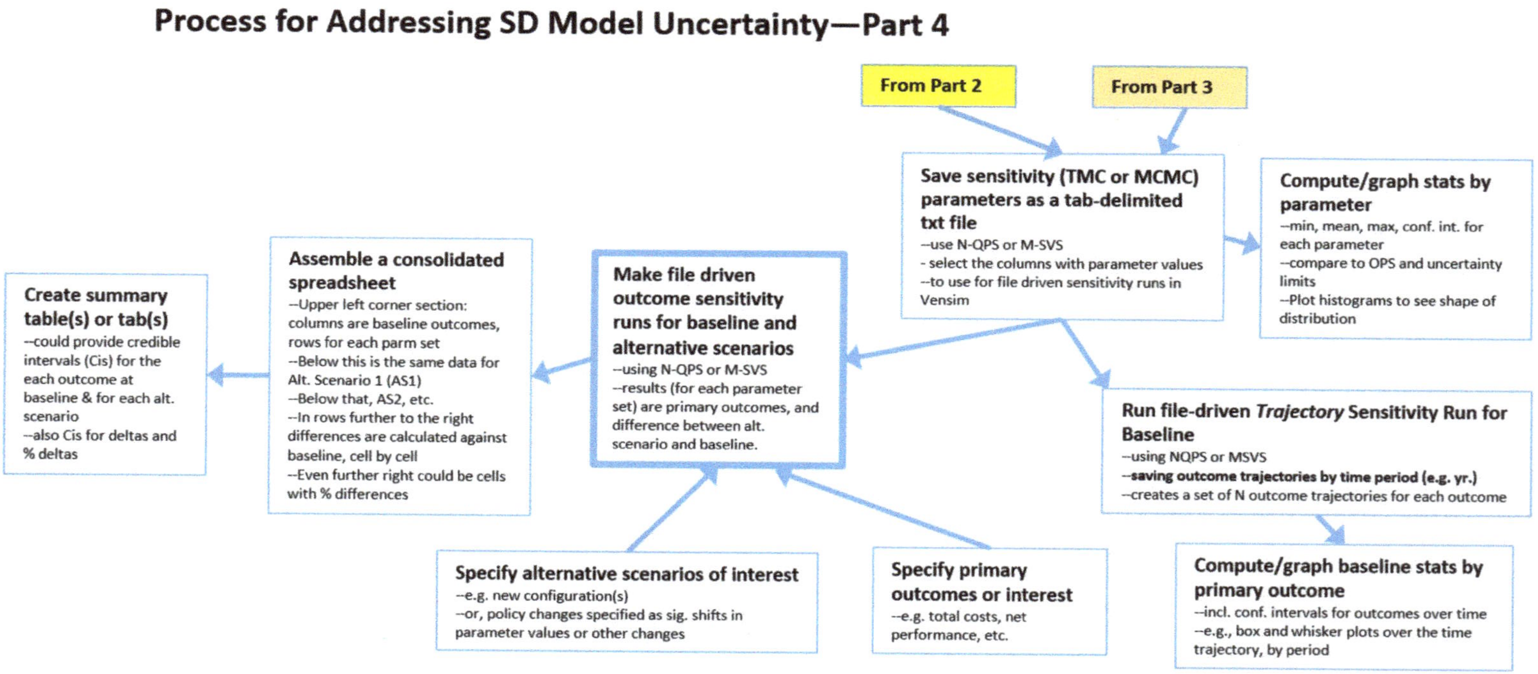

Process for Addressing SD Model Uncertainty—Part 4

From Part 2 → **Save sensitivity (TMC or MCMC) parameters as a tab-delimited txt file**
- use N-QPS or M-SVS
- select the columns with parameter values to use for file driven sensitivity runs in Vensim

From Part 3 → **Compute/graph stats by parameter**
- min, mean, max, conf. int. for each parameter
- compare to OPS and uncertainty limits
- Plot histograms to see shape of distribution

Make file driven outcome sensitivity runs for baseline and alternative scenarios
- using N-QPS or M-SVS
- results (for each parameter set) are primary outcomes, and difference between alt. scenario and baseline.

Run file-driven *Trajectory* Sensitivity Run for Baseline
- using NQPS or MSVS
- saving outcome trajectories by time period for each outcome
- creates a set of N outcome trajectories for each outcome

Compute/graph baseline stats by primary outcome
- incl. conf. intervals for outcomes over time
- e.g., box and whisker plots over the time trajectory, by period

Specify primary outcomes or interest
- e.g. total costs, net performance, etc.

Specify alternative scenarios of interest
- e.g. new configuration(s)
- or, policy changes specified as sig. shifts in parameter values or other changes

Assemble a consolidated spreadsheet
- Upper left corner section: columns are baseline outcomes, rows for each parm set
- Below this is the same data for Alt. Scenario 1 (AS1)
- Below that, AS2, etc.
- In rows further to the right differences are calculated against baseline, cell by cell
- Even further right could be cells with % differences

Create summary table(s) or tab(s)
- could provide credible intervals (CIs) for the each outcome at baseline & for each alt. scenario
- also CIs for deltas and % deltas

Figure 4. Final steps of the process.

Next, the N-QPS (or M-SVS) file can be used in two primary ways. One is the *Run file-driven Trajectory Sensitivity Run for Baseline*, for which the user can change the SAVEPER to a useful time-period, such as by year, in order to create a series of N (or M) trajectories for each outcome. The result is exported to a tab-delimited file that can be imported into Excel to *Compute/graph baseline statistics by primary outcome*, including uncertainty intervals for the model calculated outcome at each time period, since there is now a sample of N model-calculated values at each time point. Excel can also be used to create box and whisker plots at each time point, with or without outliers. However, we found it more expedient to create these plots using Python.

For the other primary use of the N-QPS (or M-SVS) file, explained below, the user first needs to *Specify primary high-level outcomes of interest* such as total cost and net performance. The previous sensitivity run was focused on behavior over time for all outcome time series, but to compare alternative scenarios in an overall sense, a few key end-of-run metrics are needed. In addition, one also needs to *Specify alternative scenarios of interest*; these might be different configurations or policy changes that could be implemented in the model as switches that are used in conjunction with magnitude-of-impact parameters and timing parameters linked to specific model constants.

Using the N-QPS or M-SVS, the user will change the SAVPER back to the End of Run and then *Make file driven sensitivity runs for baseline and each alternative scenario*. The results, for the baseline and for each scenario, are matched pairs of data points (where all of the uncertain parameter values are the same for baseline and the alternative). This means that the distributions of the differences can be used to determine, in a statistically valid fashion, the credible interval estimates (a term from Bayesian statistics), for the mean of the difference by outcome between baseline and the alternative, that can be attributed to parameter uncertainty.

We suggest that one *Assemble a consolidated spreadsheet* to perform these analyses. In the upper left corner, is O × N, where O is the number of overall outcomes and N is the number of runs. Note that the raw sensitivity results file has columns for all the parameters as well as columns for each outcome. The user selects and copies only the end columns for each outcome into the consolidated sheet. The data for Alternative 1 is placed below the Baseline results; Alternative 2 below Alternative 1, etc. Then, starting at the first row of Alternative 1, columns will be added to compute the differences between the Alternative 1 numbers and baseline number, one column for each outcome. Similarly for Alternative 2 vs. baseline, and so forth. Columns for percentage differences can also be added.

Finally, *Create summary table(s) or tab(s)* is used to provide the results of relevant calculations, such as means and their credible intervals for each outcome at baseline and for each alternative. In addition, the results for the differences by outcome between baseline and Alternative 1, baseline and Alternative 2, etc., may be compiled. Similarly, for the percentage differences.

2.5. About the Opioid Epidemic Model

To illustrate the process and results, the TMC method was applied to an SD model of significant complexity that explored the opioid epidemic in the United States from 1990 to 2030 including the impacts of alternative policies (hereafter the Opioid Epidemic Model) [2,21]. SD has been frequently applied to drug abuse and other areas of public health and social policy [22–26]. The current model adopts the basic scientific approach and some of the same elements as these forerunner models, but the current model was completely redeveloped to address current needs.

A committee of the National Academies of Sciences/Engineering/Medicine considered the complexities of the opioid epidemic and stated that for informed decision making "a true systems model, not just simple statistics" was needed because "decisions made about complex systems with endogenous feedback can be myopic in the absence of a formal model" [27]. The NAS cited the system dynamics model by Wakeland et al. [24] as an example of a true systems model.

Best practices for model development, testing, and reporting are well documented [4,28–30]. The model building process for the Opioid Epidemic Model involved amassing evidence from many different sources and developing a dynamic structure that reproduces historical trends and is sufficiently parsimonious to allow explanation. Uncertainties are addressed through sensitivity testing and the multivariate TMC testing described previously that allows results to be reported with rigorous credible intervals.

A complete list of the approximately 340 interacting model equations (including about 80 input constants, 17 time series for input and validation, and 240 output variables) is available in the model's reference guide [21]. This guide also provides stock and flow diagrams for each sector of the model and describes how model constants and time series were estimated, including data sources. The model time horizon was 1990–2030. Figure 5 shows the basic model structure.

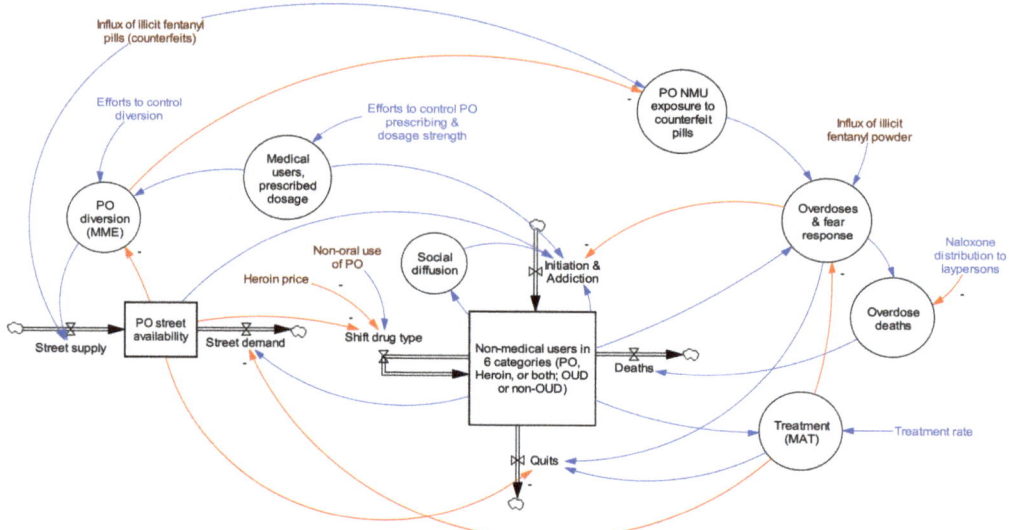

Figure 5. Opioid Epidemic Model diagram showing high level stocks, flows, and primary feedback structures. Red lines are causal links with negative valence, while blue lines have positive valence. Reproduced by permission from Homer and Wakeland 2020 [2].

3. Results

3.1. Error Metrics

As the first step in the TMC approach, error metrics were created, in this case, MAEM (mean absolute error over mean) for multiple outcome time series with historical data counterparts. We used the Vensim SSTATS macro provided by Professor John Sterman at MIT; see Supplement Part S2. This code was inserted via text editor (we used Notepad) at the top of the model file starting at the second line. Supplement Part S3 presents the model code for calculating the statistics, which was also inserted into the model file via text editor, typically after the Control block, which is located after the user-defined model variables/constants section. We utilized an Excel workbook that included a worksheet with Time in Row 1 and historical time series data in the rows below. In some cases, there were data only for some of the historical years. The SSTATS macro calculations are designed to handle this correctly. An example Vensim equation for reading one these data time series is GET XLS DATA ('model RBP data.xlsx', 'RBP', '1', 'B2').

Another step to prepare the model for analysis was to add a custom graphs file via the Control Panel and add custom tables that display the variables calculated by the SSTATS macro (R2, MAPE, MAEM, RMSE, Um, Us, Uc, and Count), one table for each Outcome variable. I/O Objects were added to a model view to display the custom tables.

Figure 6 shows a sample of these statistical parameter displays created using the SSTATS macro, with the MAEM statistics on the left and R-squared statistics on the right. These outputs were from the optimized parameter set (OPS) version of the Opioid Epidemic Model; see discussion below. In addition to the weighted average of all the MAEMs of 8.9% (bottom left 2020 column), it is clear that OD death-related trajectories were reproduced more accurately than, for example, heroin-related trajectories. The MAEM for *OD deaths total* was 3.6%, whereas for *H initiates* it was 18%. This large difference was due mostly to noise in the data representing the actual values. OD death data are the actual data collected by the CDC, and the changes from year to year are modest. Data on persons initiating heroin in a given year is based on a small sample of a difficult-to-access population and the resulting estimates by year vary dramatically. In fact, the difference between the data and the corresponding three-period moving average was 12.5%, suggesting that most (70%) of the 18% model-calculated MAEM was due to noise in the data.

Time (Year)	2020	Time (Year)	2020
MAEM PO Abusers	0.0635467	R2 PO abusers	0.920513
MAEM Addicted PO Abusers	0.0904467	R2 Addicted PO abusers	0.792607
MAEM Addicted frac PO Abusers	0.0565265	R2 Addicted frac PO abusers	0.797944
MAEM PO abuse initiates	0.108133	R2 PO abuse initiates	0.822349
MAEM H users	0.121204	R2 H users	0.865612
MAEM Addicted H users	0.0900014	R2 Addicted H users	0.896018
MAEM Addicted frac H users	0.0569164	R2 Addicted frac H users	0.293248
MAEM H initiates	0.18316	R2 H initiates	0.292869
MAEM frac H users also PO	0.138318	R2 frac H users also PO	0.691761
MAEM frac H initiates also PO	0.1005	R2 frac H initiates also PO	0.0539205
MAEM street price PO	0.179008	R2 street price PO	0.69684
MAEM OD deaths from PO	0.0509725	R2 OD deaths from PO	0.956034
MAEM OD deaths from illicits	0.0392809	R2 OD deaths from illicits	0.998476
MAEM OD deaths total	0.0363724	R2 OD deaths total	0.997179
Simple avg of all MAEM	0.0938847		
Weighted avg of all MAEM	0.0892688		

Figure 6. Selected SSTATS displays (MAEM and R-squared for outcome variables).

3.2. Optimized Parameter Set (OPS)

Before using optimization to estimate uncertain parameter values, the user must specify an appropriate range for each parameter to be used by the Powell search algorithm. Supplement Part S4 provides an example Vensim optimization control file (.voc) which specified the uncertain parameters to be varied. Table 1 shows the first few rows of the model parameter spreadsheet by parameter, including the minimum and maximum values. Many of the 80 model parameters had empirical support from the literature, which helped to reduce the uncertainty ranges for these parameters.

In addition, weights must be specified for the objective function, informed by the relative magnitudes and variances of the outcome variables. In this example, weights were set so that metrics with solid empirical data were given more weight than those for which empirical data were scant or less reliable.

The optimization runs using the CG (calibration Gaussian) option ran for several minutes on a laptop computer. A blend of modeler judgment and optimization results was used iteratively to select the values for the optimized parameter set. The MAEMs for many of the outcomes were reduced compared with a purely manual calibration process. The weighted (based on the amount of data available for each outcome) average of the MAEMs was 8.9%, with the largest individual MAEM being 17.9%.

Table 1. Portion of the opioid model parameter spreadsheet showing parameter name, units, value (central estimate), source (or optimized), and the minimum and maximum values used during optimization runs.

Parameter	Units	Value	Sources	Min Value	Max Value
Addicted frac of H users initial	fraction	0.65	Optimized; our NSDUH analysis showed 60.8% 2000, 61.1% 2005.	0.6	0.7
Addicted frac of PONHA initial	fraction	0.123	Optimized; our NSDUH analysis showed 11.4% 2000, 14.2% 2005.	0.1	0.15
Addicted H user OD death rate initial	1/year	0.010	Optimized	0.005	0.015
Addicted H user quit rate initial	1/year	0.138	Optimized	0.07	0.21
Addicted opioid abuser misc death rate	1/year	0.0045	Ray et al. 2016 [31] determined a mortality hazard ratio of 1.94 vs. general popn for high dose users (>60 mg ME). Multiplied by general popn: average of NVSR death rates for [age 25–34, 35–44, 45–54] = 0.0023 for 2000–2010 × 1.94 = 0.0045.		
Addicted PONHA move to heroin rate initial	1/year	0.021	Optimized	0.01	0.03
Addicted PONHA OD death rate initial	1/year	0.0059	Optimized	0.004	0.007
Addicted PONHA quit rate initial	1/year	0.149	Optimized	0.08	0.22

Figure 7 shows the trajectories for two example outcomes calculated by the model using the optimized parameter set compared with the available historical data for these metrics. The MAEMs for the two outcomes in Figure 7 were 9% and 4%. The calculated *Persons with Addiction* trajectory was somewhat biased downward, whereas the *OD Deaths* trajectory matched very well. One possible reason could be the amount of data available: the standardized errors for the first variable may carry somewhat less weight than the second one. Additionally, note that measurement uncertainty was greater for the first variable than the second one.

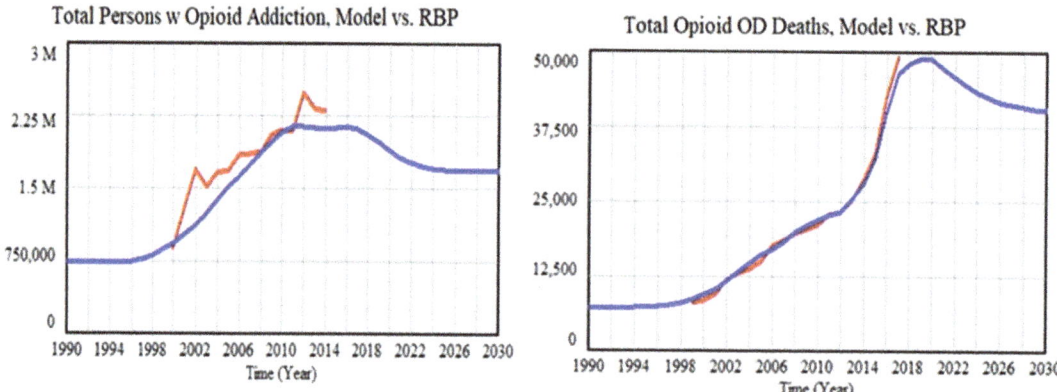

Figure 7. Model fit to two key outcomes using the optimized parameter set.

3.3. Qualified Parameter Sets (N-QPS)

Creating a large Monte Carlo run is easy using the sensitivity feature in Vensim, which uses or creates a .vsc file. One option for exploring parameter space could be to use Uniform distributions between thoughtfully chosen minima and maxima. These values could be the same as those used during calibration, or perhaps narrowed somewhat. Another option could be to use a Triangular distribution with the optimum value as the mode, which would increase samples near the optima. For this illustration, Triangular distributions were used. The user also needs to specify a .lst file that lists which variables are to be saved for each run. Sensitivity runs automatically save the varied parameters used for each run, and in addition, it is useful to know the maximum MAEM and average MAEM (to be used to select which runs are qualified). Since we do not need to know the time trajectories, we set the model SAVEPER to 40. This kept the output file modest in size. Supplement Part S5 shows the .vsc and .lst files.

The simulation was set to create one million runs, which took about seven hours on a laptop. Ten such runs were made, changing the random seed for each run, creating a total sample of ten million runs. Each resulting data output file (.vdf) was exported (via the model menu) to a tab-delimited file and read into Excel using data/get external data/from text (switch to All Files to see .tab files). This was sorted by weighted average of MAEMs. The weighted average MAEM was below 0.11 for 300–600 runs in each of the one million runs, and these rows were kept. The other rows were deleted.

The file was then sorted by maximum MAEM, and 100–130 runs were less than 0.20 and kept. The rest were deleted. These ten spreadsheets were combined, yielding a sample of 1119 runs that accomplished <11% weighted average error and <20% maximum error. Rows were added below the sample to calculate useful statistics about the sample, regarding both the distributions of the input parameters and the how well each run performed. Table 2 shows the first and last few rows of the spreadsheet.

Table 2. First and last few rows and columns of the file used to create the N-QPS.

	Uncertain Parameters				MAEM Statistics	
	Addicted Frac H Users	Addicted Frac PONHA	Addicted H User OD Death Rate		Simple	Weighted
Simulation Number	Initial	Initial	Initial	Max	Average	Average
681,526	0.6303	0.1269	0.0121	0.1994	0.1002	0.0958
376,905	0.6913	0.1186	0.0126	0.1975	0.1019	0.0969
131,761	0.6460	0.1180	0.0098	0.1967	0.1055	0.0980
67,350	0.6841	0.1172	0.0078	0.1713	0.1013	0.0982
726,864	0.6501	0.1246	0.0108	0.1838	0.1018	0.0983
736,791	0.6538	0.1236	0.0109	0.1904	0.1150	0.1100
358,518	0.6887	0.1224	0.0100	0.1849	0.1147	0.1100
MIN all sims	0.6012	0.1003	0.0059	0.1612	0.1002	0.0958
MIN allowed	0.6	0.1	0.005			
MAX all sims	0.6998	0.1488	0.0145	0.2000	0.1191	0.1100
MAX allowed	0.7	0.15	0.015			
MEAN all sims	0.6487	0.1247	0.0105			
OPS value	0.650	0.123	0.010	0.1795	0.0994	0.0935
STD DEV all sims	0.0204	0.0100	0.0015			

We next examined the properties of the parameter samples contained in the N-QPS. The rows at the bottom of Table 2 show the minimum, maximum, mean, and standard deviation of each parameter. For more detail, histogram plots were created, with examples shown in Figure 8. The parameter shown on the left, *Addicted PONHA move to heroin rate initial*, was limited to be in the 0.01 to 0.03 range. As the histogram shows, nearly all of this allowed range was included in the N-QPS. The mode was about 0.0235, which was slightly higher than its value of 0.021 in the optimized parameter set. The parameter on the right, *Consumption mgs ME per addicted PO abuser per month initial*, was limited to be in the range of 2000 to 5000; the values in the N-QPS were well inside these limits (2092 to 4566). The mode was 3330, very slightly higher than its value of 3200 in the optimized parameter set. One can examine all of the parameter histograms in this fashion to build confidence in the sample.

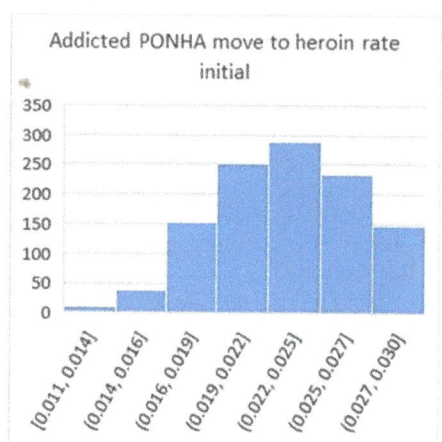 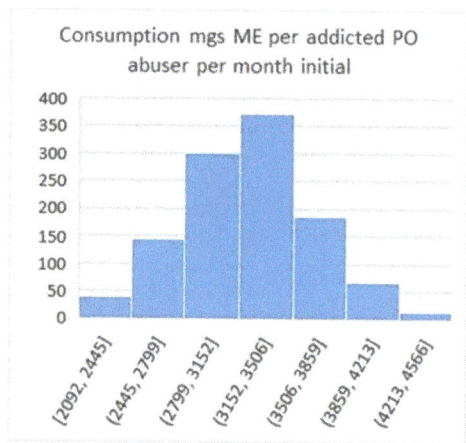

Figure 8. Histograms for two uncertain parameters resulting from the TMC approach.

For comparison, Figure 9 shows a histogram that results from using the MCMC algorithm rather than TMC, again considering the parameter that was on the left side of Figure 8. For MCMC, nearly all of the samples fell in the range from 0.02 to 0.0216 with a width of 0.0016, whereas the range for same parameter in Figure 8 is from 0.014 to 0.03 with a width of 0.026 (greater by 16x), and the shape has a sharp rather than rounded peak. We found that nearly all of the parameter distributions from testing MCMC on the Opioid Epidemic Model had this narrow and pointed characteristic. The problem was not skewness, but the implausibly high degree of precision in the estimated parameter value, within just a few percentage points.

Using different settings for the MCMC algorithm yielded similar very narrow and pointed samples, prompting the decision to rely on the TMC-based method that tests a much broader range of potential values for these parameters. However, other researchers have reported successful use of the MCMC method [15–19], indicating that the MCMC approach may be preferred in many cases.

3.4. Sensitivity Runs for the Baseline Scenario

To put the N-QPS sample from the MC-based method to use, file-driven sensitivity runs were performed. The SAVEPER was changed to 40, and the Sensitivity tool was selected. Previous settings were cleared, and the Type of sensitivity run was changed to File. The N-QPS text file was selected as the file. Next a save list was created. The previous save list (with the statistical variables) was cleared, and three primary outcome variables were entered: *Total opioid addicts, Opioid overdoses seen at ED, and Total opioid OD deaths*. This run took just a minute to complete, and the data output file (.vdf) it produced was exported via Vensim and imported into Excel.

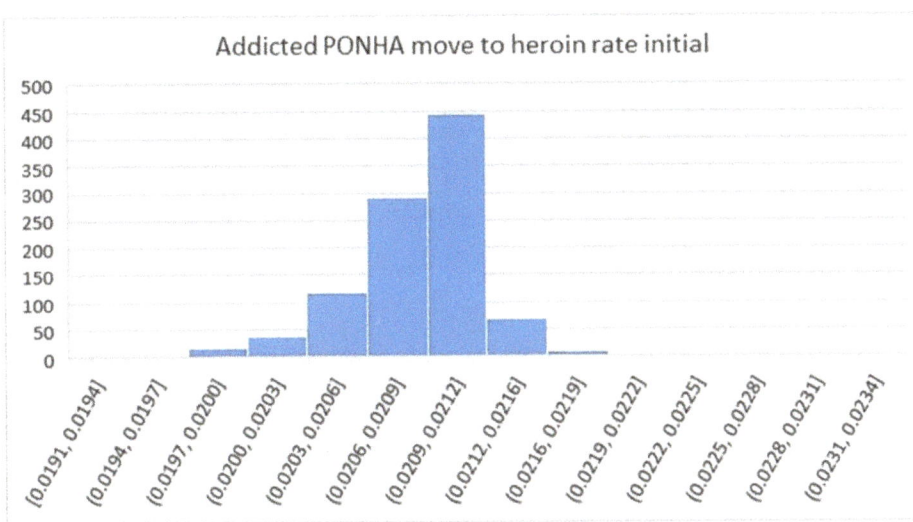

Figure 9. Histogram for an uncertain parameter resulting from the MCMC approach. Note that all of the bars in this diagram are contained within the fourth bar on the left side of Figure 8.

The first 50 columns of this trajectory spreadsheet provided the run number (1–1119) and the values of the 49 uncertain parameter values used for each specific run. The remaining 41 columns were values from time 1990 to 2030 for the three outcome variables. Figure 10 shows the trajectory under uncertainty for *Overdoses Seen at ED* using a box-and-whiskers plot. One can also use the data in the spreadsheet to report useful sample statistics, such as mean and standard deviation.

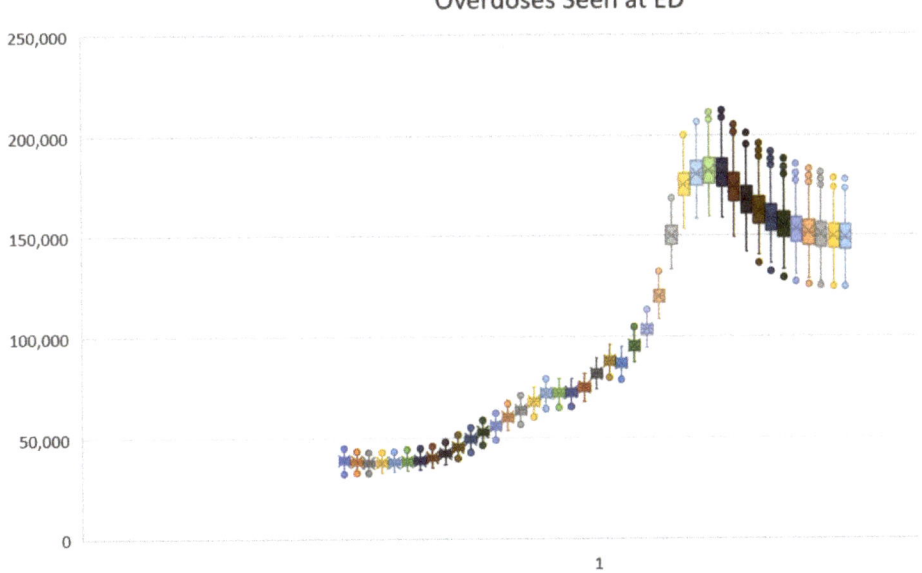

Figure 10. Excel box-and-whisker time series plot for *Overdoses Seen at ED* under the baseline scenario.

Unfortunately, there was no easy way using Excel to superimpose the historical data on this plot. Python software could be used to create such a plot as needed. Figure 11 shows the plot produced using Python for *Total opioid OD deaths*, showing the credible interval trajectory overlaid with green dots for the historical data. The credible interval was similar in spirit to the confidence intervals used to characterize statistical samples from actual populations.

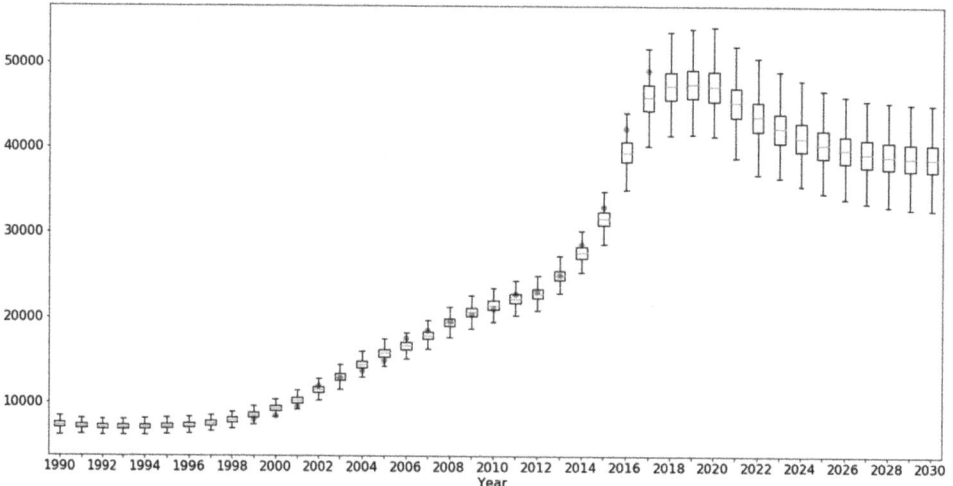

Figure 11. Python box-and-whisker time series plot for *Total Opioid OD Deaths* under the baseline scenario, overlaid with historical data (green dots).

To prepare the file needed by Python, a version of the trajectory spreadsheet was created, named Outcome Trajectory Data for Python Plotting (OTDPP), in which the columns for run number and the parameter values were deleted. Additionally, two rows were added below the first row. Row 2 should contain the actual data to be overlaid. For each outcome variable, the appropriate row of the RBP spreadsheet was copied above its corresponding section in OTDPP. Since the RBP data spreadsheet contained up to 30 values of historical data for each outcome trajectory, and since the data sections for each outcome in OTDPP were oriented horizontally, it was a simple copying process, even for several outcomes. Row 3 in OTDPP should provide the time values, which was easily created in Excel or could be copied from the historical data spreadsheet (41 cells copied once and pasted N times in the OTDPP, where N is the number of outcome variable, 3 for this example).

3.5. Sensitivity Runs for Alternative Scenarios (Policy Testing under Uncertainty)

Another use of the N-QPS is to compare a baseline case with policy runs, to determine how much impact parameter uncertainty may have with respect to the most important outcome indicators. In the case of the Opioid Epidemic Model, three key indicators were the number of people with opioid addiction (also known as opioid use disorder or OUD), opioid overdose events, and opioid overdose deaths. These metrics are saved for each of the parameter sets in the N-QPS, for the baseline condition and for each alternative. The net change in outcome, and policy vs. baseline, were calculated run by run, in both absolute and percentage terms.

The Opioid Epidemic Model was run using the file-driven sensitivity tool reading in the 1119-QPS parameter sets, and for five potential policies aside from the baseline. The final values for the three key metrics were saved for each of the 1119 runs, and a spreadsheet was created to compute the differences in outcome metrics, run by run. This spreadsheet had 1119 rows and 48 columns. The first three columns were the final baseline values for each of the three metrics. Then, nine columns were created for each of the five policies. These were the three columns of raw outcomes, plus three columns that calculated the change, and three more that calculated the percentage change. A row was added at the bottom to compute the mean percentage change in each outcome due to each policy. Two more rows computed minimum change in each metric and the maximum change in each metric.

Table 3 presents a summary of the parameter uncertainty analysis of the impacts of the various policies. The *% change vs. Baseline* under OPS may be compared with the *Mean %Δ* and the range (min, max) of percentage changes under the QPS 1119. Even though the mean of the QPS-driven change was generally close to the results using the OPS, seeing the uncertainty interval provides more information to inform policy decisions. Three examples are highlighted in yellow, as follows:

- *Treatment rate 65% (from 45%)* policy and the outcome Persons with OUD: The model projected a modest unfavorable impact for the OPS and a modest favorable impact for the QPS. The QPS sample interval contained zero, so this policy should perhaps be considered not to impact Persons with OUD;
- *All four policies combined* and the outcome Overdoses Seen at ED: a mean beneficial outcome was predicted by both, but the credible interval again included zero, indicating that the net effect of all four policies on overdose events could be neutral;
- *Diversion control policy* and the outcome OD Deaths: The uncertainty interval again included zero, suggesting that for a significant number of the qualified parameter sets, the impact was unfavorable. This was likely due to persons switching to more dangerous drugs. This hypothesis could be examined directly by studying the uncertainty analysis results to find the specific parameter values which render the policy ineffective.

Table 3. Impact of parameter uncertainty on the simulated results of policy changes.

Outcome Measure	Test Condition	Optimized Parameter Set		QPS 1119 MC Result			QPS 1119 MC, % Change vs. Baseline		
		Result	% Change vs. Baseline	Mean	Credible Interval		Mean %Δ	Credible Interval	
					Min	Max		Min	Max
Persons with OUD (thou)	Baseline	1694		1593	1111	2084			
	Avg MME dose down 20%	1510	−10.9%	1416	1035	1823	−11.1%	−25.7%	−3.4%
	Diversion Control 30%	1428	−15.7%	1339	1007	1716	−15.9%	−37.4%	−4.6%
	Treatment rate 65% (from 45%)	1713	1.1%	1585	1054	2130	−0.5%	−9.0%	5.0%
	Naloxone lay use 20% (from 4%)	1728	2.0%	1624	1150	2111	1.9%	1.3%	2.3%
	All four policies combined	1285	−24.1%	1189	905	1560	−25.4%	−60.2%	−6.5%
Overdoses seen at ED (thou)	Baseline	155		149	124	179			
	Avg MME dose down 20%	153	−1.3%	145	118	176	−2.7%	−8.2%	3.8%
	Diversion Control 30%	153	−1.1%	144	116	175	−3.4%	−11.6%	6.0%
	Treatment rate 65% (from 45%)	150	−3.0%	144	118	171	−3.7%	−11.3%	−0.3%
	Naloxone lay use 20% (from 4%)	159	2.9%	154	128	187	3.1%	2.2%	5.1%
	All four policies combined	148	−4.1%	139	111	168	−7.3%	−19.6%	6.1%
Overdose deaths (thou)	Baseline	40.3		39.0	32.5	46.7			
	Avg MME dose down 20%	39.8	−1.3%	37.9	30.9	46.0	−2.7%	−8.2%	0.6%
	Diversion Control 30%	39.9	−1.1%	37.6	30.3	45.5	−3.4%	−11.6%	6.0%
	Treatment rate 65% (from 45%)	39.2	−3.0%	37.5	30.8	44.6	−3.7%	−11.3%	−0.3%
	Naloxone lay use 20% (from 4%)	35.3	−12.5%	34.2	28.4	41.4	−12.3%	−18.6%	−8.1%
	All four policies combined	32.9	−18.4%	30.7	24.5	31.2	−21.1%	−36.4%	−6.9%

4. Discussion

Here we have demonstrated a practical method for analyzing the effects of parameter uncertainty on simulated model projections, using a health policy example. The process summarized in Figures 1–4 (and Supplement Part S1) provides two alternative approaches: traditional Monte Carlo (TMC) and Markov Chain Monte Carlo (MCMC). We featured the former in this paper, because of its greater familiarity and ease of understanding.

However, it should be noted that, despite our difficulties with MCMC (specifically, the overly narrow parameter distributions we observed), it is the theoretically superior and less time-consuming of the two approaches. Tom Fiddaman at Ventana Systems (the makers of Vensim) has suggested that a better choice of likelihood function for MCMC might have produced better dispersed parameter distributions.

Indeed, other research teams have had success with MCMC [15–19]. Although MCMC yields theoretically superior results, further examination and characterization of the parameter distributions resulting from MCMC seems to be in order. Garfazadegan and Rahmandad [17] note in their Appendix A "rather tight confidence intervals coming from MCMC methods directly applied to large nonlinear models," which they address via heuristics that scale the likelihood function.

A possible limitation of both TMC and MCMC is their reliance on the goodness of fit to historical data. Forrester [32] warned that "the particular curves of past history are only a special case." The implication is that this method should not be used to make claims of precision in predicted outcomes, but rather to better appreciate the range of possible outcomes and, especially, the uncertainty in projected policy impacts.

5. Conclusions

We have presented a step-by-step approach to assessing the degree of uncertainty in simulation model outcomes related to uncertainty in the model's input parameters. Our flowchart summarizes two ways to perform this, and we have demonstrated one of these in detail with a concrete health policy example. Providing uncertainty intervals for the range of possible outcomes from contemplated policy options, as we have described here, could increase the value of simulation models to decision makers.

Supplementary Materials: The following supporting information can be downloaded at: https://www.mdpi.com/article/10.3390/systems10060225/s1, Supplement Part S1: Complete process for addressing simulation model uncertainty (uniting Figures S1 to S4) and Supplement Parts S2 to S5.

Author Contributions: W.W. and J.H. have met authorship requirements, and contributed to every part of the manuscript. All authors have read and agreed to the published version of the manuscript.

Funding: The original Opioid Epidemic Model was developed under contract in 2019 (see [2]), but the uncertainty analysis described here was performed subsequently and received no funding.

Institutional Review Board Statement: Not applicable.

Informed Consent Statement: Not applicable.

Data Availability Statement: All data presented in this article were extracted from publicly available data sources (see [2]).

Acknowledgments: The authors wish to thank Kevin Stoltz who wrote the Python code for graphing uncertainty interval time series, as well as John Sterman and Tom Fiddaman for their advice.

Conflicts of Interest: The authors declare no conflict of interest.

References

1. Wakeland, W.; Hoarfrost, M. The case for thoroughly testing complex system dynamics models. In Proceedings of the 23rd International Conference of the System Dynamics Society, Boston, MA, USA, 17–21 July 2005.
2. Homer, J.; Wakeland, W. A dynamic model of the opioid drug epidemic with implications for policy. *Am. J. Drug Alcohol. Abuse.* **2020**, *47*, 5–15. [CrossRef] [PubMed]

3. Ford, A. Estimating the impact of efficiency standards on the uncertainty of the northwest electric system. *Oper. Res.* **1990**, *38*, 580–597. [CrossRef]
4. Sterman, J.D. *Business Dynamics: Systems Thinking and Modeling for a Complex World*; Irwin McGraw-Hill: Boston, MA, USA, 2000.
5. Helton, J.C.; Johnson, J.D.; Sallaberry, C.J.; Storlie, C.B. Survey of sampling-based methods for uncertainty and sensitivity analysis. *Reliab. Eng. Syst. Saf.* **2006**, *91*, 1175–1209. [CrossRef]
6. Dogan, G. Confidence interval estimation in system dynamics models: Bootstrapping vs. likelihood ratio method. In Proceedings of the 22nd International Conference of the System Dynamics Society, Oxford, UK, 25–29 July 2004.
7. Dogan, G. Bootstrapping for confidence interval estimation and hypothesis testing for parameters of system dynamics models. *Syst. Dyn. Rev.* **2007**, *23*, 415–436. [CrossRef]
8. Cheung, S.H.; Beck, J.L. Bayesian model updating using hybrid Monte Carlo simulation with application to structural dynamic models with many uncertain parameters. *J. Eng. Mech.* **2009**, *135*, 243–255. [CrossRef]
9. Ter Braak, C.J.F. A Markov Chain Monte Carlo version of the genetic algorithm Differential Evolution: Easy Bayesian computing for real parameter spaces. *Stat. Comput.* **2006**, *16*, 239–249. [CrossRef]
10. Vrugt, J.A.; ter Braak, C.J.F.; Diks, C.G.H.; Robinson, B.A.; Hyman, J.M.; Higdon, D. Accelerating Markov Chain Monte Carlo Simulation by differential evolution with self-adaptive randomized subspace sampling. *Int. J. Nonlinear Sci. Numer. Simul.* **2009**, *10*, 271–288. [CrossRef]
11. Fiddaman, T.; Yeager, L. Vensim calibration and Markov Chain Monte Carlo. In Proceedings of the 33rd International Conference of the System Dynamics Society, Cambridge, MA, USA, 19–23 July 2015.
12. Osgood, N. Bayesian parameter estimation of system dynamics models using Markov Chain Monte Carlo methods: An informal introduction. In Proceedings of the 31st International Conference of the System Dynamics Society, Cambridge, MA, USA, 21–25 July 2013.
13. Osgood, N.D.; Liu, J. Combining Markov Chain Monte Carlo approaches and dynamic modeling. In *Analytical Methods for Dynamic Modelers*; Rahmandad, H., Oliva, R., Osgood, N.D., Eds.; MIT Press: Cambridge MA, USA, 2015; Chapter 5; pp. 125–169.
14. Andrade, J.; Duggan, J. A Bayesian approach to calibrate system dynamics models using Hamiltonian Monte Carlo. *Syst. Dyn. Rev.* **2021**, *37*, 283–309. [CrossRef]
15. Jeon, C.; Shin, J. Long-term renewable energy technology valuation using system dynamics and Monte Carlo simulation: Photovoltaic technology case. *Energy* **2014**, *66*, 447–457. [CrossRef]
16. Sterman, J.D.; Siegel, L.; Rooney-Varga, J.N. Does replacing coal with wood lower CO_2 emissions? Dynamic lifecycle analysis of wood bioenergy. *Environ. Res. Lett.* **2018**, *13*, 015007. [CrossRef]
17. Ghaffarzadegan, N.; Rahmandad, H. Simulation-based estimation of the early spread of COVID-19 in Iran: Actual versus confirmed cases. *Syst. Dyn. Rev.* **2020**, *36*, 101–129. [CrossRef]
18. Lim, T.Y.; Stringfellow, E.J.; Stafford, C.A.; DiGennaro, C.; Homer, J.B.; Wakeland, W.; Jalali, M.S. Modeling the evolution of the US opioid crisis for national policy development. *Proc. Natl. Acad. Sci. USA* **2022**, *119*, e2115714119. [CrossRef]
19. Rahmandad, H.; Lim, T.Y.; Sterman, J. Behavioral dynamics of COVID-19: Estimating underreporting, multiple waves, and adherence fatigue across 92 nations. *Syst. Dyn. Rev.* **2021**, *37*, 5–31. [CrossRef]
20. Menzies, N.A.; Soeteman, D.I.; Pandya, A.; Kim, J.J. Bayesian methods for calibrating health policy models: A tutorial. *Pharmacoeconomics* **2017**, *35*, 613–624. [CrossRef]
21. Homer, J. Reference Guide for the Opioid Epidemic Simulation Model (Version 2u); February 2020. Available online: https://pdxscholar.library.pdx.edu/cgi/viewcontent.cgi?filename=0&article=1154&context=sysc_fac&type=additional (accessed on 7 November 2022).
22. Levin, G.; Roberts, E.B.; Hirsch, G.B. *The Persistent Poppy: A Computer-Aided Search for Heroin Policy*; Ballinger: Cambridge, MA, USA, 1975.
23. Homer, J.B. A system dynamics model of national cocaine prevalence. *Syst. Dyn. Rev.* **1993**, *9*, 49–78. [CrossRef]
24. Homer, J.; Hirsch, G. System dynamics modeling for public health: Background and opportunities. *Am. J. Public Health* **2006**, *96*, 452–458. [CrossRef]
25. Wakeland, W.; Nielsen, A.; Schmidt, T.; McCarty, D.; Webster, L.; Fitzgerald, J.; Haddox, J.D. Modeling the impact of simulated educational interventions in the use and abuse of pharmaceutical opioids in the United States: A report on initial efforts. *Health Educ. Behav.* **2013**, *40*, 74S–86S. [CrossRef]
26. Wakeland, W.; Nielsen, A.; Geissert, P. Dynamic model of nonmedical opioid use trajectories and potential policy interventions. *Am. J. Drug Alcohol. Abuse* **2015**, *41*, 508–518. [CrossRef]
27. Bonnie, R.J.; Ford, M.A.; Phillips, J.K. (Eds.) *Pain Management and the Opioid Epidemic: Balancing Societal and Individual Benefits and Risks of Prescription Opioid Use*; National Academies Press: Washington, DC, USA, 2017.
28. Homer, J.B. Why we iterate: Scientific modeling in theory and practice. *Syst. Dyn. Rev.* **1996**, *12*, 1–19. [CrossRef]
29. Richardson, G.P. Reflections on the foundations of system dynamics. *Syst. Dyn. Rev.* **2011**, *27*, 219–243. [CrossRef]
30. Rahmandad, H.; Sterman, J.D. Reporting guidelines for system dynamics modeling. *Syst. Dyn. Rev.* **2012**, *8*, 251–261.
31. Ray, W.A.; Chung, C.P.; Murray, K.T.; Hall, K.; Stein, C.M. Prescription of long-acting opioids and mortality in patients with chronic noncancer pain. *JAMA* **2016**, *315*, 2415–2423. [CrossRef] [PubMed]
32. Forrester, J.W. System dynamics—The next fifty years. *Syst. Dyn. Rev.* **2007**, *23*, 359–370. [CrossRef]

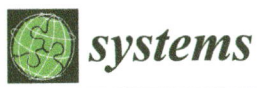

Article

Enabling Mobility: A Simulation Model of the Health Care System for Major Lower-Limb Amputees to Assess the Impact of Digital Prosthetics Services

Jefferson K. Rajah [1], William Chernicoff [2], Christopher J. Hutchison [3], Paulo Gonçalves [4] and Birgit Kopainsky [1,*]

1. System Dynamics Group, Department of Geography, University of Bergen, 5020 Bergen, Norway
2. Toyota Mobility Foundation, Plano, TX 75024, USA
3. ProsFit Technologies JSC, 1407 Sofia, Bulgaria
4. Facoltà di Scienze Economiche, Università della Svizzera Italiana, 6900 Lugano, Switzerland
* Correspondence: birgit.kopainsky@uib.no

Abstract: The World Health Organization estimates that 5 to 15% of amputees in any given population have access to a prosthesis. This figure is likely to worsen as the amputee population is expected to double by 2050, straining the limited capacity of prosthetics services. Without proper and timely prosthetic interventions, amputees with major lower-limb loss experience adverse mobility outcomes, including the loss of independence, lowered quality of life, and decreased life expectancy. Presently, the use of digital technology in prosthetics (e.g., 3D imaging, digital processing, and 3D printed sockets) is contended as a viable solution to this problem. This paper uses system dynamics modeling to assess the impact of digital prosthetics service provision. Our simulation model represents the patient-care continuum and digital prosthetics market system, providing a feedback-rich causal theory of how digital prosthetics impacts amputee mobility and the corollary socio-health-economic outcomes over time. With sufficient resources for market formation and capacity expansion for digital prosthetics services, our work suggests an increased proportion of prosthesis usage and improved associated health-economic outcomes. Accordingly, our findings could provide decision support for health policy to better mitigate the accessibility problem and bolster the social impact of prosthesis usage.

Keywords: prosthetics; major lower-limb amputations; prosthesis usage; amputee mobility; system dynamics; simulation model; health care system; health policy

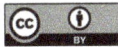

1. Introduction

The World Health Organization (WHO) estimates that around 0.5% of any given population require prosthetics and orthotics services [1]. This figure is expected to double by 2050 as a result of ageing populations and rising rates of medical conditions, such as diabetes mellitus, peripheral arterial disease (PAD), and sepsis [1,2]. Particularly for major lower-limb amputations (i.e., above ankle), over 90% of cases in industrialized countries are attributed to PAD (either primary or secondary to diabetes); whereas traumatic injuries make up most cases in developing countries [3–5]. PAD is a progressive vascular disease that commonly causes arterial obstruction in the lower extremities. Known PAD risk factors include cigarette smoking, diabetes mellitus, hypertension, and dyslipidemia, with incidence sharply rising for populations above age 50 [6,7]. PAD progresses to the more severe critical limb ischemia, if not effectively managed at an earlier stage, which could lead to amputation [8].

Major lower-limb amputation, without timely prosthetic intervention, leads to a loss of mobility, which has several ripple effects at both the individual and societal level. It worsens individual health and psychosocial outcomes, including the loss of independence, increased depression and self-esteem issues, lowered quality of life, and increased risk of comorbidities and mortality [9–11]. There is also high economic burden on patients, families (increased caregiving), health and welfare systems, as well as the workforce (lower rates of return to work) [1,12,13]. Such negative externalities can be alleviated with the use of prostheses to regain mobility and functional independence [14]. However, WHO estimates that only 5 to 15% of amputees have access to prosthetics services [1]. Even then, approximately 50% of amputees in prosthetics care abandon the process or their prosthetic devices [15,16]. Barriers include high financial costs for treatment, poor health care coverage, prosthetics service capacity constraints, limits in prosthetics technology and fitting, lack of proximity to services, and inadequate continuity of care [14–17].

The recent introduction of digital technology in prosthetics is seen as a viable solution to the accessibility problem [16,18,19]. Digital solutions to prosthesis fitting (henceforth, digital prosthetics) involve a streamlined process of scanning the limb and using a digital software to create a model of the socket for three-dimensional printing. Digital technology reduces the delays, patient time and travel burden, and labor involved in traditional prosthetics. Using traditional methods, the prosthetist must handcraft the socket using plaster casts and test the fittings several times before a definitive socket is manufactured and assembled [19]. With digital prosthetics, this manufacturing delay can be more than halved. In turn, this reduces the chances of the patient's limb and/or weight having changed before receiving the prosthesis device—the main cause of discomfort and pain [16]. The fit challenges are a primary cause for the 50% abandonment [15,16]. Hence, digital prosthetics could lead to higher success rates since the digital design is more accurate, precise, and enables direct translation of a prosthetist's skill-level over a minimum baseline in place; has a much shorter timeframe such that there is little time for limb changes; and results in a more comfortable fit for patients [16].

Moreover, digital prosthetics could improve accessibility by expanding service capacity. With a more streamlined and effective fitting process, each prosthetist can fit more patients in their schedule than it otherwise would have been possible with conventional techniques and processes. Digital technology also frees the prosthetist from their clinic and gives them the flexibility to bring the service to patients through distributed care networks [20]. Accordingly, proponents of digital prosthetics anticipate several positive externalities for amputees, their families, and the economy more broadly. This paper seeks to assess this impact of digital prosthetics service provision on total amputee mobility. Mobility, here, is measured by the proportion of medically eligible amputees who are fitted with a prosthesis and have regained functional mobility. The benefit of digital prosthetics can be further measured by the health-related socio-economic consequences of such mobility; namely, the surplus economic productivity from returning to work and the net economic costs incurred or avoided (health care, family opportunity cost, social and welfare payments).

The purpose of this study is to explore how the adoption of digital prosthetics impact amputee mobility and associated outcomes over time. To assess such changes, we model the key causal mechanisms found in the health care system, including the patient-care continuum and prosthetic service provision. For this purpose, we build and analyze a dynamic simulation model to identify high-leverage points that can enhance the effects of digital prosthetics service provision on mobility outcomes. This paper describes the structure, empirical foundation, illustrative results, and strategic insights from the prototype prosthetic service provision model, as well as how it might be further refined. The results reported in this paper result from two activities: First, we use an in-depth review of the existing knowledge (from literature and expert interviews) coupled with causal loop diagramming [21] to identify core feedback mechanisms driving prosthetic service provision. Second, we developed a formal system dynamics simulation model to characterize the range of outcomes that these processes generate, even in a data-poor context. The end result is an internally consistent theory that provides insights into the determinants of success and failure of digital prosthetics service provision.

2. Materials and Methods

This study employs the system dynamics (SD) method, using compartment models, for conducting model-based hypothesis testing. SD models seek to simulate and explain problem behaviors by modeling the underlying system structure [21]. Importantly, they offer an "endogenous or feedback perspective" to structural problems [22] (p. 1) that can aid "theory building, policy analysis, and strategic decision support" [23] (p. 11). This endogenous perspective relates to two fundamental methodological tenets: (1) problem behaviors arise from the complex interaction of interrelated components within a closed boundary of a system, and (2) the system components are connected in feedback loops (circular chains of causal relationships), which endogenously generate the observed system behavior [24,25]. In this sense, the SD method "helps construct a causal-loop theory of system behavior in terms of feedback linkages" [26] (p. 400).

SD modeling is well-suited to domains in public health and medicine, with over 300 applications to date – for a review, see [27,28]. The "dynamic complexity in public health" (particularly due to nonlinear effects of multiple interacting variables within the system that affect health outcomes) makes it "difficult to know how, where, and when to intervene" [29] (p. 452). SD simulation modelling can effectively address this challenge and "elucidate the counterintuitive behavior of complex healthcare problems" [28] (p. 1). Particularly for prosthetics provision and related health care policy, SD modelling can support decision-making under uncertainty. The domain of prosthetics services is mired by the lack of robust data collection, contributing to a high level of uncertainty surrounding policy planning [1,16]. SD models, however, can "admit more variables on the basis of logic or expert opinion and for which solid statistical estimates may not be available" [29] (p. 453) and still generate useful insights under such uncertainty.

2.1. Literature Review

To our knowledge, apart from the two preliminary versions of this work [30,31], there has been no other application of SD to prosthetic service provision or major lower limb amputations in the academic literature. However, this work builds on existing SD literature on emerging medical technologies and innovation diffusion more generally. Paich, Peck and Valant present a model on pharmaceutical product strategy that integrates patient flows, product diffusion and adoption by physicians, and treatment attractiveness to patients [32]. Homer developed a model for medical technology adoption based on demand-side (user dispositions to accept or abandon based on social exposure and evaluation of product performance) and supply-side (R&D for product performance improvement and investment in promotional activities) dynamics [33]. These models are extensions of the Bass Diffusion generic structure that includes a word-of-mouth diffusion process (social exposure and imitation) and external adoption from advertising, which enhance the realism of innovation diffusion [21].

In their systematic review of SD models on innovation systems, Uriona and Grobbelaar point to a "promising stream of research" based on Technological Innovation Systems (TIS) theory, that departs from the innovator-imitator structure of Bass Diffusion [34] (p. 34). TIS theory posits that the formation of a new technological innovation system requires seven key interacting elements: (1) entrepreneurial activities, (2) knowledge development, (3) knowledge diffusion, (4) guidance of search, (5) market formation, (6) mobilization of resources, and (7) creation of legitimacy [35–37]. The complex interactions of these elements determine the growth prospects of a new technology. Subsequently, Walrave and Raven operationalized the theory into a conceptual SD simulation model [36,38]. The main advantage of the TIS framework is its explanatory power for the market formation of new technologies—a "complex non-linear interactive process" that involves several actors and institutions [34] (p. 28). Indeed, market formation requires collective market-oriented action to develop "shared market infrastructure" for "supporting the functioning of a stable market" [39] (p. 244).

Our work contributes to existing knowledge by synthesizing the TIS model with medical technology adoption models. Similar to Paich, Peck and Valant, we represent the patient flow of the health care and prosthetics care system for amputees. Like Homer, we represent the demand-side dispositions of amputees to adopt or abandon the emerging digital prosthetic device based on performance evaluation and word-of-mouth diffusion. We then captured the supply-side conditions of digital prosthetics using the TIS framework. In doing so, we present a feedback perspective to digital prosthetics market formation prospects and the corollary effects on product adoption as well as on the socio-economic and health indicators for the amputee population.

2.2. Data Collection

The iterative model building process, from conceptualization, quantification, to validation, was conducted in collaboration with Toyota Mobility Foundation—expert in system dynamics and human centered design for promoting mobility (second author) and ProsFit Technologies—digital prosthetics service provider (third author). It is tradition in SD to include problem owners and experts in the model building process who possess important domain expertise, experiential knowledge, and mental models of the system under investigation [40–42]. During this process, several iterations of the model were presented to the collaborators for validation. In terms of model parameterization, ProsFit provided numerical estimates for some parameter values where existing data was not available. In such instances, ProsFit relied on its network of prosthetists and other experts in the field to corroborate their assumptions and understanding. Estimates and comments from these domain experts were anonymized and shared via email correspondence. Such estimates represent the best available data and expert judgement at the time of the model development.

Apart from expert opinion, existing peer-reviewed literature was utilized extensively for model conceptualization—especially so for the conceptual market formation subsystem in the model. As for quantification, parameter values were obtained either from epidemiological data reported in the literature or from secondary datasets (Table 1). The model is calibrated to data from the United Kingdom (UK), since expert knowledge and literature pertaining to the country is more readily available, but it can nevertheless be calibrated to other contexts.

Table 1. Data sources used for model parameterization.

Data Source	Description
UK Office for National Statistics [43–48]	UK population estimates for fertility rate and mortality rate
Healthcare Quality Improvement Partnership [49–54]	UK National Vascular Registry statistics on PAD-related major lower limb amputations and clinical outcomes
Global Burden of Disease Collaborative Network [55]	UK estimates for yearly prevalence and incidence estimates on PAD as well as lower limb amputations from injuries as a cause between 2010 and 2019
ProsFit Technologies [56]	UK health economics data for estimating economic costs and net benefit of prosthetic service provision

2.3. Model Description

In this section, we present a simplified stock-and-flow representation of the model. The simplified structure is split into the top-level Health Care System (Figure 1) and the Market Subsystem (Figure 2). We then briefly describe the key feedback processes involved (see Appendix A for a more detailed description of each feedback loop).

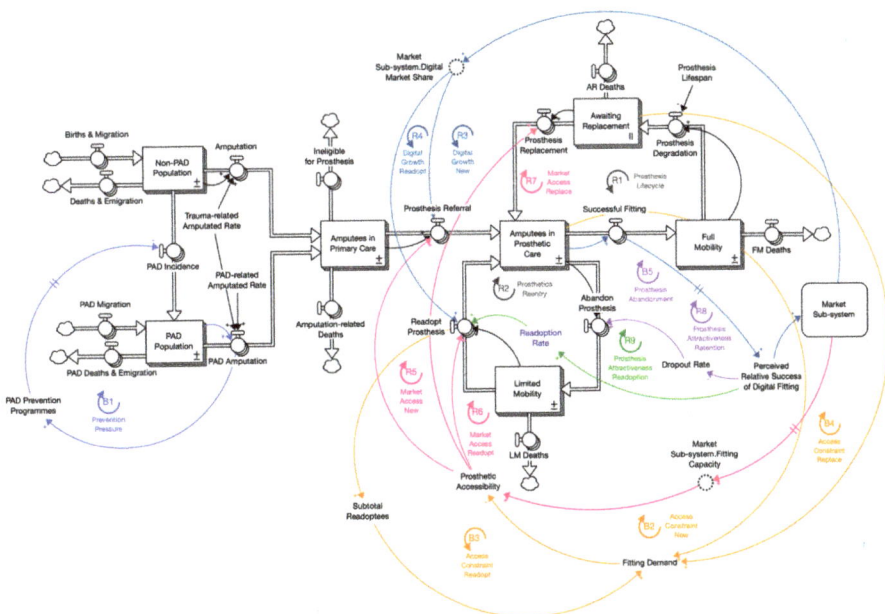

Figure 1. Simplified feedback structure of the amputee health care system. The sign on each link (+/−) indicates the polarity of the relationship between the connected two variables.

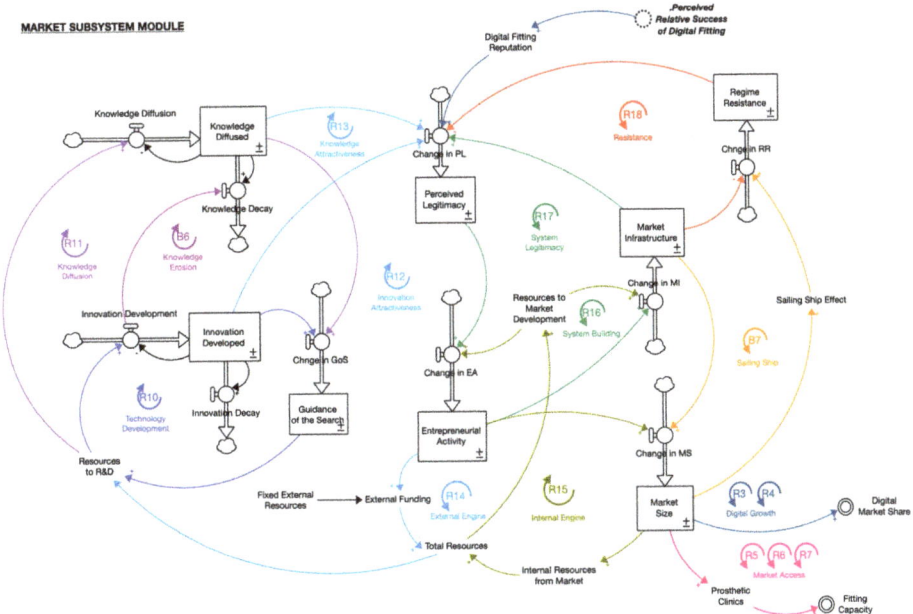

Figure 2. Simplified feedback structure of market subsystem. The sign on each link (+/−) indicates the polarity of the relationship between the two connected variables.

2.3.1. Health Care System

The health care system for amputees is represented as an aging chain that captures the flow of people across different stages or compartments. This structure is further arrayed to better capture and represent the characteristics and choices of different population groups (e.g., age and prosthesis type). Aging chains, commonly used in SD health models, can help identify accumulations and key bottle-necks in patient flows [27]. Figure 1 captures the flow of people from the general population and the PAD population stocks to acute care for either trauma-related or PAD-related amputation. At this stage, the *Prevention Pressure* loop (B1) works to reduce the PAD incidence rate over the long-term as the PAD-related amputations increase over time. This balancing feedback loop represents the prevention pressure faced by public health agencies to address the prevalence of PAD by stepping up efforts towards primary prevention, including early screening, smoking cessation, nutritional and activity programs [57,58]. A decline in PAD incidence would lead to a reduction of the PAD prevalence over time, which would eventually decrease major lower-limb amputations from PAD.

Amputees then flow into the prosthetic care stage, either into traditional prosthetics or digital prosthetics depending on the respective market share, from the primary care stage. They may achieve full mobility if successfully fitted with a prosthesis. However, both prosthesis types need to be replaced every three years on average [59]. As more amputees enter the prosthetics care stage, prosthesis degradation over time increases the number of amputees awaiting replacement of their devices before re-entering the prosthetic fitting process again. In this regard, the *Prosthesis Lifecycle* loop (R1) could result in a growing pressure for prosthetics demand, emanating from our best efforts to successfully fit new amputees with a prosthesis. Alternatively, amputees may dropout from the prosthesis fitting process altogether or abandon the device due to an unsuccessful fit [16,60]. These individuals flow into the limited mobility stock. However, amputees with limited mobility may later decide to readopt a prosthesis and therefore re-enter the prosthetic care stage again. This process is captured in the *Prosthetics Re-entry* loop (R2). Both loops engender a reinforcing mechanism that moves amputees through different stages of prosthetics care. They do not independently multiply the number of amputees in the loop beyond those already within the closed aging chain.

With the introduction of a digital prosthetics market, amputees are probabilistically referred to a digital prosthetist dependent on the market share. The perceived success of digital prosthetics is then conceptualized as the ratio of the rate of successful digital fitting relative to traditional fitting. When the rate of digital fittings surpass the incumbent traditional technology, we can expect a stronger favorable word-of-mouth diffusion about the success or reputation of digital prosthesis [61,62]. Over time, we expect the reputation of digital technology to reinforce the growth of the digital market size and thus the market share of the digital prosthetics through the *Digital Growth* loops (R3 and R4). With a higher market share, even more amputees are more likely to be referred to a digital prosthetist or may seek out one themselves if they are re-adoptees. Concurrently, the *Prosthesis Attractiveness* loops (R8 and R9) encourage stronger uptake of digital prosthesis devices. Word-of-mouth diffusion about the relative success of digital technology could motivate individuals to stick to the process and thus translate to a lower drop-out rate. It could also motivate those who have previously abandoned the process to re-enter the fitting the process, consequently increasing the re-adoption rate. Here, the diffusion processes are driven by evaluations of the relative performance of digital prosthetics (successful digital fitting rates vs. traditional), similar to the adoption structure in Homer's model [33].

While the digital growth and prosthesis attractiveness loops drive the accumulation of amputees in the digital prosthetics care sector, the *Access Constraint* loops (B2, B3 and B4) counteract their reinforcing effects. Amputees' access to the prosthetics care stage is limited by the capacity of the sector (number of fittings that can be accommodated by available prosthetists). Fitting demand is driven by new amputees, those seeking to replace their degraded device, and re-adoptees who previously abandoned the fitting process. When the fitting demand outweighs the fitting capacity, prosthetic accessibility reduces and thus limits amputees from entering the stage even if so desired. Over the longer term, however, the *Market Access* loops (R5, R6 and R7) work to improve accessibility for digital prosthetics by expanding capacity. A higher market share of digital technology would lead to an expansion of digital prosthetic clinics, which enables the sector to accommodate a larger number of patients. This effect, however, is delayed as it takes time to assess the market and set up new clinics.

As for the incumbent traditional prosthetics, they compete with the growing digital prosthetics market for referrals from the primary care stage. This is captured in the patient flow between the two stages, where entry to traditional prosthetics is determined by the inverse of the digital market share (i.e., 1–"Digital Market Share"). However, in the model, traditional prosthetics is assumed to be unaffected by the diffusion processes of digital technology. Should digital technology gain dominance, one might expect the incumbent's reputation to diminish and, as a result, more amputees might dropout and fewer might re-adopt a traditional prosthesis. Moreover, traditional prosthetics sector might also face a capacity contraction. Yet, these effects were not modeled for a more conservative estimate of digital prosthetics' impact since, without concrete data, this could add to further uncertainty of the model. Instead, the patient flows within the traditional prosthetics care sector were held at constant fractional rates, apart from new amputee referrals.

2.3.2. Market Subsystem

In the top-level health care system, we sought to explain the effects of digital prosthetics market growth on the prosthetics care sector. The complexity involved in market formation within the market subsystem is represented in Figure 2.

The process of technological knowledge development is described by the synergistic interaction of the *Technology Development* loop (R10) and *Knowledge Diffusion* loop (R11). Innovation development and diffusion of knowledge is required for any TIS to grow, and this is dependent on the level of resources available for R&D [35,63]. As innovation is developed and diffused through the exchange of knowledge between various actors in the system, the guidance of search for the new technology increases. Guidance of search refers to the "visibility and clarity" of the state of the art [35] (p. 423) that reflects the "promises and expectations of the emerging technology" [63] (p. 56). This helps in the priority-setting of that technology and directing more resources for further R&D, which would enable even more technological knowledge development and diffusion.

This process, in turn, attracts new entrepreneurs into the emerging market through the *Innovation Attractiveness* loop (R12) and *Knowledge Attractiveness* loop (R13). Entrepreneurs are central to any TIS for carrying out market-oriented action [63]. As more innovation is developed and diffused, the technological legitimacy of the technology increases and accumulates the perceived legitimacy of innovation system. [36]. This encourages more entrants to enter the market and grow the level of market-oriented entrepreneurial activity. Since entrepreneurial activities indicate the health and sustainability of an innovation system [35], this would bring in more external funding/resource stream into the system from private or public actors [36,63]. External funding further reinforces the growth of entrepreneurial activities through the *External Engine* loop (R14). External backing reduces the perceived entrepreneurial risks involved, and consequently is better able to attract further entry into the market [36,63]. Moreover, the external funding stream increases the total resources available in the system, which spurs more development of innovation that increases the legitimacy of the technology even further.

While the external engine stimulates entrepreneurial activity initially, the *System Legitimacy* loop (R17) endogenously generates internal ("financial, material, human capital") resources over the longer term for market sustainability [63] (p. 57). This loop comprises the two smaller *Internal Engine* loop (R15) and the *System Building* loop (R16), and is capable of driving the entire system [37]. Entrepreneurs contribute to the "development of formal market rules, establishment of intermediary networks, the building of infrastructure, or the development of formal regulations" [36] (p. 1837). The developed market infrastructure generates market legitimacy for the TIS, which reduces market formation uncertainty and the perceived cost to participation [39]. Hence, more entrepreneurs are willing to overcome perceived risks and enter the market, contributing to further infrastructure development (R16). Moreover, these established market structures, mediated by entrepreneurial activities, "contribute to the creation of a demand for the emerging technology" [63] (p. 56). This increases the market size for the technology that generates internal resources from the market (R15). The synergy of the loops, reflected in R17, thus drives the self-reinforcing growth of entrepreneurial activities, market infrastructure, market legitimacy, and market size.

The formation of a niche market for the emerging technology, however, precipitates "resistance from actors with interests in the incumbent" regime [63] (p. 57). For instance, "when regime actors try to influence public discourses, or lobby against favourable support" [36] (p. 1837). This process is captured in the *Resistance* loop (R18). Regime resistance decreases the market legitimacy of the emerging technology, which disincentivizes entrants due to higher perceived risks. In turn, there will be less market infrastructure development to counter the regime resistance. As the niche market grows and competes with the incumbent regime, resistance could also come in the form of innovation. Given the new threat, regime actors would "increase their efforts to improve the performance of the existing regime through innovation" [36] (p. 1838). This is referred to as the sailing ship effect [64,65] and is represented in the *Sailing Ship* loop (B7). It contributes to a stronger regime resistance and counteracts the effects of the System Legitimacy loop.

Finally, the top-level health care system is connected to market subsystem through the *Digital Growth* loops and *Market Access* loops. As the reputation of digital fittings grow, we expect it to bolster the technological legitimacy of digital prosthetics. This would lend strength to the System Legitimacy loop, which ultimately increases the market size. With a larger market size, the market share of digital prosthetics rises relative to the incumbent traditional prosthetics. Importantly, the number of digital prosthetic clinics also increases to expand the fitting capacity. This improves the digital prosthetics accessibility, which enables more amputees to be fitted with a prosthesis and achieve mobility.

2.4. Model Validation

The described feedback structure was operationalized into a SD simulation model. The model was built in Stella Architect version 3.0 (SD modelling software from isee systems) using Euler Integration with a time-step of 1/16 of a month, or about 2 days, which is less than half of the smallest time constant of 7 days (0.23 months) for the pre-operation hospital stay in the primary care sector. The model is simulated over a time horizon of 480 months, representing January 2010 to January 2050. Simulation modelling facilitates the visualization of the impact of digital prosthetics on the health care system and, more importantly, experimentations to better understand the dynamic complexity of the system [21,29]. Here, we summarize the results of the model validation procedure as proposed by Forrester and Senge [66] and Barlas [67] to build confidence in the simulation results. A more detailed validation report is available in a previous iteration of this work [30].

The model structure is supported by relevant literature and input from stakeholders. As a digital prosthetics service provider (ProsFit) and a double lower-limb amputee, the third author of this paper was heavily consulted during the iterative process of model building to validate the structures in the health care system. Parameterization of the health care system was based on empirical data sources (Table 1). In instances where data was not available, the values were estimated from expert opinion. This pertains to the fractional dropout and readoption rates, which are estimates from ProsFit and their network of prosthetists. Parameter verification for the market subsystem, however, was challenging given the conceptual nature of the model. Thus, the parameter values set in the original model [38] was kept and subject to further sensitivity tests. All parameters and variables in the model were assigned units of measurement that are both mathematically and conceptually consistent. The model documentation provided in the Supplementary Materials details the above for each variable in the model.

Moreover, direct- and indirect-extreme conditions tests were performed to ensure robustness of structural formulations. There were no computational errors detected in the model and the results conform to values that are within bounds. We further conducted sensitivity analysis for all parameters in the model. Each parameter was varied over 100 sensitivity runs. The variation is based on a uniform distribution random draw using Sobol Sequence sampling method [68]. The results of the sensitivity analysis are summarized in Table 2. Expectedly, the model was mostly sensitive to parameters in the conceptual market subsystem. As a result, it introduces uncertainty to the relatively empirical top-level model. This means that this model cannot produce accurate numerical estimations. Nevertheless, it was deemed more useful to represent the complexity of market formation than the alternative: a simplistic table function with high levels of sensitivity. Understanding how digital prosthetic market formation may plausibly occur from a feedback perspective could be useful to decision-makers seeking to improve mobility outcomes and maximize the impact of limited resources.

Table 2. Parameters resulting in model sensitivity.

Model Sector	Parameter	Range	Sensitivity
Prosthetic Care	Reference Dropout Fraction (Eligible for Prosthesis)	0.01–0.50	Numerical
	Reference Dropout Fraction (Initial Device)	0.01–0.50	Numerical
	Reference Dropout Fraction (Matured Limb)	0.01–0.50	Numerical
	Reference Readoption Fraction	0.01–0.50	Numerical
Market Formation	Market Size Threshold	0.025–0.075	Behavioral *
	Relative External Resources Size	0–9	Behavioral *
	Sensitivity of Clinics to Market Size	0.25–0.75	Numerical
	Sensitivity of Resources to Market Size	0.5–1.5	Behavioral *
	Steepness Effect of Total Resources on EA	1.25–3.75	Numerical
	Steepness Effect of EA on Market Infrastructure	0.2–0.6	Numerical
	Steepness Effect of Legitimacy on EA	0.2–0.6	Numerical
	Steepness Effect of Total Resources on Infrastructure	1.25–3.75	Numerical
	Time to Adjust Clinics	12–36	Numerical
	Time to Adjust Entrepreneurial Activity	6–18	Numerical
	Time to Adjust Market Infrastructure	30–90	Numerical
	Time to Adjust Market Size	12–36	Numerical
	Time to Perceive Legitimacy	6–18	Numerical
	Weight of Entrepreneurial Activity	0.25–0.75	Behavioral *
	Weight of Perceived Legitimacy	0.25–0.75	Numerical
Innovation Diffusion	Time to Decay	30–90	Numerical

* Refer to Appendix B for the confidence plots of the model's sensitivity.

3. Simulation Results

3.1. Baseline Setup

The model was initialized in equilibrium to produce the baseline simulation results. In a previous iteration, we attempted to initialize the stocks at the obtained or calculated initial values [30]. However, there are virtually no numerical estimates for individuals in the various transitory stages of the primary care continuum and prosthetic care continuum. Consequently, we opted to initialize the stocks in their long-term equilibrium values to prevent transient stock adjustments. Moreover, initializing the model in equilibrium enables us to observe the full effects of any shocks exogenously introduced to the model—in our case, the formation of a niche digital prosthetics market.

To set the model in equilibrium, we held the total population of the UK constant at about 61.1 million individuals over the time horizon and initialized the population stocks in their long-term equilibrium values. The equilibrium switch in the market subsystems initializes the innovation diffusion stocks at zero and cuts off the exogenous input of relative resources. This ensures there are no dynamics in the market subsystem, thus representing a scenario wherein the prosthetics sector is solely serviced by the traditional prosthetics service providers at their existing capacity.

3.2. Baseline Results

The baseline results provide the estimated equilibrium values of the respective key indicators for the system (see Table 3). With a constant population size of 61.1 M people, we estimate a total of 84.8 K major lower-limb amputees, with about 85% of them being deemed medically eligible for a prosthetic device (71.9 K people). Of those eligible, only 5.5 K amputees are estimated to be fitted with a (traditional) prosthesis, thus resulting in a mobility proportion of over 7%. The amputee mobility proportion represents the proportion of eligible amputees who have achieved full mobility through a successful prosthesis fitting, which is determined by three factors. First, the accessibility of prosthetics services, which represents the percentage of demand that is met by the existing service capacity. The model estimates this to be just under 12%, indicating a bottleneck in the prosthetic care system. This is also within range of the WHO global estimate—that only 5 to 15% of amputees have access to prostheses [1]. Second, individual dispositions to drop out from the fitting process (estimated by experts to be about 10% for each stage of the process prior to the final device) and to readopt it (about 20%) at a later time. Third, the probability of final device fit success, which is about 50% for traditional devices [15,16].

Table 3. Baseline results of key indicators.

Indicator	Result	Units
Total Amputee Population	84.8 K	People
Medically Eligible Amputee Population	71.9 K	People
Amputees fitted with Prosthesis	5.5 K	People
Amputee Mobility Proportion	0.07	Dimensionless
Prosthetics Accessibility	0.12	Dimensionless
Economic Productivity	14 M	USD/Month
Economic Cost	210 M	USD/Month
Prosthesis Reimbursement	1.94 M	USD/Month

Furthermore, health-related economic indicators were calculated based on the inputs from the endogenous processes in the health and prosthetics care systems. The monthly economic productivity of amputees is estimated to be about USD14 M per month. This indicator represents the economic participation of amputees from returning to work and reintegrating into the workforce. It is conceptualized as the product of the estimated number of employed amputees with the gross domestic product per capita. Amputees not fitted with prostheses are excluded from workforce participation given their limited mobility. This is a gross simplification that does not completely reflect the economic contribution of amputees from other measures such as individual consumption. The total economic cost incurred, on the other hand, is estimated to be USD210 M per month. This includes the differentiated health care costs, unemployment and social payments, and the opportunity costs borne by families for caretaking. Lastly, the estimated total cost of prosthesis provision is about USD1.94 M per month, which includes both successful and failed prosthesis fittings. Reimbursements for prosthesis costs are assumed to be fully covered by national insurance mechanisms, which would otherwise be borne as out-of-pocket payments.

3.3. Experimental Setup

To simulate and investigate the impact of digital prosthetics on the baseline behavior, we introduced dynamics in the market subsystem module. This was done by setting the parameter value of Relative External Resources (RER) Size above 0 from month 96 for an assumed duration of 180 months (year 2018 to 2033) to exogenously kick start the dynamics. This simulates the deployment of external funding streams to support initial market growth prior to self-sufficiency. Moreover, the Innovation Developed and Knowledge Diffused stocks were initialized at 0.01 to push them out of unstable equilibrium.

As mentioned, given the conceptual nature of the market subsystem, we have introduced several assumptions in the parameter values that would result in estimation errors. Therefore, we ran a global sensitivity analysis with combined variations in all the parameters that the model is sensitive to (as identified in Table 2). The experimental results, in turn, show the confidence intervals (up to 95%) of the key indicators from 1000 runs based on Sobol Sequence sampling method [68]. A total of 1000 runs was sufficient to fully explore the state space of the stocks in the market subsystems. This experiment gives us the full range of possibilities for digital prosthetics market growth and thus enables us to observe the corollary effects on the more empirical prosthetics care system.

3.4. Experimental Results

Given its known sensitivity, the model produces a range of market growth for digital prosthetics, from 0.03% to 96% market share by 2050 with a mean of 43.6% (Figure 3). In general, with a RER size of more than 0, the External Engine loop (R14) powers the endogenous market formation processes that allows the Digital Market Share to start growing. However, as R14 loop is cut off by year 2033, we observe three behavioral patterns: (1) steady decline, (2) a much slower albeit continued growth, or (3) sustained growth. The sustainability of market growth is ultimately dependent on the strength of the Internal Engine (R15) and the System Legitimacy (R17) loops in endogenously generating sufficient internal market resources.

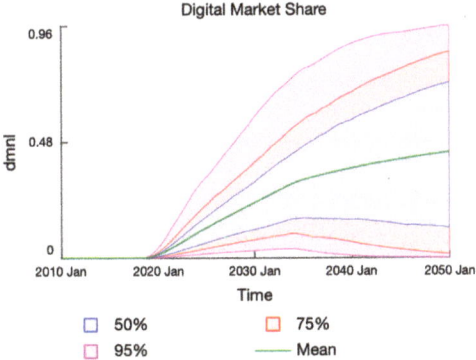

Figure 3. Confidence plot of the market share of the digital prosthetics service.

Nevertheless, we can observe the impact of digital prosthetics market growth on the amputee population and mobility outcomes. As digital prostheses are introduced to the prosthetics care system, Figure 4a shows an increase in the mobility proportion from the baseline of 7% to a mean of 23% by 2050 (range: 6.2–50%). The introduction of digital prosthetics not only increases the existing service capacity, but also results in more successful fittings—a synergistic product of the Digital Growth (R3 and R4) and Prosthetics Attractiveness (R8 and R9) loops. The Digital Growth loops enable more amputees to enter the prosthetics care system either as a new entrant or a re-adoptee, whereas the Prosthetics Attractiveness loops discourages amputees in the fitting process from dropping out and encourages previous dropouts to re-adopt a device. In turn, more amputees achieve mobility. The increased mobility further leads to improved health outcomes, including a lower mortality risk. In this sense, the expansion of digital prosthetics prevents more deaths, which accounts for the increase in the amputee population from the baseline of 84.8 K to an average of 87.6 K individuals by 2050 (range: 83.2 K–94 K) as seen in Figure 4b.

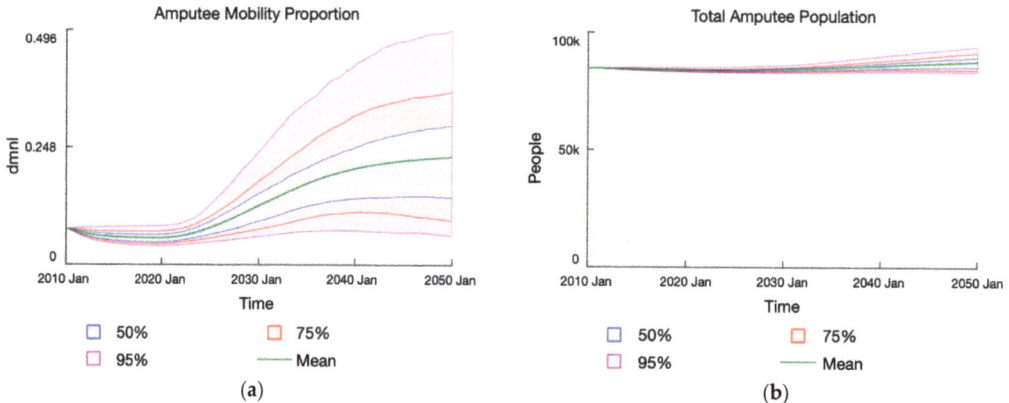

Figure 4. (a) Confidence plot of the proportion of eligible amputees who are fitted with a prosthesis; (b) Confidence plot of the total amputee population.

Additionally, we observe that the mobility proportion develops similarly to the digital market share; if the market share were to decline after year 2033, so would the mobility proportion. However, the mobility proportion develops at slower pace and changes to a smaller extent. This is due to (1) the multiple delays involved in the aging chains of the fitting process and (2) the effect of the Access Constraint loops (B2, B3 and B4) from prosthetics accessibility that limits the number of amputees according to available service capacity.

As for the prosthetics accessibility, it increases for the first of half the simulation duration before declining again, which consequently limits the growth of the mobility proportion. With reference to Figure 5, the peak of the mean accessibility is about 44% some time in 2028 (range: 13.6% to 100%), which eventually declines to 20% by 2050 (range: 2.8% to 93.6%). In general, the accessibility ratio increases as the digital market grows and adds additional service capacity to the existing level. In conditions where there is limited market growth, we observe that the accessibility declines around the time when the exogenous funding is cut-off in year 2033. However, under more optimistic market growth conditions, we observe that the accessibility peaks prior to the cut-off time and declines thereafter. This is due to the higher volume of demand for replacing degraded prostheses generated by the Prosthesis Lifecycle loop (R1). Prostheses have a lifecycle of 3 years on average, and hence there is a captive consumer base that will continue to shore up fitting demand—more so when the proportion of fitted amputees is high. As seen in Figure 5, the total accessibility may increase to the maximum (100%) in instances where parameters enable a rapid and large expansion of digital clinics (e.g., Sensitivity of Clinics to Market Size) to meet the demand for fittings. Even then, it declines by the tail end of the simulation for the reasons described.

As a result of the developments in the prosthetics care system, we can further assess the impact on the health-related economic indicators. The economic productivity of amputees follows a similar development to the mobility proportion since employed amputees make up a fraction of those who are mobile. Figure 6a shows and increase in the monthly productivity of amputees from an average of USD14 M to USD43 M by year 2050 (range: USD11.5 M to USD97.7 M). Again, these figures are underestimates that only partially captures the true economic contribution of amputees. Whereas Figure 6b shows a reduction in the monthly economic cost incurred, decreasing from USD210 M to USD202 M on average (range: USD289 M to USD211 M). The economic cost per capita reduces as the mobility proportion increases because mobile amputees incur smaller health care costs, social payments, and opportunity costs for their families. However, note that effect from the per capita cost reduction has been counteracted by the overall increase in amputee population size from improved health outcomes (less deaths). In this sense, the reduction in total economic cost is not as pronounced as the per capita reduction in economic cost. Based on these figures, we can further anticipate the net benefit of digital prosthetics service provision: the sum of the additional economic productivity and the amount of reduction in economic cost. The average net social benefit is then calculated to be a mean of USD37 M per month.

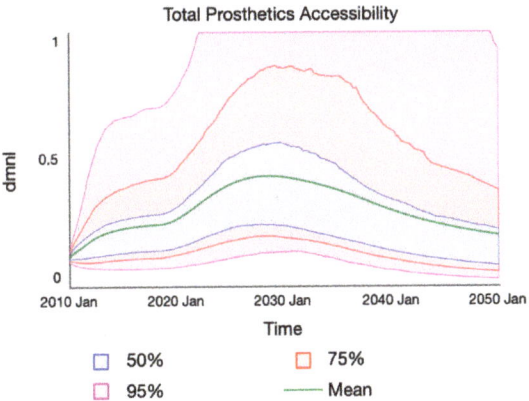

Figure 5. Confidence plot of the total accessibility of prosthetics services in terms of ability to meet total demand.

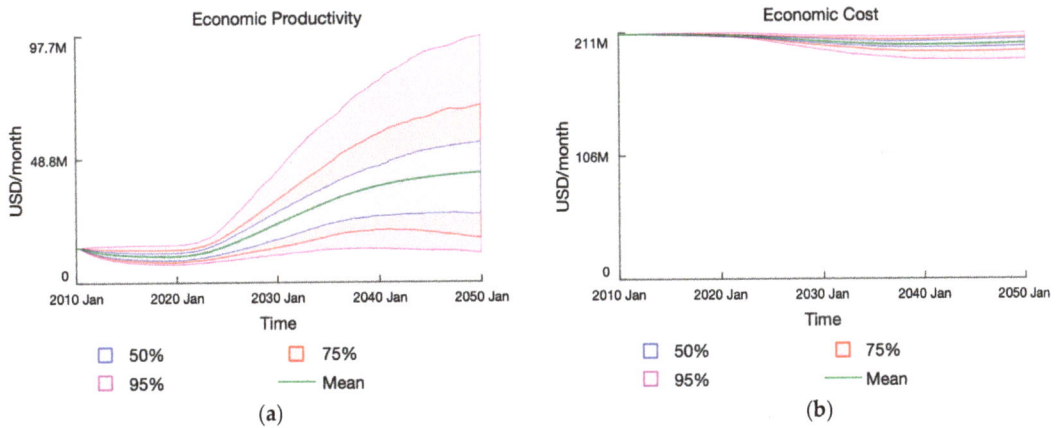

Figure 6. (a) Confidence plot of the undiscounted monthly economic productivity rate in terms of GDP per capita from amputees returning to work; (b) Confidence plot of the undiscounted monthly economic cost incurred for the total amputee population.

3.5. Scenario Setup

The experimental results have shown that there are three fundamental behavior modes within the range of possibilities for digital market growth. To better visualize the differentiated impact on the prosthetics care system, we developed three hypothetical scenarios for digital market growth. First, a pessimistic scenario to represent the growth and steady decline. Second, a realistic scenario wherein the digital market experiences a much slower rate of growth after external funding is cut off. Third, an optimistic scenario to represent the sustained market growth throughout the simulation duration.

To this end, we conducted a sensitivity analysis with only the parameters that the model is behaviorally sensitive to (see Table 2) for a total of 50 runs. From these runs, we selected the set of parameter values that produced the appropriate behavior mode for each of the scenarios. These values are reported in Table 4.

Table 4. Behaviorally sensitive parameters and corresponding values for each scenario.

Parameter	Pessimistic	Realistic	Optimistic	Remarks
Relative External Resources Size	1.27	4.78	8.02	The higher the figure, the larger the size of the external resources brought in from entrepreneurial activity relative to a certain normal size.
Market Size Threshold	0.04	0.05	0.05	The threshold is the base value of the Relative Market Size, which determines how much the internal resources generated by market grows beyond the normal amount. A higher threshold means that the nascent market must grow to a larger extent before becoming profitable.
Sensitivity of Resources to Market Size	1.20	0.72	0.95	A sensitivity of less than 1 results in a less than proportional change in the Relative Internal Resources to changes in the Relative Market. Conversely, a sensitivity of more than 1 results in a more than proportional relative change.
Weight of Entrepreneurial Activity	0.65	0.32	0.27	The smaller the value, the more weight is placed on the effect of total resources available for market development on market infrastructure than on the effect of entrepreneurial activities, vice versa.

The set of parameter values for the pessimistic scenario results in a condition where there is a low level of resources flowing in the market subsystem. With a relatively lower RER size, the External Engine loop (R14) has a weaker reinforcing effect in the pessimistic scenario as compared to the other two. The weight of entrepreneurial activity modulates the level of market infrastructure development. A higher weight implies that infrastructure development is more dependent on the level of entrepreneurial activity in the system than the volume of resources available for market formation. Not only is there a low level of resources to begin with, but the market infrastructure development is also not as reactive to those resources in the pessimistic scenario. On the other end, in the optimistic scenario there are ample of resources in the system for market formation. A relatively lower weight on entrepreneurial activity further implies that market development is stimulated by the resources available. The realistic scenario represents a more likely median between the two extremes.

3.6. Scenario Results

We reproduced the three behavior patterns representing the varied conditions for digital prosthetics market growth (see Figure 7a). Under pessimistic market growth conditions, the market share of digital prosthetics growths to a maximum of about 5% before declining to 0.5% by 2050. Under the realistic scenario, the digital market share increases to 36% in 2033 and thereafter increases gradually to 43% by 2050. Whereas digital prosthetics experiences sustained growth in the optimistic scenario, capturing 80% of the market share by 2050.

Based on these three hypothetical market growth scenarios, we can observe the relative impact on the amputee mobility outcome in Figure 7b. In general, the mobility proportion follows the same behavioral pattern as the digital market share. The proportion increases as market share increases and vice versa. The gap between the realistic and optimistic scenarios for amputee mobility is disproportionately smaller than the gap for the digital prosthetics market share. This is due to the dampening effect of the Access Constraint loops (B2, B3 and B4) as explained before. Amputee mobility is being constrained by the fitting capacity that is unable to meet the demand. By further expanding digital fitting capacity, we can strengthen the effect of the Market Access loops (R5 and R6) to better counteract the constraint loops. In this sense, we can anticipate an even higher mobility proportion in the optimistic scenario than the 32% mobility observed in Figure 7b.

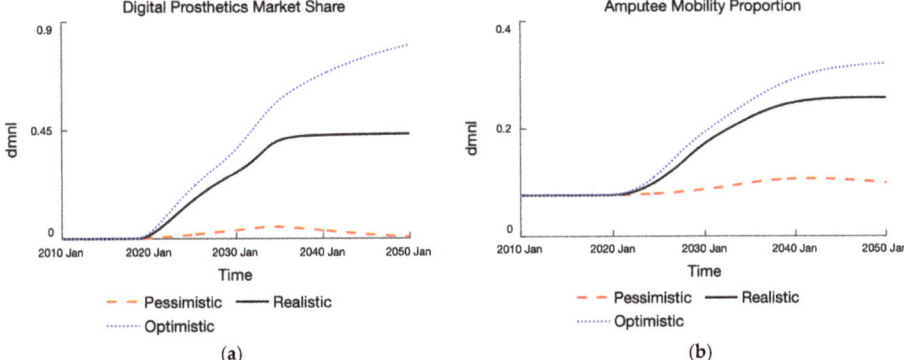

Figure 7. (**a**) Comparative graphs of the digital prosthetics market share under three growth scenarios; (**b**) Comparative graphs of the proportion of eligible amputees who are fitted with a prosthesis under three scenarios.

As for the health-related economic indicators, we can now graphically represent the net benefit of digital prosthetics service provision compared to the baseline behavior (Figure 8a). In all three scenarios, the introduction of digital prosthetics results in a positive net benefit. A 0.5% digital market share in 2050 still yields a net benefit of USD5 M per month in the pessimistic scenario. This figure is USD41 M and USD53 M for the realistic and optimistic scenario, respectively. Moreover, we can compare the scale of the net benefit to that of the additional prosthesis reimbursement (Figure 8b). The additional reimbursement is the difference between the total costs for prosthesis services and the baseline costs. In contexts where prosthetics services are covered by national health care systems, digital market growth increases the total costs borne by the state in terms of insurance reimbursements as the volume fittings increases over time. Nevertheless, additional costs incurred in that instance is far outweighed by the net benefit accrued—on average by a factor of 15 across all scenarios.

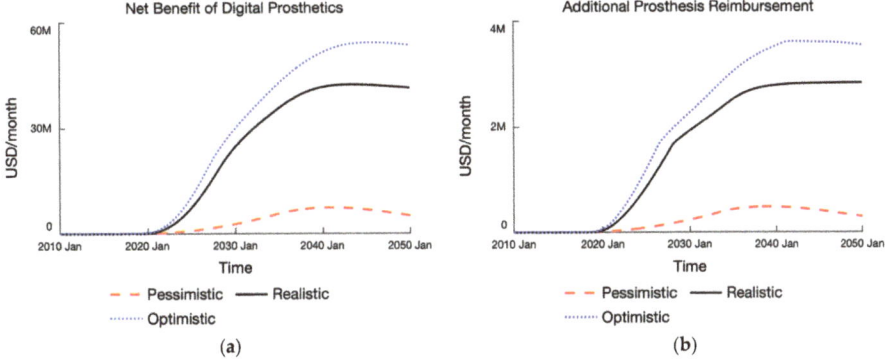

Figure 8. (**a**) Comparative graphs of the undiscounted net benefit of digital prosthetics under three growth scenarios; (**b**) Comparative graphs of the undiscounted additional prosthesis reimbursement cost incurred under three scenarios.

4. Discussion

In summary, our simulation model allows exploring the range of mobility outcomes for the amputee population given different market growth conditions for digital prosthetics. We observed in all experimental scenarios that an increase in digital prosthetics market share was associated with improved mobility outcomes. Specifically, there was an increase in the mobility proportion, an increase in total economic productivity, a decrease in total economic costs and an overall positive net benefit from digital prosthetics even under pessimistic conditions. Our model could, thus, serve as a tool for health policy planners to explore a shift in prosthetics service provision to better mitigate the accessibility problem and bolster the social impact of prosthesis usage.

Furthermore, our model contributes to the growing body of public health modeling literature within the system dynamics field. To the best of our knowledge, this model is the first application of simulation modeling to the domain of amputee patient-care continuum and prosthetics service provision. Our work builds on and integrates elements of existing SD models on TIS and medical technologies diffusion and adoption [32,33,36], which we have adapted to anticipate the growth of the emerging digital prosthetics. In doing so, our model presents an internally consistent theory of the complex interactions between the health care system and the market formation subsystem and provides a feedback-rich explanation for the dynamics of prosthetics service provision and amputee mobility.

4.1. Strategic Insights

The main insights from our work can be summarized as follows:

- While the *External Engine* loop provides the initial fuel for the various endogenous market formation processes, the *System Legitimacy* loop ultimately determines the trajectory of market growth for digital prosthetics. This loop generates internal resources from the market to sustain the growth in entrepreneurial activities, market infrastructure, perceived legitimacy of digital prosthetics, and its market size.
- The *Digital Growth* loops and *Prosthesis Attractive* loops are the key drivers for improving prosthetic accessibility and enabling mobility. With a higher market share of digital prosthetics, more amputees can receive prosthetics services and are incentivized to remain in or re-adopt prosthetics care.
- The *Market Access* loops are particularly important for driving the expansion of prosthetics clinics and service capacity, thus improving prosthetics accessibility over time. The strength of this loop determines the extent of the counteracting effect on the *Access Constraint* loops, which limits the mobility proportion.
- To best ensure the sustainability of the digital prosthetics market over the longer term, investment is needed in this emerging technological system to garner sufficient resources and momentum for sustained market growth. As seen in the sensitivity analyses, the model is behaviorally sensitive to parameters related to the internal and external resources in the market subsystem. High-leverage policies would thus seek to influence the resource flows in the system.
- Investments in digital prosthetics could improve accessibility and ameliorate the underuse of prosthesis amongst amputees, which enables mobility. Importantly, this results in a positive net benefit for society in terms of higher economic productivity and reduced economic costs.
- Besides the economic value of individuals, improving mobility appears to improve health, also preventing more amputee deaths over time.
- To maximize the impact on the mobility outcomes and net benefit of prosthetics services, policy planning must ensure that service capacity is expanded to meet fitting demand. The scenario analysis revealed that prosthetics accessibility is limited by service capacity even under optimistic market growth conditions. Policy planners should be cognizant of the effect of *Prosthesis Lifecycle* loop, which drives the pressure on fitting demand as the mobility outcomes improve over time.

4.2. Limitations and Further Research

The main limitation of the top-level health care system pertains to modelling individual predispositions or decision points. Specifically, the propensity to dropout from the fitting process or readopt a prosthesis. They remain as simplifications (estimated average fractional rates) that could benefit from further work. Such predispositions are not simply functions of attractiveness, but also dependent on a broad array of individual factors, including mental health state, level of social support, and occurrence of limb pain [69]. In addition, we have excluded individual factors related to quality of life for amputees [70]—which is particularly difficult to operationalize without the involvement of amputees in the model building process. Including groups of amputees, through Group Model Building [71], could be a potent avenue for further research in this field. This could lead to a more robust model boundary that includes individual predispositions as well as quality of life measures.

The partially conceptual nature of the model further precludes it from generating numerically accurate estimates of indicators. Though numerical estimation is beyond the scope of this paper, further modelling work could be carried out to improve the model's ability to do so. Here, a much larger research scope is required to empirically study the digital prosthetics market growth that should involve robust data collection for parameterization. Additionally, the boundary of the subsystem could be expanded to include fitting capacity adjustment structures that are more responsive to market dynamics (demand, supply, profits, etc.).

Nevertheless, our model in its current iteration provides a structural explanation for digital prosthetics growth and reasonable projected developments under different conditions. It further generates qualitatively and directionally indicative results of digital prosthetics' impact on key amputee mobility and health-related socio-economic outcomes. The strategic insights from our findings could further provide decision support for health policy planning. To that end, further work should expand on these insights in a more accessible language for relevant decision makers.

Supplementary Materials: The following supporting information can be downloaded at: https://www.mdpi.com/article/10.3390/systems11010022/s1, File S1: Model Documentation.

Author Contributions: Conceptualization, J.K.R., W.C., C.J.H., P.G. and B.K.; methodology, J.K.R.; validation, J.K.R., W.C., C.J.H., P.G. and B.K.; formal analysis, J.K.R.; investigation, J.K.R.; data curation, J.K.R.; writing—original draft preparation, J.K.R.; writing—review and editing, J.K.R., W.C., C.J.H., P.G. and B.K.; visualization, J.K.R.; supervision, P.G. and B.K.; project administration, J.K.R. All authors have read and agreed to the published version of the manuscript.

Funding: This research received no external funding.

Data Availability Statement: Data is contained within the article or Supplementary Material.

Acknowledgments: The authors would like to thank Christina Gkini, Claudiu Eduard Nedelciu, and Derek Chan for their review of earlier iterations of this work.

Conflicts of Interest: The third author, C.J.H., is the chief technology officer (CTO) of ProsFit Technologies with a vested interest in digital prosthetics service provision. Nevertheless, research independence of the primary researcher (J.K.R.) has been codified in the collaboration agreement and no compensation is provided for this research. C.J.H. had no input in the formal analysis and conclusions drawn from the simulation results.

Appendix A. Feedback Loop Descriptions

Here, we present the detailed feedback loop descriptions extracted from an earlier version of this work [30]. Each description includes the causal pathway of the feedback loop. The arrow symbol (à) represents a causal link between two variables. (+) indicates a positive polarity, while (−) indicates a negative polarity. Polarities simply indicate the directionality of the correlation. For instance, "A à(−) B à(+) C" should be interpreted as such: when A increases, B decreases, and in turn C decreases. Here, the positive polarity between B and C indicates that both vary in the same direction.

Prevention Pressure (B1): PAD Amputation à(+) PAD Prevention Programs à(-) PAD Incidence à(+) PAD Population à(+) PAD Amputation

This balancing feedback loop represents the prevention pressure faced by public health agencies to address the prevalence of PAD. As PAD-related amputation rates increases over time, we expect reporting from medical professionals to raise the alarms for stepping up efforts towards primary prevention. This is observed, for instance, in trend studies of PAD incidence and risk factors, calling for better detection and prevention interventions [57,58]. With increased reporting, we can expect more resources directed towards prevention interventions such as screening, smoking cessation, nutritional and activity programs [57]. In the long run, such interventions could lead to a decrease in PAD incidence rate. Indeed, there is evidence that PAD incidence have declined in the UK, which have been attributed to the uptake of prevention strategies [58]. A declining PAD incidence would lead to a reduction of the PAD Population over time, which would eventually decrease the PAD Amputation Rate. Since an initial increase in amputation rate ends up with an eventual decrease in amputation rate, this feedback loop has a negative polarity overall and is thus described as a balancing loop.

Prosthesis Lifecycle (R1): Amputees in Prosthetic Care à(+) Successful Fitting à(+) Full Mobility à(+) Prosthesis Degradation à(+) Awaiting Replacement à(+) Prosthesis Replacement à(+) Amputees in Prosthetic Care

This loop describes the lifecycle that is part of the lifelong holistic care for amputees successfully fitted with a prosthesis [59]. As more amputees enter the prosthetic care continuum from the primary care sector, there will be more people who are successfully fitted with a prosthesis thus increasing the number of amputees with full mobility. However, the prosthesis device has an average lifespan of three years [16,59]. Hence, over time, prosthesis degradation increases the number of amputees awaiting replacement of their devices before re-entering the prosthetic care continuum to be fitted for a new device again. In this regard, this loop represents a growing pressure emanating from our best efforts to successfully fit individuals with a prosthesis. While this closed aging chain engenders a reinforcing mechanism, that transitions amputees through different stages of prosthetic care, it does not endogenously accumulate the stocks without an exogenous inflow to the Amputees in Prosthetics Care stock. As more amputees enter the prosthetics fitting stage from elsewhere, the more the other stocks in this aging chain get filled.

Prosthetics Re-entry (R2): Amputees in Prosthetic Care à(+) Abandon Prosthesis à(+) Limited Mobility à(+) Readopt Prosthesis à(+) Amputees in Prosthetic Care

R2 represents the Prosthetic Care Re-entry process for amputees. Not all amputees who enter the care continuum end up with a prosthesis; some individuals dropout from the fitting process or some abandon the device due to an unsuccessful fit [16,60]. Hence, with more people in the continuum abandoning prosthesis, there will be more people who are left with limited mobility due to the lack of a prosthesis device. However, more amputees might later decide to readopt a prosthesis, thus re-entering the prosthesis fitting process. Similarly, the reinforcing effect of this loop is dependent on an exogenous inflow of amputees entering the closed aging chain.

Digital Growth (R3): Amputees in Digital Prosthetic Care à(+) Successful Fitting à(+) Perceived Relative Success of Digital Fitting à(+) Digital Market Size à(+) Digital Market Share à(+) Digital Prosthesis Referral à(+) Amputees in Digital Prosthetic Care

R3 is a reinforcing loop that represents the hypothesis for the market growth of digital prosthetics. As more amputees get referred to a digital prosthetic clinic and more people become successfully fitted with a prosthesis with better outcomes, we expect favorable word-of-mouth diffusion about the success of digital prosthesis [61]. This is captured with the Perceived Relative Success of Digital Fitting, which represents the mental perceptions of people's comparison of success between the digitally fitted prosthesis and traditional plaster-casted device. Over time, we expect the attractiveness of digital fitting to grow the digital market size and thus the market share of the digital prosthetics relative to traditional.

With a higher market share, more amputees are probabilistically to be referred to a digital prosthetist and thus driving up the number of amputees in the digital prosthetic care continuum as opposed to the traditional one.

Digital Growth (R4): Amputees in Digital Prosthetic Care à(+) Successful Fitting à(+) Perceived Relative Success of Digital Fitting à(+) Digital Market Size à(+) Digital Market Share à(+) Digital Prosthesis Readoption à(+) Amputees in Digital Prosthetic Care

Similarly, the R4 loop drives up the number of amputees in Digital Prosthetic Care by way of readoption. As the digital market share increases, potential re-adoptees looking to restart their prosthetic fitting journey are more likely to seek out a digital prosthetist. The assumption here is that as digital fittings experience more success, people are more likely to be motivated to try the digital process and experience a similar success as others [61,62]. Thus, more re-adoptees enter the digital prosthetic care continuum as opposed to the traditional one.

Access Constraint—B2, B3 and B4 Loops

Access Constraint (B2): Amputees in Prosthetic Care à(+) Fitting Demand à(-) Prosthetic Accessibility à(+) Prosthesis Referral à(+) Amputees in Prosthetic Care

The balancing feedback loop B2 counteracts the reinforcing Digital Growth loops. As more Amputees in Prosthetic Care are attracted to the digital prosthesis fitting process, the Fitting Demand for digital prosthesis increases. In turn, this limits availability of resources and limits Prosthetic Accessibility if demand outweighs the fitting capacity, which then reduces the amount of people who can enter the prosthesis fitting process. Hence, the Amputees in Prosthetic Care declines to a level lower than it otherwise would have been. Through this balancing feedback, B2 dampens the strength of the R3 and R4 loops.

Access Constraint (B3): Prosthesis Readoption à(+) Subtotal Re-adoptees à(+) Fitting Demand à(-) Prosthetic Accessibility à(+) Prosthesis Readoption

Access Constraint (B4): Amputees Awaiting Replacement à(+) Fitting Demand à(-) Prosthetic Accessibility à(+) Prosthesis Replacement à(+) Amputees Awaiting Replacement

Fitting Demand is not solely determined by the number of Amputees in Prosthetic Care. Amputees who have previously abandoned the fitting process and those seeking to replace their degraded prosthesis device also make up the demand. Hence, B3 captures a similar mechanism whereby more Prosthesis Readoption brings up the demand and consequently reduces the Prosthetic Accessibility. B4, on the other hand, reduces the Accessibility through the Prosthesis Replacement process. All three balancing loops work in concert to counteract the reinforcing loops seeking to increase the demand for digital prosthesis fitting.

Market Access (R5): Amputees in Prosthetic Care à(+) Successful Fitting à(+) Perceived Relative Success of Digital Fitting à(+) Digital Market Size à(+) Fitting Capacity à(+) Prosthetic Accessibility à(+) Prosthesis Referral à(+) Amputees in Prosthetic Care

The Market Access loops, however, interplay with the balancing Access Constraint loops described above. In the longer term, these loops work to increase the Fitting Capacity so as to improve the Prosthetic Accessibility that was driven down by increased demand. With reference to R5 loop, when more Amputees in Prosthetic Care get successfully fitted with the prosthesis and the perceived success of digital prosthesis relative to traditional increases, the digital market share grows. The growth in market share is likely to lead to the expansion of digital prosthetic clinics, which in turn drives up the Fitting Capacity. Hence, with more capacity, more people have access to prosthetic services, and thus the care continuum can accommodate a larger number of new amputees seeking a prosthesis.

Market Access (R6): Amputees in Prosthetic Care à(+) Successful Fitting à(+) Perceived Relative Success of Digital Fitting à(+) Digital Market Size à(+) Fitting Capacity à(+) Prosthetic Accessibility à(+) Readopt Prosthesis à(+) Amputees in Prosthetic Care

Market Access (R7): Amputees in Prosthetic Care à(+) Successful Fitting à(+) Perceived Relative Success of Digital Fitting à(+) Digital Market Size à(+) Fitting Capacity à(+) Prosthetic Accessibility à(+) Prosthesis Replacement à(+) Amputees in Prosthetic Care

Likewise, R6 enables a larger number of people seeking to readopt the prosthesis fitting process to enter the Prosthetic Care, whereas R7 enables more people waiting to replace their old prosthesis to re-enter the care continuum at any one point in time. However, it must be noted that increasing capacity involves a delay as it takes time to assess the market and set up new clinics. Hence, the effects of Market Access loops are delayed.

Prosthesis Attractiveness (R8): Amputees in Prosthetic Care à(+) Successful Fitting à(+) Perceived Relative Success of Digital Fitting à(-) Dropout Rate à(+) Abandon Prosthesis à(-) Amputees in Prosthetic Care

Prosthesis Attractiveness (R9): Amputees in Prosthetic Care à(+) Successful Fitting à(+) Perceived Relative Success of Digital Fitting à(+) Re-adoption Rate à(+) Readopt Prosthesis à(+) Amputees in Prosthetic Care

As previously described, when people perceive digital prosthesis to be more successful than traditional ones, the attractiveness of digital prosthesis is expected to increase through word-of-mouth diffusion. However, a negative experience with the new technology would reduce the consideration and available market. [61]. Hence, R8 captures the process by which a higher attractiveness translates to a lower dropout rate as individuals might be more motivated to see through the process and experience a similar success as others. This could lead to fewer people abandoning the prosthesis fitting process and therefore increasing the number of Amputees in Prosthetic Care to a level higher than it otherwise would have been. Concurrently, R9, works to increase the re-adoption rate amongst those who have previously abandoned the process. The higher attractiveness of digital fitting would then increase the number of people readopting a prosthesis and thus re-entering the prosthetic care continuum.

Prosthesis Abandonment (B5): Amputees in Prosthetic Care à(+) Successful Fitting à(+) Perceived Relative Success of Digital Fitting à(-) Dropout Rate à(+) Abandon Prosthesis à(+) Limited Mobility à(+) Readopt Prosthesis à(+) Amputees in Prosthetic Care

This balancing feedback loop counteracts the effects of R2 and R9, by draining the number of people available for entering readoption process. When more amputees enter the digital prosthetics care stage, more individuals are fitted with a digital prosthesis. As a result, the perceived attractiveness of digital prosthetics increases. Amputees are therefore less likely to dropout from digital prosthetics fitting. In turn, the Limited Mobility stock does not accumulate as much as it otherwise would have. This takes away the effect of R2 and R9 since fewer amputees are available for the re-adoption process. Regardless, this is a constructive effect that reduces rates of prosthesis abandonment and yields better overall mobility outcomes.

Technology Development (R10): Innovation Developed à(+) Guidance of Search à(+) Resources to R&D à(+) Innovation Development à(+) Innovation Developed

This feedback loop represents the process of technological knowledge development, typical of research and development (R&D), required for any TIS to grow [35,63]. As more innovation is developed, the Guidance of Search for the technology increases. Guidance of search refers to the "visibility and clarity" of the state of the art [35] (p. 423) that reflects the "promises and expectations of the emerging technology" [63] (p. 56). It helps in the priority-setting process for R&D resource allocation and "thus the direction of technological change" [35] (p. 423). Hence, in this context, increased Guidance of Search for the digital solutions in prosthetic fittings, would help increase the Resources to R&D, which would enable further Innovation Development that increases the Innovation Developed even more [62].

Knowledge Diffusion (R11): Knowledge Diffused à(+) Guidance of Search à(+) Resources to R&D à(+) Knowledge Diffusion à(+) Knowledge Diffused

Knowledge Diffusion, R11 loop, refers to process by which various actors in the TIS interact and exchange knowledge and thus establish "a mutual understanding" that enables institutions to gradually adjust to new technologies [63] (p. 55). Since Guidance of Search is also "an interactive and cumulative process of exchanging ideas" [35] (p. 423), it increases with more Knowledge Diffused [36]. In turn, this works to increase the Resources to R&D, which further enables more Knowledge Diffusion.

Knowledge Erosion (B6): Knowledge Diffused à(+) Guidance of Search à(+) Resources to R&D à(+) Innovation Development à(+) Knowledge Decay à(-) Knowledge Diffused

B6 loop represents the process of Knowledge Erosion, which counteracts R11. Knowledge Diffused can become "obsolete over time (due to new technological developments, etc.)" [38] (p. 4). When knowledge diffusion increases guidance of search, and thus secures more resources for R&D to further develop innovation, previously diffused knowledge become outdated, and thus increases the Knowledge Decay. In turn, this drains the body of Knowledge Diffused.

Innovation Attractiveness (R12): Innovation Developed à(+) Perceived Legitimacy à(+) Entrepreneurial Activity à(+) External Funding à(+) Total Resources à(+) Resources to R&D à(+) Innovation Development à(+) Innovation Developed

According to Hekkert et al. [35] and Surrs [63], entrepreneurs are central to any TIS. Entrepreneurs refer to actors within the system whose "actions are directed at conducting market-oriented experiments with an emerging technology" [63] (p. 54). The Innovation Attractiveness loop represents the process of attracting new entrepreneurs to the system through innovation. When the Innovation Developed increases, technological legitimacy of the innovation system increases [36]. As potential entrants perceive the legitimacy of the emerging technology positively, they are more willing to enter the market, thus increasing the Entrepreneurial Activity. Entrepreneurial activities indicate the health and sustainability of an innovation system [35]. Higher levels of Entrepreneurial Activity thus increase the Total Resources in the system by way of attracting more External Funding or resources from private or public actors [36,63]. In turn, more resources become available for R & D, which spurs further development of innovation that increases the attractiveness to entrepreneurs even more.

Knowledge Attractiveness (R13): Knowledge Diffused à(+) Perceived Legitimacy à(+) Entrepreneurial Activity à(+) External Funding à(+) Total Resources à(+) Resources to R&D à(+) Knowledge Diffusion à(+) Knowledge Diffused

R13 loop works in a similar mechanism in attracting entrepreneurs. Technological legitimacy is a function of both Innovation Developed and Knowledge Diffused. The more knowledge about the technological innovation diffused in various networks, the higher the perceived legitimacy of the technology. Loops R12 and R13, thus, work concurrently and in concert to shore up the attractiveness of the emerging technology to potential market actors.

External Engine (R14): Entrepreneurial Activity à(+) External Funding à(+) Total Resources à(+) Resources to Market Development à(+) Entrepreneurial Activity

The External Engine loop represents the effect of external funding in reinforcing the growth of entrepreneurial activity within the emerging market. As explained previously, Entrepreneurial Activity can build confidence in the prospect of investment, thus increasing funding and resources from external actors, either private funders or governmental bodies. This increases the Total Resources available for market development. External backing reduces the perceived entrepreneurial risks involved, and consequently is better able to attract further entry into the market to spur even more Entrepreneurial Activity [36,63].

Internal Engine (R15): Entrepreneurial Activity à(+) Market Infrastructure à(+) Market Size à(+) Internal Resources from Market à(+) Total Resources à(+) Resources to Market Development à(+) Entrepreneurial Activity

While the external engine stimulates entrepreneurial activity temporarily, the Internal Engine endogenously generates internal ("financial, material, human capital") resources over the longer term through market formation to become self-sufficient [63] (p. 57). With reference to R15, increased Entrepreneurial Activity leads to the development of Market Infrastructure [39]. Entrepreneurs contribute to the "development of formal market rules, establishment of intermediary networks, the building of infrastructure, or the development of formal regulations" [38] (p. 1837). Through establishing the Market Infrastructure for market formation, entrepreneurial activity "contribute to the creation of a demand for the emerging technology" [63] (p. 56). This increases the Market Size for the technology that generates Internal Resources from the Market. In turn, with more Total Resources in the innovation system, Entrepreneurial Activity can further flourish by attracting more entrants to the system.

System Building (R16): Perceived Legitimacy à(+) Entrepreneurial Activity à(+) Market Infrastructure à(+) Perceived Legitimacy

Previously, we discussed how innovation diffusion increases the technological legitimacy of the emerging technology. Here, we consider market legitimacy, which stems from established market structures [36]. When market infrastructure is developed, it reduces market formation uncertainty and the perceived cost to participation [39]. With reference to R16, as the Perceived Legitimacy of the emerging technology increases, more entrepreneurs are willing to overcome perceived risks and enter the market. Consequently, the development of Market Infrastructure increases with the growth of Entrepreneurial Activity. This feeds back into increasing the market legitimacy of the emerging technology.

System Legitimacy (R17): Entrepreneurial Activity à(+) Market Size à(+) Internal Resources from Market à(+) Total Resources à(+) Resources to Market Development à(+) Market Infrastructure à(+) Perceived Legitimacy à(+) Entrepreneurial Activity

The System Legitimacy loop, R17, encompasses the aforementioned smaller loops R15 and R16, and "constitutes the most powerful self-reinforcing loop, potentially able to drive the whole system" [36] (p. 1838). Following the previous explanations provided for the individual links between variables, we observe that when Entrepreneurial Activity increases Market Size through market formation, Internal Resources from the Market burgeon and increase the Total Resources. This translates to more Resources for Market Development, which enables further development of Market Infrastructure. Consequently, the market legitimacy of the technological innovation flourishes, and thus begets even more Entrepreneurial Activity.

Resistance (R18): Regime Resistance à(-) Perceived Legitimacy à(+) Entrepreneurial Activity à(+) Market Infrastructure à(-) Regime Resistance

Market formation of a new technology is bound to precipitate "resistance from actors with interests in the incumbent" regime [63] (p. 57). This Resistance is captured in R18. Regime Resistance decreases the market legitimacy of the emerging technology, for instance "when regime actors try to influence public discourses, or lobby against favourablefavorable support" [36] (p. 1837). In turn, entrepreneurs might be less willing to enter the market due to higher perceived risks, thus reducing the Entrepreneurial Activity to a lower level than it otherwise would have been. In turn, there will be less Market Infrastructure development to counter Regime Resistance, which further emboldens resistance given the inverse relationship. The underlying mechanism for the negative link is supported by the fact that market infrastructure enables the system "to become less dependent on external dynamics and counter-balance regime-resistance" [36] (p. 1838). Importantly, R18 could work in a virtuous or vicious manner, depending on whosever perspective, either working to reinforce more resistance or reduce it.

Sailing Ship (B7): Perceived Legitimacy à(+) Entrepreneurial Activity à(+) Market Infrastructure à(+) Market Size à(+) à(+) Regime Resistance à(-) Perceived Legitimacy

As the emerging market grows and competes with the incumbent regime, resistance could also come in the form of innovation. Given the new threat, regime actors would "increase their efforts to improve the performance of the existing regime through innovation" [36] (p.1838). This "response aimed at improving the incumbent technology" is referred to as the sailing-ship effect [64,65] (p. 593). The Sailing Ship effect is thus represented in the balancing loop, B7. When the Perceived Legitimacy of the emerging technology increases, which attracts more entrepreneurial activity and thus market formation, the Sailing Ship Effect increases. This contributes to a stronger Regime Resistance, which consequently reduces the Perceived Legitimacy of the emerging technology. This loop thus seeks to counteract the effect of the System Legitimacy loop, R17.

In the top-level health care system, we assumed that the Perceived Relative Success of Digital Fitting will lead to an increase in Digital Market Size, thus masking the underlying structure between that link. Here, we consider the conceptual model in the Market Formation subsystem that could possibly explain how exactly the two variables are linked. Since R3 and R4 share a similar pathway in the subsystem, we only comment on R3.

Digital Growth (R3): Amputees in Digital Prosthetic Care à(+) Successful Fitting à(+) Perceived Relative Success of Digital Fitting à(+) Digital Fitting Reputation à(+) Perceived Legitimacy à(+) Entrepreneurial Activity à(+) Market Infrastructure à(+) Digital Market Size à(+) Digital Market Share à(+) Digital Prosthesis Referral à(+) Amputees in Digital Prosthetic Care

When the perceived relative success of digital fittings increases, we expect the emerging digital technology for prosthesis fitting to start amassing a reputation. This formed reputation improves technological legitimacy, which would attract more Entrepreneurial Activity to the emerging technological innovation system. Hence, the System Legitimacy loop works to increase the Market Infrastructure as well as Market Size for digital prosthetics. Consequently, the Digital Market Share rises to compete with the traditional prosthetics industry. The Digital Growth loops and the System Legitimacy loop thus work in tandem to increase the number of Amputees in Digital Prosthetic Care.

Market Access (R5): Amputees in Prosthetic Care à(+) Successful Fitting à(+) Perceived Relative Success of Digital Fitting à(+) Digital Fitting Reputation à(+) Perceived Legitimacy à(+) Entrepreneurial Activity à(+) Market Infrastructure à(+) Digital Market Size à(+) Prosthetic Clinics à(+) Fitting Capacity à(+) Prosthetic Accessibility à(+) Prosthesis Referral à(+) Amputees in Prosthetic Care

Similarly, we expect the interaction of the Market Access loops and the System Legitimacy loop. As Digital Fitting Reputation forms over time and builds the Digital Market Size, through the same pathway described above, we expect the expansion of digital prosthetic clinics that increases the Fitting Capacity. This improves the Market Access in the digital prosthetic continuum, which enables more people to be fitted with a prosthesis and improves the overall mobility outcomes.

Appendix B. Sensitivity Analysis Results

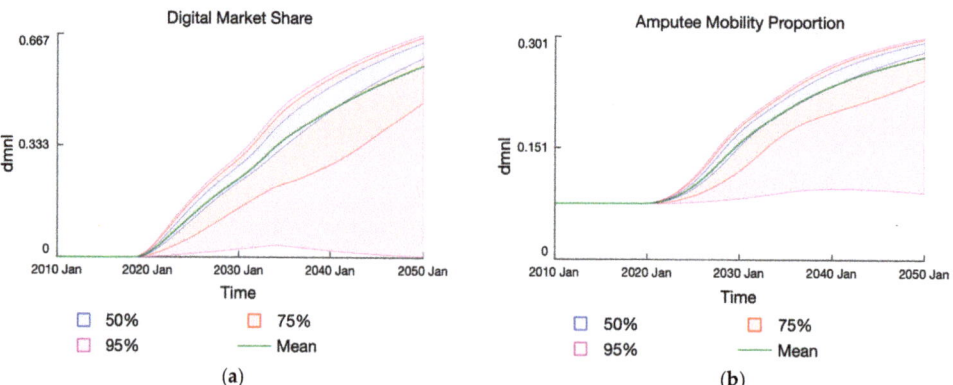

Figure A1. Confidence plots of (**a**) digital prosthetics market share and (**b**) amputee mobility proportion sensitivity to variations in Relative External Resources Size (range: 1–9).

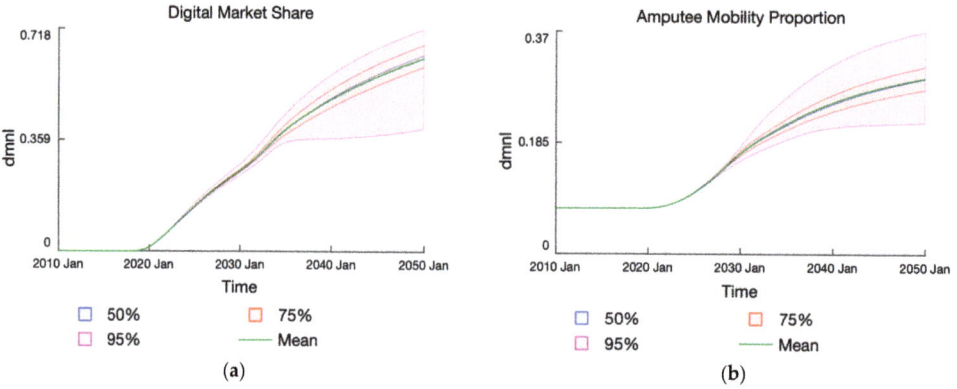

Figure A2. Confidence plots of (**a**) digital prosthetics market share and (**b**) amputee mobility proportion sensitivity to variations in Market Size Threshold (range: 0.025–0.075).

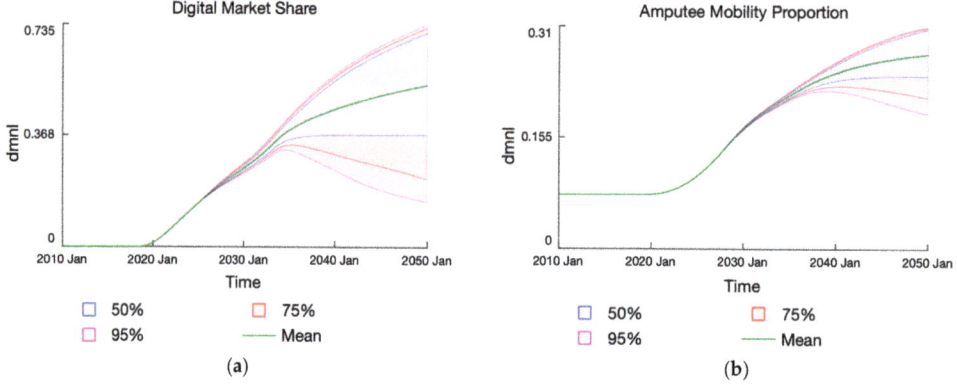

Figure A3. Confidence plots of (**a**) digital prosthetics market share and (**b**) amputee mobility proportion sensitivity to variations in Sensitivity of Resources to Market Size (range: 0.5–1.5).

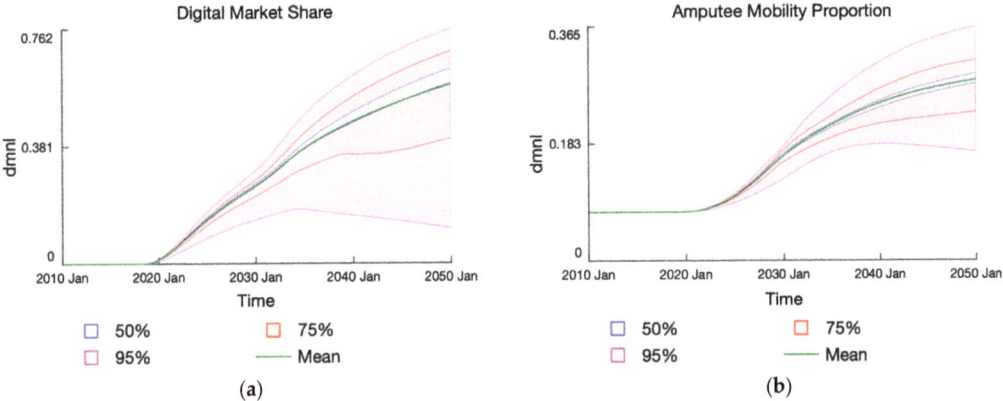

Figure A4. Confidence plots of (**a**) digital prosthetics market share and (**b**) amputee mobility proportion sensitivity to variations in Weight of Entrepreneurial Activity (range: 0.25–0.75).

References

1. World Health Organization. *WHO Standards for Prosthetics and Orthotics: Part 1*; World Health Organization: Geneva, Switzerland, 2017.
2. Moxey, P.W.; Gogalniceanu, P.; Hinchliffe, R.J.; Loftus, I.M.; Jones, K.J.; Thompson, M.M.; Holt, P.J. Lower Extremity Amputations—A Review of Global Variability in Incidence: Lower Extremity Amputations-a Global Review. *Diabet. Med.* **2011**, *28*, 1144–1153. [CrossRef] [PubMed]
3. Ahmad, N.; Thomas, G.N.; Gill, P.; Torella, F. The Prevalence of Major Lower Limb Amputation in the Diabetic and Non-Diabetic Population of England 2003–2013. *Diabetes Vasc. Dis. Res.* **2016**, *13*, 348–353. [CrossRef] [PubMed]
4. Geertzen, J.; van der Linde, H.; Rosenbrand, K.; Conradi, M.; Deckers, J.; Koning, J.; Rietman, H.S.; van der Schaaf, D.; van der Ploeg, R.; Schapendonk, J.; et al. Dutch Evidence-Based Guidelines for Amputation and Prosthetics of the Lower Extremity: Amputation Surgery and Postoperative Management. Part 1. *Prosthet. Orthot. Int.* **2015**, *39*, 351–360. [CrossRef] [PubMed]
5. Kohler, F.; Cieza, A.; Stucki, G.; Geertzen, J.; Burger, H.; Dillon, M.P.; Schiappacasse, C.; Esquenazi, A.; Kistenberg, R.S.; Kostanjsek, N. Developing Core Sets for Persons Following Amputation Based on the International Classification of Functioning, Disability and Health as a Way to Specify Functioning. *Prosthet. Orthot. Int.* **2009**, *33*, 117–129. [CrossRef] [PubMed]
6. Criqui, M.H.; Aboyans, V. Epidemiology of Peripheral Artery Disease. *Circ. Res.* **2015**, *116*, 1509–1526. [CrossRef] [PubMed]
7. Meffen, A.; Pepper, C.J.; Sayers, R.D.; Gray, L.J. Epidemiology of Major Lower Limb Amputation Using Routinely Collected Electronic Health Data in the UK: A Systematic Review Protocol. *BMJ Open* **2020**, *10*, e037593. [CrossRef]
8. Belch, J.J.F. Critical Issues in Peripheral Arterial Disease Detection and ManagementA Call to Action. *Arch. Intern. Med.* **2003**, *163*, 884. [CrossRef]
9. Akarsu, S.; Tekin, L.; Safaz, I.; Göktepe, A.S.; Yazıcıoğlu, K. Quality of Life and Functionality after Lower Limb Amputations: Comparison between Uni- vs. Bilateral Amputee Patients. *Prosthet. Orthot. Int.* **2013**, *37*, 9–13. [CrossRef]
10. Horgan, O.; MacLachlan, M. Psychosocial Adjustment to Lower-Limb Amputation: A Review. *Disabil. Rehabil.* **2004**, *26*, 837–850. [CrossRef]
11. Roberts, T.L.; Pasquina, P.F.; Nelson, V.S.; Flood, K.M.; Bryant, P.R.; Huang, M.E. Limb Deficiency and Prosthetic Management. 4. Comorbidities Associated With Limb Loss. *Arch. Phys. Med. Rehabil.* **2006**, *87*, 21–27. [CrossRef]
12. Darter, B.J.; Hawley, C.E.; Armstrong, A.J.; Avellone, L.; Wehman, P. Factors Influencing Functional Outcomes and Return-to-Work After Amputation: A Review of the Literature. *J. Occup. Rehabil.* **2018**, *28*, 656–665. [CrossRef] [PubMed]
13. Stewart, C.C.; Berhaneselase, E.; Morshed, S. The Burden of Patients With Lower Limb Amputations in a Community Safety-Net Hospital. *J. Am. Acad. Orthop. Surg.* **2022**, *30*, e59–e66. [CrossRef] [PubMed]
14. Pasquina, P.F.; Carvalho, A.J.; Sheehan, T.P. Ethics in Rehabilitation: Access to Prosthetics and Quality Care Following Amputation. *AMA J. Ethics* **2015**, *17*, 535–546. [CrossRef] [PubMed]
15. Raichle, K.A.; Hanley, M.A.; Molton, I.; Kadel, N.J.; Campbell, K.; Phelps, E.; Ehde, D.; Smith, D.G. Prosthesis Use in Persons with Lower- and Upper-Limb Amputation. *JRRD* **2008**, *45*, 961–972. [CrossRef] [PubMed]
16. ProsFit Technologies. *Solution to Mobility and Quality of Life for Millions of Amputees at Scale*; ProsFit Technologies JSC: Sofia, Bulgaria, 2022; (Unpublished).
17. Wyss, D.; Lindsay, S.; Cleghorn, W.L.; Andrysek, J. Priorities in Lower Limb Prosthetic Service Delivery Based on an International Survey of Prosthetists in Low- and High-Income Countries. *Prosthet. Orthot. Int.* **2015**, *39*, 102–111. [CrossRef] [PubMed]
18. Silva, K.; Rand, S.; Cancel, D.; Chen, Y.; Kathirithamby, R.; Stern, M. Three-Dimensional (3-D) Printing: A Cost-Effective Solution for Improving Global Accessibility to Prostheses. *PMR* **2015**, *7*, 1312–1314. [CrossRef]

19. Kozbunarova, A. ProsFit: The Startup That Aims To Democratize the Prosthetic Industry. *Trending Topics* **2019**. Available online: https://www.trendingtopics.eu/prosfit-prosthetic-industry-democratization-pandofit/ (accessed on 28 December 2022).
20. Hutchison, A. Distributed Care: The Third Dimension! *LinkedIn* **2020**. Available online: https://www.linkedin.com/pulse/distributed-care-third-dimension-alan-hutchison/ (accessed on 28 December 2022).
21. Sterman, J. *Business Dynamics: Systems Thinking and Modeling for a Complex World*; Irwin/McGraw-Hill: Boston, MA, USA, 2000; ISBN 978-0-07-231135-8.
22. Hovmand, P.S. *Community Based System Dynamics*; SpringerLink; Springer: New York, NY, USA, 2014; ISBN 978-1-4614-8763-0.
23. Richardson, G.P. Core of System Dynamics. In *Encyclopedia of Complexity and Systems Science*; Meyers, R.A., Ed.; Springer: Berlin, Heidelberg, 2019; pp. 1–10. ISBN 978-3-642-27737-5.
24. Forrester, J.W. *Principles of Systems*; Pegasus Communications, Inc.: Waltham, MA, USA, 1968; ISBN 978-1-883823-41-2.
25. Richardson, G.P. Reflections on the Foundations of System Dynamics: Foundations of System Dynamics. *Syst. Dyn. Rev.* **2011**, *27*, 219–243. [CrossRef]
26. Sohn, T.-W.; Surkis, J. System Dynamics: A Methodology for Testing Dynamic Behavioral Hypotheses. *IEEE Trans. Syst. Man. Cybern.* **1985**, *SMC-15*, 399–408. [CrossRef]
27. Darabi, N.; Hosseinichimeh, N. System Dynamics Modeling in Health and Medicine: A Systematic Literature Review. *Syst. Dyn. Rev.* **2020**, *36*, 29–73. [CrossRef]
28. Davahli, M.R.; Karwowski, W.; Taiar, R. A System Dynamics Simulation Applied to Healthcare: A Systematic Review. *IJERPH* **2020**, *17*, 5741. [CrossRef] [PubMed]
29. Homer, J.B.; Hirsch, G.B. System Dynamics Modeling for Public Health: Background and Opportunities. *Am. J. Public Health* **2006**, *96*, 452–458. [CrossRef] [PubMed]
30. Rajah, J.K. Enabling Mobility for Persons with Major Lower-Limb Amputations: A Model-Based Study of the Impact of Digital Prosthetics Service Provision on Mobility Outcomes. Master Thesis, University of Bergen, Bergen, Norway, 2022.
31. Rajah, J.K.; Hutchison, C.; Chernicoff, W.; Gonçalves, P. The Dynamics of Prosthetics Care Continuum for Persons with Amputation. In Proceedings of the International Conference of the System Dynamics Society 2022, Frankfurt, Germany, 19 July 2022.
32. Paich, M.; Peck, C.; Valant, J.J. *Pharmaceutical Product Strategy*; CRC Press: Boca Raton, FL, USA, 2004; ISBN 978-0-203-49252-9.
33. Homer, J.B. A Diffusion Model with Application to Evolving Medical Technologies. *Technol. Forecast. Soc. Change* **1987**, *31*, 197–218. [CrossRef]
34. Uriona, M.; Grobbelaar, S.S. Innovation System Policy Analysis through System Dynamics Modelling: A Systematic Review. *Sci. Public Policy* **2019**, *46*, 28–44. [CrossRef]
35. Hekkert, M.P.; Suurs, R.A.A.; Negro, S.O.; Kuhlmann, S.; Smits, R.E.H.M. Functions of Innovation Systems: A New Approach for Analysing Technological Change. *Technol. Forecast. Soc. Change* **2007**, *74*, 413–432. [CrossRef]
36. Walrave, B.; Raven, R. Modelling the Dynamics of Technological Innovation Systems. *Res. Policy* **2016**, *45*, 1833–1844. [CrossRef]
37. Wicki, S.; Hansen, E.G. Clean Energy Storage Technology in the Making: An Innovation Systems Perspective on Flywheel Energy Storage. *J. Clean. Prod.* **2017**, *162*, 1118–1134. [CrossRef]
38. Walrave, B.; Raven, R. Modelling the Dynamics of TIS-Model Appendix. *Res. Policy* **2016**, *45*, 1833–1844.
39. Lee, B.H.; Struben, J.; Bingham, C.B. Collective Action and Market Formation: An Integrative Framework. *Strat Mgmt. J.* **2018**, *39*, 242–266. [CrossRef]
40. Forrester, J.W. *Industrial Dynamics*; M.I.T. Press: Cambridge, MA, USA, 1961; ISBN 978-0-262-06003-5.
41. Király, G.; Miskolczi, P. Dynamics of Participation: System Dynamics and Participation-An Empirical Review. *Syst. Res. Behav. Sci.* **2019**, *36*, 199–210. [CrossRef]
42. McCardle-Keurentjes, M.H.F.; Rouwette, E.A.J.A.; Vennix, J.A.M.; Jacobs, E. Potential Benefits of Model Use in Group Model Building: Insights from an Experimental Investigation. *Syst. Dyn. Rev.* **2018**, *34*, 354–384. [CrossRef]
43. *Office for National Statistics Population Estimates and Deaths by Single Year of Age for England and Wales and the United Kingdom, 1961 to 2014*; UK Statistics Authority: London, UK, 2015.
44. Office for National Statistics. *Long-Term International Migration 2.07, Age and Sex, UK and England and Wales*; UK Statistics Authority: London, UK, 2020.
45. *Office for National Statistics United Kingdom Population Mid-Year Estimate*; UK Statistics Authority: London, UK, 2021.
46. *Office for National Statistics 2020-Based Interim National Population Projections*; UK Statistics Authority: London, UK, 2022.
47. *Office for National Statistics Age-Specific Fertility Rates (ASFRs) and Total Fertility Rates (TFRs) for UK-Born and Non-UK-Born Women Living in the UK, Scotland and Northern Ireland: 2004 to 2020*; UK Statistics Authority: London, UK, 2022.
48. Office for National Statistics. *Mortality Rates (Mx), 2020-Based Principal Projection, UK (Ages 0 to 125 Years, 1961 to 2120)*; UK Statistics Authority: London, UK, 2022.
49. Vascular Services Quality Improvement Programme. In *2015 Annual Report of the National Vascular Registry*; Healthcare Quality Improvement Partnership: London, UK, 2015.
50. Vascular Services Quality Improvement Programme. In *2016 Annual Report of the National Vascular Registry*; Healthcare Quality Improvement Partnership: London, UK, 2016.
51. Vascular Services Quality Improvement Programme. In *2017 Annual Report of the National Vascular Registry*; Healthcare Quality Improvement Partnership: London, UK, 2017.

52. Vascular Services Quality Improvement Programme. In *2018 Annual Report of the National Vascular Registry*; Healthcare Quality Improvement Partnership: London, UK, 2018.
53. Vascular Services Quality Improvement Programme. In *2019 Annual Report of the National Vascular Registry*; Healthcare Quality Improvement Partnership: London, UK, 2019.
54. Vascular Services Quality Improvement Programme. In *2020 Annual Report of the National Vascular Registry*; Healthcare Quality Improvement Partnership: London, UK, 2020.
55. Global Burden of Disease Collaborative Network. *Global Burden of Disease Study 2019 (GBD 2019) Results*; Institute for Health Metrics and Evaluation: Seattle, WA, USA, 2020.
56. Hutchison, C. *ProsFit Health Economics Model*; ProsFit Technologies JSC: Sofia, Bulgaria, 2021; (Unpublished Data Set).
57. Farndon, L.; Stephenson, J.; Binns-Hall, O.; Knight, K.; Fowler-Davis, S. The PodPAD Project: A Podiatry-Led Integrated Pathway for People with Peripheral Arterial Disease in the UK—A Pilot Study. *J. Foot Ankle. Res.* **2018**, *11*, 26. [CrossRef] [PubMed]
58. Cea-Soriano, L.; Fowkes, F.G.R.; Johansson, S.; Allum, A.M.; García Rodriguez, L.A. Time Trends in Peripheral Artery Disease Incidence, Prevalence and Secondary Preventive Therapy: A Cohort Study in The Health Improvement Network in the UK. *BMJ Open* **2018**, *8*, e018184. [CrossRef] [PubMed]
59. Rheinstein, J.; Carroll, K.; Stevens, P. Prosthetic Care for the Mangled Extremity. In *The Mangled Extremity*; Pensy, R.A., Ingari, J.V., Eds.; Springer International Publishing: Cham, Switzerland, 2021; pp. 257–283. ISBN 978-3-319-56647-4.
60. Davie-Smith, F.; Hebenton, J.; Scott, H. *A Survey of the Lower Limb Amputee Population in Scotland: 2015 Full Report*; Scottish Physiotherapy Amputee Research Group: Scotland, UK, 2018.
61. Chernicoff, W.; Naumov, S.; Sarkani, S.; Holzer, T. Modeling Market Dynamics in a Super Octane Ethanol Fuel Blend-Vehicle Power-Train System: Understanding the Role of Consumer Perception in Ethanol Market Growth. *JPCS* **2014**, *1*, 110–137. [CrossRef]
62. Nieuwenhuijsen, J.; de Almeida Correia, G.H.; Milakis, D.; van Arem, B.; van Daalen, E. Towards a Quantitative Method to Analyze the Long-Term Innovation Diffusion of Automated Vehicles Technology Using System Dynamics. *Transp. Res. Part C Emerg. Technol.* **2018**, *86*, 300–327. [CrossRef]
63. Suurs, R.A.A. *Motors of Sustainable Innovation: Towards a Theory on the Dynamics of Technological Innovation Systems*; Utrecht University: Utrecht, the Netherlands, 2009.
64. De Liso, N.; Arima, S.; Filatrella, G. The "Sailing-Ship Effect" as a Technological Principle. *Ind. Corp. Change* **2022**, *30*, 1459–1478. [CrossRef]
65. De Liso, N.; Filatrella, G. On Technology Competition: A Formal Analysis of the 'Sailing-Ship Effect'. *Econ. Innov. New Technol.* **2008**, *17*, 593–610. [CrossRef]
66. Senge, P.M.; Forrester, J.W. Tests for Building Confidence in System Dynamics Models. In *System Dynamics*; Legasto, A.A., Forrester, J.W., Lyneis, J.M., Eds.; North-Holland Publishing Company: Amsterdam, the Netherlands, 1980; pp. 209–228.
67. Barlas, Y. Formal Aspects of Model Validity and Validation in System Dynamics. *Syst. Dyn. Rev.* **1996**, *12*, 183–210. [CrossRef]
68. Burhenne, S.; Jacob, D.; Henze, G.P. Sampling Based on Sobol' Sequences for Monte Carlo Techniques Applied to BuildingSimulations. In Proceedings of the Proceedings of the Building Simulation 2011: 12th Conference of International Building Performance SimulationAssociation, Sydney, Australia, 14 November 2011; pp. 1816–1823.
69. Webster, J.B.; Hakimi, K.N.; Williams, R.M.; Turner, A.P.; Norvell, D.C.; Czerniecki, J.M. Prosthetic Fitting, Use, and Satisfaction Following Lower-Limb Amputation: A Prospective Study. *JRRD* **2012**, *49*, 1493. [CrossRef]
70. Pell, J.P.; Donnan, P.T.; Fowkes, F.G.R.; Ruckley, C.V. Quality of Life Following Lower Limb Amputation for Peripheral Arterial Disease. *Eur. J. Vasc. Surg.* **1993**, *7*, 448–451. [CrossRef] [PubMed]
71. Andersen, D.F.; Richardson, G.P.; Vennix, J.A.M. Group Model Building: Adding More Science to the Craft. *Syst. Dyn. Rev.* **1997**, *13*, 187–201. [CrossRef]

Disclaimer/Publisher's Note: The statements, opinions and data contained in all publications are solely those of the individual author(s) and contributor(s) and not of MDPI and/or the editor(s). MDPI and/or the editor(s) disclaim responsibility for any injury to people or property resulting from any ideas, methods, instructions or products referred to in the content.

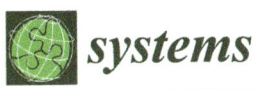

Article

Using a System Dynamics Simulation Model to Identify Leverage Points for Reducing Youth Homelessness in Connecticut

Gary B. Hirsch [1,*] and Heather I. Mosher [2]

[1] Independent Consultant and Creator of Learning Environments, 7 Highgate Road, Wayland, MA 01778, USA
[2] Institute for Community Research (ICR), 146 Wyllys Street, Hartford, CT 06106, USA; heather.mosher@icrweb.org
* Correspondence: gbhirsch@comcast.net

Abstract: Youth homelessness is a significant problem in most United States communities. Health problems are both a contributor to and a consequence of homelessness. Responses to youth homelessness are typically fragmentary. Different agencies deal with various causes and consequences of the problem. Stakeholders in Connecticut sought a more coherent approach. This article describes the development and use of a system dynamics simulation model as a decision-support tool that: (1) brings stakeholders together from diverse service sectors and allows them to see the system as a whole, (2) enables them to explore how delivery systems interact to affect homeless and unstably housed youth, (3) lets them test the impact of different intervention alternatives on reducing the problem, and (4) helps develop insights about coherent approaches to youth homelessness. The model's development is described as a phased process including stakeholder engagement, causal mapping, and creation of the quantitative simulation model. The resulting model is presented along with an interface that enables stakeholders to use the model in a Learning Lab setting. Results of an initial set of Learning Labs are presented, including types of insights gained by participants from using the simulation model. Conclusions include limitations of the model and plans for its future use.

Keywords: youth homelessness; system dynamics; child welfare; juvenile justice; mental health

Citation: Hirsch, G.B.; Mosher, H.I. Using a System Dynamics Simulation Model to Identify Leverage Points for Reducing Youth Homelessness in Connecticut. *Systems* **2023**, *11*, 163. https://doi.org/10.3390/systems11030163

Academic Editor: Wayne Wakeland

Received: 18 January 2023
Revised: 11 March 2023
Accepted: 18 March 2023
Published: 22 March 2023

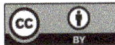

Copyright: © 2023 by the authors. Licensee MDPI, Basel, Switzerland. This article is an open access article distributed under the terms and conditions of the Creative Commons Attribution (CC BY) license (https://creativecommons.org/licenses/by/4.0/).

1. Introduction

1.1. Magnitude of Youth Homelessness as a Problem

Most communities across the United States are struggling to address the complex and persistent problem of youth homelessness. In 2017, an estimated 4.3% of teens (13–17 years old) and 12.5% of young adults (18–25 years old) experienced some form of homelessness [1]. Homelessness among youth is typically defined as unaccompanied youth between 14- and 24-years old who are living apart from parents/guardians and who lack a fixed, regular, and adequate residence (e.g., living in shelters, on the streets, in cars or vacant buildings, or who are "couch surfing" or living in other unstable circumstances) [2]. Young people find themselves without homes for many reasons, including family conflicts, mental health and substance use problems, early pregnancy and parenting, coping with the effects of sexual and/or gender minority status, fleeing domestic or sexual violence, and leaving child welfare or juvenile justice systems without adequate skills or support [3–5]. The impact of homelessness on youth and society is extensive. Evidence suggests that periods of homelessness lead to higher rates of substance use, sexual risk behaviors, early parenthood, unemployment, incarceration, mental illness, suicide, injury due to physical violence, and poor educational and health outcomes [6–16].

Young people experiencing homelessness have histories of contact with multiple systems—education, child welfare, mental health, and juvenile/criminal justice—yet no entity has ongoing responsibility for them. For example, approximately 44% of homeless youth in a national study indicated that they had been in foster care [17]. A study following a sample of adolescents who left the foster care system two years prior found that 43% endured housing instability since their exit from foster care, and 20% experienced chronic homelessness [18]. These young people experiencing housing instability reported having spent time in foster care, inpatient mental health settings, juvenile detention, or jail [18]. Effective solutions to addressing youth homelessness will involve coordination and collaboration among multiple system stakeholders and a holistic understanding of the factors and dynamics that influence the issue.

1.2. Case Study: Connecticut's Mission to Address Youth Homelessness

This article describes a system dynamics simulation model developed in partnership with a cross-sector coalition of youth-serving providers and young people with lived experience of homelessness in Connecticut (CT). The coalition has been meeting since 2012 with the mission to end youth homelessness across the state. At the time of model development, the total population projection by 2015 in CT was nearly 3.6 million people, with 191,056 minors (ages 14–17) and 348,167 young adults (ages 18–24) [19]. In 2019, an estimated 28.7% of young people (ages 14–24) had reported experiencing a form of homelessness in CT, which is greater than the national prevalence estimate [1,20]. Of those who were experiencing housing instability or homelessness, approximately half had experienced literal homelessness (e.g., sleeping outside, in a shelter, or other places not meant for human habitation) while the remaining individuals had been living in precarious housing situations, such as staying with others and moving frequently from place to place while unaccompanied by a parent [20]. Over half of the young adults experiencing housing instability and homelessness had a history of criminal justice involvement (56.7%), and over 80% had been involved in foster care [20]. To prevent this ongoing cycle between homelessness and involvement in state systems, the coalition hoped to develop a coordinated response that would address the varied and unique needs of young people who are at risk of or experiencing homelessness.

Connecticut's goals aligned with the United States Interagency Council on Homelessness (USICH) national strategic plan to prevent and end homelessness by making youth homelessness rare, brief and non-recurring [21,22]. This means: (a) driving down the number of youth experiencing housing instability/homelessness to as close to zero as possible; (b) enhancing and coordinating systems and interventions to prevent new youth from entering into housing instability/homelessness; (c) quickly identifying and rapidly providing necessary assistance when a youth does fall into housing instability/homelessness; and (d) ensuring formerly homeless youth have the tools to remain in stable housing.

A number of problems interfered with developing a coherent approach to youth homelessness in CT. One was simply a lack of consensus about definitions of homelessness, complicated by different definitions used by Federal programs. Another was the lack of compatible data systems and protocols which prevented sharing of data needed to provide a complete picture of youth homelessness. There also was not a history of coordination among agencies that were dealing with the same population of at-risk and housing-unstable youth. Finally, there was an acknowledged shortage of housing and other resources that resulted in too many youths not receiving the help they needed and suffering more serious and long-lasting consequences as a result. It was hoped that the modeling effort would highlight these problems and point the way to practical solutions.

1.3. Role of System Dynamics in Addressing Youth Homelessness in Connecticut

Connecticut stakeholders sought the use of a system dynamics simulation model as a decision-making tool that would bring stakeholders together from diverse service sectors and allow them to see the system as a whole, explore how intervention delivery systems interact, and determine the impact that state policy might have on solving the problem. The aims were to help stakeholders develop and use the simulation model to identify the best combination of interventions and avoid unintended impacts, coordinate services across systems, and garner support for resource allocation and policy change. Due to the geographic diversity (urban, rural, and suburban) and differences in available resources across the state, stakeholder planning and coordination occurred both at the regional and statewide levels. Therefore, a model was needed that can be used in planning statewide efforts and also adapted to particular regions.

Prior to initiating the modeling process, the coalition had been using an Excel spreadsheet to estimate the number of housing resources that would be needed based on a population of young people with diverse needs. However, they expressed a desire for a tool that would allow them to project the dynamics of movement into and out of homelessness for young people, visually map the intersections between systems of care (e.g., child welfare, justice, mental health), and assess how specific policies and prevention strategies could reduce the inflow of young people into homelessness and result in a reduced need for housing resources. The purpose of this paper is to describe the processes by which stakeholders came together and formed a core modeling and data team (CMDT), developed an initial causal map that embodied their understanding of the system of forces responsible for youth homelessness, created a simulation model based on that understanding along with an interface that enabled stakeholders to use the model themselves, and derived insights from using the simulation model in a series of Learning Labs.

2. Methodology

Solving a complex problem such as youth homelessness requires collaboration in a community setting and across multiple sectors. We used a community-based group model building (GMB) approach to engage diverse stakeholders in the process of systems thinking and developing system dynamics models [23,24]. GMB is an intentional approach to model building that is participatory and embedded in the community, involving stakeholders as partners in the modeling process from defining the problem to developing and using models to implement changes [25]. This direct involvement leads to a better model as well as enhanced capacity for the use of systems thinking, more effective collaborations, and increased ability to implement changes based on system insights gained through the process. We also used the Typology of Youth Participation and Empowerment (TYPE) Pyramid framework for effective youth–adult partnerships in the modeling process [26]. The TYPE Pyramid articulates different configurations of youth–adult control that reflect optimal participation for youth empowerment and positive youth development. Youth–adult partnerships are crucial to creating solutions that are effective, relevant, and responsive to youth needs.

The project was divided into four major phases to support the involvement of a large number of stakeholders, providing the broadest perspectives possible from many vantage points. The four phases involved: (1) forming a core modeling team to co-design a modeling process; (2) mapping the causal factors and the relationships between them; (3) co-developing a simulation model; and (4) building stakeholders' capacity to use the model for gaining system insights. The project was implemented between March 2017 to March 2023. Overall, 126 system stakeholders participated in the modeling process. Each stakeholder was selected based on their expertise with different systems that touch the lives of young people who experience homelessness. A total of 97 front-line service providers, service directors, and policymakers participated. Young people (n = 29) with lived expertise of youth homelessness and the service systems were involved in all phases of the project, including on the core modeling team.

2.1. Forming a Core Modeling Team and Engaging Stakeholders (Phase 1)

The Youth Homelessness System Dynamics Modeling project was initiated by the community, specifically, a statewide taskforce focused on addressing youth homelessness in CT. The second author, as a member of this taskforce, was approached by coalition partners to lead and facilitate the system dynamics modeling (SDM) process. All decisions regarding the SDM process were made in collaboration with taskforce members which consisted of 30–40 representatives of youth-serving institutions, community-based service providers, policymakers, and advocates.

Twelve individuals from the taskforce formed the "core modeling and data team" (CMDT) responsible for designing the causal mapping process. The CMDT consisted of four young people (17–24 years old) with lived experience of youth homelessness, a senior-level representative from the CT Department of Housing and one from the CT Department of Children and Families, a director of a social service organization, a director of a community-based organization, two housing/homelessness policy analysts, an attorney/legislative advocate for homeless youth, and a researcher/system scientist (second author HM). The CMDT met six times between March and July 2017 to select stakeholders to participate in all phases of the modeling process, to plan, design, and co-facilitate the GMB workshops and to review synthesized causal maps. The CMDT defined the goals of phase 1 as: (a) build strong collaborations across systems, (b) develop a shared problem definition and language, (c) build systems thinking, and (d) create a shared understanding of causal pathways driving youth homelessness by using causal mapping.

As an initial step in identifying stakeholders to participate in the modeling process (e.g., GMB workshops, model review sessions, simulation model workshops), the team identified seven areas of stakeholder expertise needed for creating a holistic understanding of the causal pathways involved in youth homelessness and for building confidence in the model. These areas of expertise included: housing, health/mental health, education, employment, child welfare, juvenile/criminal justice, and parenting as a teen/young adult. The group carried out stakeholder analysis using a power/interest grid stakeholder mapping tool [27] to strategically plan who and how different stakeholders were to be meaningfully engaged in the project and modeling process. To increase diversity, additional factors were considered in the selection process, including stakeholder demographics (race, ethnicity, gender, and sexual orientation), geographic expertise within CT, and role/perspective (e.g., service-user, front-line service providers, director/management, policymakers, data expert).

2.2. Causal Mapping (Phase 2)

Over a hundred (n = 108) system stakeholders from across the state—including 29 young people (14–24 years old) who had experienced housing instability/homelessness—participated in the causal mapping process. The process involved thirteen separate GMB workshops (with different stakeholders) and three model review sessions (same stakeholders across the three sessions) to map and validate the structural dynamics that drive the problem of youth homelessness in CT, and to build systems thinking and collaboration among stakeholders. Professionals did not receive monetary incentives for participating in the modeling process. However, service users (young adults who had experienced homelessness) received $50 each to participate in a GMB session.

Each GMB workshop was 4 h long and consisted of short orientation presentations and a sequence of structured small group activities called "scripts" [28] that focus on different goals of the modeling process and support team decision making that results in useful products and insights for community stakeholders by the end of the workshop. The workshop sequence started with a "Hopes and Fears" activity to understand group expectations for the GMB sessions and products [29] and then a variable elicitation activity called "Connection Circles" to elicit information about the factors that affect or are affected by youth homelessness. These variables were used in "Causal Mapping in Small Groups" where subgroups worked together to map key causal factors and their relationships in a causal loop diagram. Time was set aside for breaks, discussion, and model reflections between scripted activities to identify and understand the main feedback loops in the diagrams. The "Action Ideas" and "Dots" activities were used at the end of the workshop to brainstorm, prioritize potential actions to impact variables, and emphasize connections between variables. Detailed procedures for executing each script can be viewed online from Scriptapedia [30].

During the GMB sessions, the CMDT served as presenters, reflectors, runners, and wall-builders. HM functioned as a community facilitator and three staff researchers at the Institute for Community Research served as ethnographers/notetakers. GMB experts from Washington University in St. Louis supported HM and the CMDT in the design and facilitation of the GMB workshops and in developing systematic procedures for model synthesis and review/refinement.

Raw data (small group causal maps) from GMB sessions were synthesized by HM into a causal map that integrated key variables and feedback relationships found in participants' maps. The synthesis involved transferring individual hand-drawn causal maps into STELLA Architect [31], identifying the most common variables and links among variables across the maps using content analysis [32], and then creating a synthesized causal diagram that included the variables in common that had the most links [24]. Validation occurred iteratively in stakeholder model review sessions [33], which were used to seek participant feedback on synthesized maps, insights and stories, and to check researcher interpretation. The review involved stakeholder feedback on a synthesized map created by HM, discussing each variable and causal link to ensure it had face validity and was supported by stakeholders' knowledge and the literature. Synthesized maps were revised through feedback from subsequent GMB and model review sessions, and consultation with the existing literature. The process resulted in 12 interconnected causal maps that visually described "stories" of stakeholders' shared understanding of what is driving the youth homelessness problem. The rich qualitative information collected through this process was used in the next phase of modeling as well as in CT's HUD Youth Homelessness Demonstration Project (YHDP) planning phase to develop collective goals, objectives, and action steps in the Coordinated Community Plan.

2.3. Developing the Simulation Model (Phase 3)

To initiate this next phase, the CMDT invited an additional six members to replace one representative of the CT Department of Children and Families, who transitioned jobs, and to address gaps in expertise. New members included a data expert at the CT Department of Mental Health and Addiction Services/Young Adult Services, a policy expert in juvenile justice systems, a researcher/scholar from the University of New Haven with expertise in justice systems, a senior-level representative from CT Court Support Services Division, and a senior level expert from the youth and adult employment sector. (See Appendix A for CMDT members' organizations.) This phase began with the co-authors facilitating a 4 h workshop with the CMDT to orient new members to the project and system dynamics concepts, practice systems thinking, and refine and expand on an initial stock-and-flow diagram seed structure. Stocks and flows in the initial diagram were identified through the co-authors' initial content analysis of the stories depicted in the qualitative maps from the previous phase that described the factors and relationships that led to youth homelessness and caused it to remain a serious problem. The workshop ended with a number of products: a parallel stock-and-flow structure that separated young people based on their age grouping (minors and young adults), shared definitions of the different stocks, and an initial list of the most important causal factors affecting each of the flows. Follow-up interviews with eight members of the CMDT were conducted to elicit more in-depth feedback on the model structure. Changes were critiqued, discussed, and refined in several subsequent CMDT meetings before settling on a final set that formed the "backbone" of the model. The causal factors determining the rates of flow were identified first by the CMDT and through analysis of the causal maps in the previous phase. Then, these factors were compared and prioritized based on an extensive review of the youth homelessness literature and feedback from our CMDT that included young people who had experienced housing instability. The estimates on the effects of these factors were extensively reviewed with the CMDT and other experts and adjusted as necessary.

The research team requested secondary quantitative data from institutions participating in the modeling process. The specific data needed for modeling was identified by stakeholders. The co-authors met with data experts from eight different institutions and submitted data sharing requests to obtain data in aggregate form with no identifying information. CMDT members helped facilitate the data request process within their agencies. Data were collected from: The Department of Housing, The Department of Corrections, The Court Support Services Division, The Department of Mental Health and Addiction Services, The Department of Education, The Department of Labor, The Department of Children and Families, and the United Way (2-1-1 helpline data).

The next task was to quantify the relationships in the model so that it could be used to simulate the impact of various interventions, by themselves and in various combinations. Some of the data assumptions in the model include:

1. Initial populations in various statuses, corresponding with stocks in the model. These come from various data sources or estimation procedures carried out by respected authorities. Some of these are further adjusted based on estimates derived from the youth homelessness literature, for example, dividing the initial population of homeless young adults into groups of those experiencing homelessness for the first time and those that endure repeated homelessness. These are presented in Table S1 in the Supplementary Materials.

2. Assumptions based on the youth homelessness literature and discussions of our CMDT that assign numerical values to concepts in the literature. Some of these numerical assumptions are not based on particular values derived from the literature as much as a sense of the relative strength of the causal relationships they represent, based on those discussions with the CMDT. These are presented in Table S2A–E in the Supplementary Materials.

3. An additional set of model parameters came from calibrating the model to produce what we believed was a reasonable baseline simulation, one that projects current trends and assumes no major new initiatives to prevent or remediate youth homelessness. We considered a number of trends in unstable housing and homelessness in youth, both locally and nationally. Some were growing, others declining. There was no definitive trend apparent. The CMDT confirmed that a stable trend going into the future was the most likely scenario. Therefore, we decided to settle on a baseline simulation that projected constant levels of unstable housing and homelessness for youth. The calibration process then consisted of calculating the fractions of minors and young adults flowing from one status to the next (e.g., from At Risk to Unstably Housed) over a given period that would maintain (relatively) stable numbers in each status as the simulation progressed over a ten-year period. These are presented in Table S3 in the Supplementary Materials for each section of the model. Table S3 also contains data derived from the CT CAN (Coordinated Access Network) Data Dashboards (ctcandata.org) on Temporary and Supportive Housing programs, the average lengths of time youth spend in those programs, and the fractions of various outcomes upon leaving those programs.

4. Data on the costs of homelessness and of various interventions to reduce homelessness, taken from various studies and used to calculate social costs and program costs, both on a monthly and cumulative basis. These are presented in Table S4 in the Supplementary Materials. Calculating these costs and resultant savings due to various interventions enables the model to project resources that can be freed up and reinvested in those interventions.

The simulation model was validated through an iterative process of model review sessions and interviews with additional experts. Data and assumptions used to quantify the model were critiqued by the CMDT over several group sessions and through member-checking with content and data experts to verify the credibility of parameters in the model. For example, we consulted with six experts outside of the CMDT to verify model assumptions related to child welfare service populations. Through these consultations, we were able to build consensus on parameters such as the proportions and relative risks of unaccompanied homelessness for minors receiving in-home services as compared to that of minors receiving out-of-home care and the proportion of out-of-home youth who have a history of behavioral health needs, among others. Validation of the model against historical data was not possible due to a lack of reliable longitudinal data on youth experiencing unstable housing and homelessness. The point-in-time counts of homeless youth most often cited significantly undercount their numbers. Estimates of actual numbers of homeless and unstably housed youth came from a methodology derived by Dr. Stephen Adair for the Connecticut Coalition to End Homelessness [20]. The CMDT and other experts supported the assumption that those numbers going forward would remain relatively constant in the absence of any additional or stronger interventions. Interventions represented in the model were tested to assure that their effects were realistic and, in the process, also indicated that the model was responding appropriately to various inputs.

2.4. Building Stakeholders' Capacity to Use the Model (Phase 4)

The CMDT hosted five virtual 1.5 h workshops, or Learning Labs, with key stakeholders via Zoom to build the stakeholders' capacity to use the model for testing and analyzing different combinations of strategies and to plan for implementing model insights. The workshop series began with an orientation on the model structure, a simulation demonstration, and time for individual hands-on play and practice with the model. Subsequent workshops involved an iterative process of structured activities for stakeholders to explore testing different scenarios and then refining strategies based on insights. The results of simulation runs were recorded by stakeholders using an intervention impact summary matrix that allowed stakeholders to analyze results by easily comparing across scenarios and creating higher order metrics to understand how different strategies performed on key objectives. Stakeholders' feedback and insights were recorded on a whiteboard and through detailed ethnographic field notes during the Learning Lab, then discussed by stakeholders to build a shared understanding of the underlying dynamics generating the observed behavior. The large number and varied simulations run during these labs provided additional opportunities to test the model and make adjustments when the results seemed questionable.

3. Results

3.1. Model Structure

Figure 1 depicts the basic flow structure of the Youth Homelessness Model. The population represented is for the entire state of Connecticut and is divided into minors (ages 14–17) and young adults (ages 18–24). Additional versions specific to regions of the state are currently being implemented using the same model structure and region-specific data. The boxes represent statuses with respect to stable housing (Stably Housed), risk (At Risk), unstable housing and homelessness (Unstably Housed and Homeless), and recovering from instability/homelessness (Stably Housed Formerly Homeless).

Horizontal arrows indicate flows among statuses as minors and young adults become at risk, become unstably housed or homeless, and potentially become stably housed again. Formerly homeless minors and young adults can also fall back into unstable housing and homelessness. Vertical arrows simply represent aging as minors reach age 18 and become young adults. Young adults age out of the youth-serving homelessness system as they reach age 25.

The majority of minors and young adults are in the two left-hand boxes and are either living with family or other guardians or are on their own in stable housing situations and considered not at risk of becoming unstably housed or homeless. These numbers come from state population data. How do we consider someone at risk of unstable housing and homelessness? How large a group do we assign to this status? There are many ways of determining risk. One that seemed appropriate was based on the experience of Adverse Childhood Experiences (ACEs). The connection between ACEs and homelessness is supported by a number of citations from the literature [34,35]. Examples of ACEs include experiencing violence within the family and living with someone who has had mental health or substance abuse problems [34]. An extensive body of literature shows that individual ACEs can impact young people's development in a dose–response manner. For example, the higher number of ACEs experienced, the greater the likelihood of poor physical and mental health outcomes, less successful educational attainment, and reduced workforce success [36–43]. Research also shows a relationship between ACEs and unstable housing and homelessness, suggesting that young people who have had three or more ACEs are at more chronic risk and have a greater likelihood of homelessness [44–49]. National prevalence research suggests that about 17% of young people in the US meet this criterion [45,46]. We applied this percentage to estimate the total number of minors and young adults at risk.

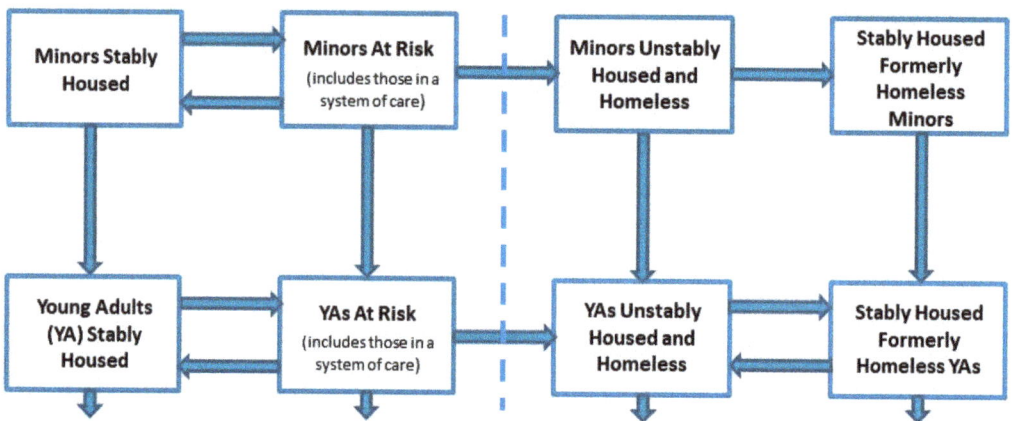

Figure 1. Overview of Model Flow Structure.

Minors and young adults at risk of housing instability or homelessness fall into two categories. One category consists of those at home with their families who are not part of an organized System of Care (SOC). An SOC is a system/institution that coherently provides services with case management or other oversight that can provide or refer clients to the services that they need (e.g., child welfare). These young people at home with their families are deemed at risk of becoming unstably housed or homeless due to family conflict, potential physical, emotional, or sexual abuse, and/or mental health and substance abuse problems suffered by themselves, their parents, or other family members. Evidence supports that these risk factors are strong predictors of youth and young adult homelessness [50–54].

The remainder of at-risk youth are in some form of SOC. Two of these SOCs are represented for minors: The Department of Children and Families (DCF) and the Juvenile Justice System. Four are represented for Young Adults: DCF, Criminal Justice, Department of Mental Health, and Department of Labor (Job Training). The numbers of minors and young adults were provided by the relevant SOCs and were subtracted from the total numbers assumed to be at risk to obtain the number of those not in an SOC. Some of the young people in SOCs may remain at home with their families, but they remain connected to the SOC under the supervision of a caseworker or probation officer; others are in residential settings. Remaining connected to an SOC with case management can serve as a protective factor for young people who are at risk of homelessness. However, these young people can become at greater risk when discharged from SOCs. Without teaching them the necessary skills and offering careful discharge planning, young people leaving systems of care can "fall through the cracks" and become unstably housed or homeless once they leave [55].

The model represents two types of housing instability for minors and three for young adults. Being unstably housed means that a young person is nominally off the street and living in a domicile fit for human habitation but is not in a secure situation and can be ejected at any time. This status is sometimes referred to as "couch surfing." While typically viewed as less dangerous than homelessness, those who are unstably housed are often at risk of abuse and exploitation from people with whom they are staying [56–60]. For minors especially, the lack of adult supervision leaves them vulnerable to additional risks.

Homelessness means having no domicile designed for human habitation (e.g., living under a bridge or in a park). This naturally exposes a young person to additional risk of harm and exploitation as well as being injurious to their physical and mental health. The impacts of homelessness feed on themselves and make it even more difficult to help a young person find stable housing [61].

A third status for young adults is repeated homelessness, which is more than one episode of homelessness. People in this status typically have accumulated more trauma and are at risk of more serious drug abuse and mental health issues and can require more extensive housing and wrap-around services [62,63].

The vertical dashed line and unidirectional arrows between at-risk and unstably housed statuses in Figure 1 indicate that young people remain at risk if they have experienced housing instability or homelessness in the past. This assumption came from a large body of literature and consensus among the CMDT. Experiencing housing instability/homelessness has long-term effects on young people's mental health, physical health, and financial and future housing stability [64–72]. These young people cannot return to the At-Risk and Stably Housed statuses that represent individuals who have not experienced housing instability. They are a different population of youth who might need a different set of interventions. As someone continues to experience homelessness, they accumulate trauma and stabilization becomes more difficult. Young people who have experienced homelessness can still become housed but remain chronically at risk due to cumulative trauma resulting from experiencing homelessness [36].

Estimating the number of youth experiencing unstable housing and homelessness is difficult [73]. "Point-in-Time (PIT) counts" are a method of trying to rigorously count numbers of people experiencing homelessness on a particular day, but are generally recognized to be undercounted because of the limited ability to accurately identify youth experiencing homelessness and unstable housing, as this population experiences more hidden forms of homelessness and tends to avoid shelters [14,74,75]. These counts also would miss many of those young people who are unstably housed. We relied instead on a Youth Outreach and Count methodology in Connecticut that added a robust element of data that addressed some of the limitations of the PIT Count by including youth from a wide variety of community contexts (e.g., schools, popular gathering spots, and youth programs) and executing the Youth Outreach and Count for a full week.

Even this more rigorous method of counting could miss some youth facing housing instability. As indicated earlier, further refinement and extension of these enhanced Point in Time Counts was based on a methodology developed by Professor Stephen Adair of Central Connecticut State University. Professor Adair started with the number of people reporting at least one night in a shelter, developed estimates of the numbers who were unstably housed and homeless for each city and town in Connecticut, and aggregated upward for the state as a whole. Detailed information on the Youth Outreach and Count and estimation methodology can be found in the 2019 PIT report on the Connecticut Coalition to End Homelessness website [20].

Formerly homeless young people who are stably housed may be placed in housing designated specifically for this population on a temporary or permanent basis or in a regular apartment with some supportive services. As suggested in Figure 1, they continue to be at risk of future homelessness and may fall back into housing instability and homelessness.

The behavior of the model is determined by the stock-and-flow structure shown in Figure 1, the model's causal structure, the magnitude of interventions applied by model users, and the places in which those interventions impact the flows of youth through the system. An overview of the causal structure affecting young adults is shown in Figure 2. It indicates that the trajectory of housing instability and homelessness is determined by a set of reinforcing loops that can worsen the problem and balancing loops that can limit or reduce its magnitude.

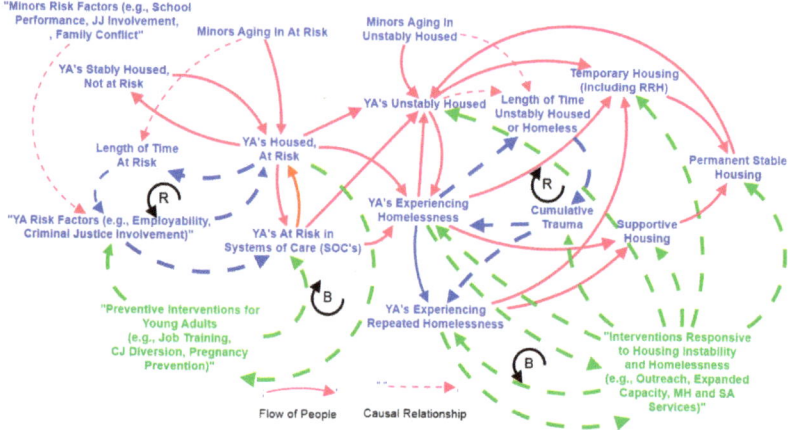

Figure 2. Overview of Model Causal Structure for Young Adults.

One set of reinforcing loops (represented by blue dotted lines) involves the numbers of young adults at risk of housing instability and the length of time they remain at risk. Longer times spent at risk increase the likelihood and severity of risk factors, such as involvement in the criminal justice system, and further lengthen the time at risk and maintain a greater at-risk number. The other set of reinforcing loops acts on young adults once they become unstably housed or homeless. Longer times spent unstably housed make it more likely that they will be exposed to risks such as mental illness and substance abuse disorders that cause them to become homeless. Once homeless, longer times on the street expose them to additional risks and increase the cumulative trauma of homelessness that can result in repeated episodes of homelessness and additional trauma. As with any reinforcing loops, efforts that reduce the lengths of time unstably housed or homeless and cumulative trauma can lead to further improvements and reductions in the number of youths dealing with these problems.

Working against these reinforcing loops are balancing loops, which reduce the risks of homelessness, the numbers of youth unstably housed and homeless, and the trauma arising from homelessness. One set of balancing loops (represented by the green dotted lines) includes interventions designed to reduce risks such as diverting young adults from criminal justice, better preparing them for jobs, or helping them deal with mental health or substance abuse conditions. These interventions can reduce the length of time and number of young adults who remain at risk. The other set of balancing loops includes services directed at young adults who have already become unstably housed or homeless. These services can reduce the number and length of time that they experience housing instability or homelessness by finding them temporary or supportive housing, or reducing cumulative trauma through care for mental health and substance abuse problems. Model users, working through an interface described below, can increase the intensity of these interventions and observe their impact on the number of youths experiencing unstable housing and homelessness. They can investigate what combinations will yield the best overall result in reducing the burden of youth housing instability. The effects of more intense interventions can be amplified by the reinforcing loops diagrammed in Figure 2 and have a greater impact.

Figure 3 indicates the full set of interventions that can be used in different combinations, where in the model they have their effect, and the assumed strength of those effects. Assumptions about the impact of various interventions were not based on single quantities derived from the literature, since there were usually multiple studies that indicated different impacts. Instead, they were estimates based on a sense of the relative impacts suggested by multiple studies. These are described further in the document "Intervention Descriptions" (Appendix B).

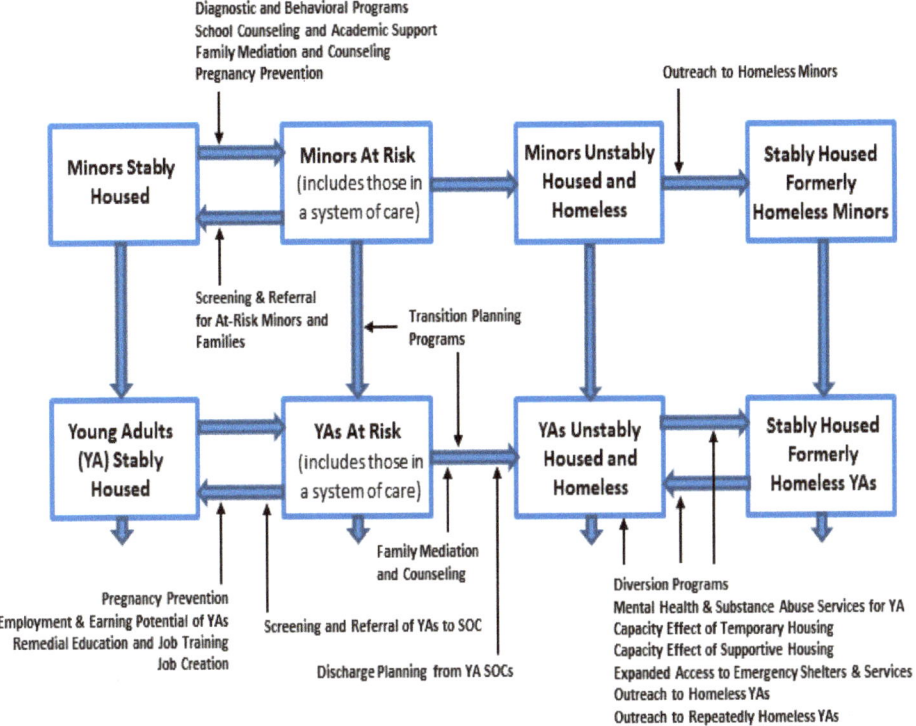

Figure 3. Interventions Available to Model Users and Their Assumed Points of Impact.

3.2. Model Interface

An interface was created to enable users to directly access the model without being familiar with the Stella modeling language. Figure 4 displays the Simulator Dashboard screen on which users can select initiatives to include in simulated strategies and compare high-level results achieved with different strategies. Figure 5 displays one of the screens with more detailed simulation results, on which users can "drill down" to better understand what is going on in the different simulations. That screen features specific results related to young adults' housing instability.

3.3. Using the Simulator

Users work from the simulator's Dashboard to set up and run scenarios with various interventions selected. They typically start by generating a baseline run to serve as a basis for comparison. As indicated earlier, the baseline simulation reflects an underlying set of assumptions that the number of minors and young adults experiencing housing instability and homelessness in Connecticut is likely to remain stable for the foreseeable future. As indicated earlier, this was supported by the CMDT and other various experts we spoke with based on recent trends and limited expected changes in exogenous factors that affect youth homelessness. This work was completed just before COVID-19 struck. COVID-19 had some immediate effects such as delays in receiving services (which was also true of a whole range of other services) and reduced access to shelters and temporary housing. The

Department of Children and Families also held off on discharging clients when they turned 18 during the quarantine. Our impression is that these effects were transitory and expect that the policy conclusions based on the types of results reported below would remain the same despite COVID-19′s impacts.

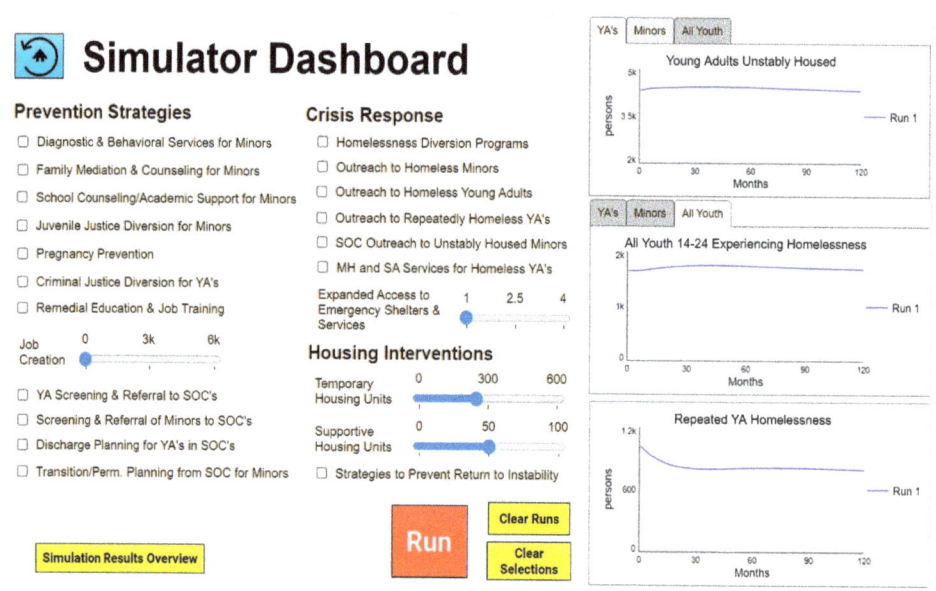

Figure 4. Simulator Dashboard Screen.

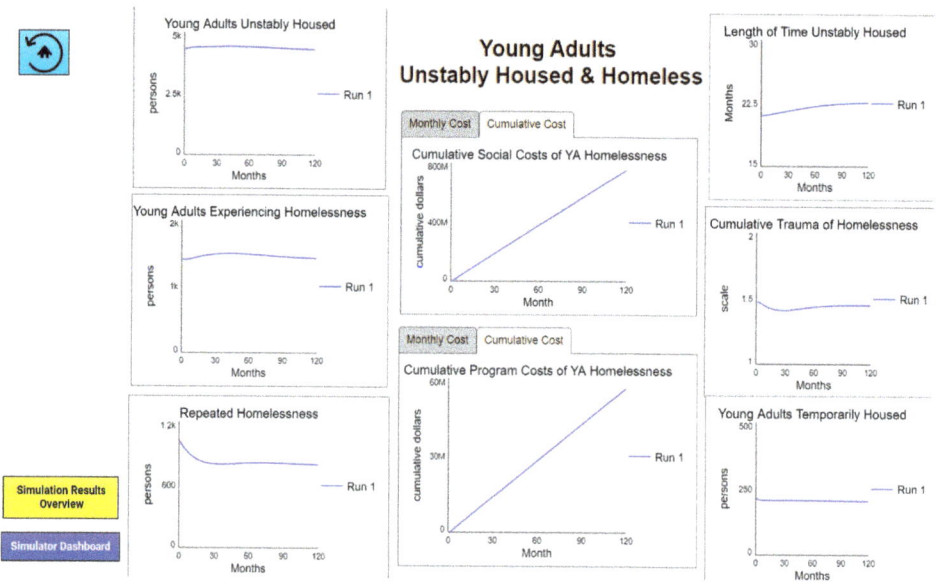

Figure 5. Detailed Results Screen for Young Adults' Housing Instability.

4. Discussion

Some of the benefits of dealing with Connecticut's youth homelessness challenge came from the model's development itself. The CMDT was a diverse group of stakeholders representing multiple state agencies and non-profit organizations concerned with various aspects of youth homelessness, as well as young adults who had experience with housing instability and homelessness. Though CMDT members were coming from different agencies that each had their own agenda, team members agreed they were seeking a holistic approach to the problem rather than representing their agencies' narrower perspectives. Seeing the problem as a coherent whole rather than in fragments and sharing insights had an immediate effect in producing a collective understanding of the need for comprehensive strategies rather than policies that focused separately on one aspect of homelessness or another.

Once developed, the model with its interface was employed in a series of Learning Labs. Approximately 20 people attended the first Learning Lab and a core group of 15 stakeholders continue to use the model to develop a strategy for addressing youth homelessness across the state of Connecticut. During the Learning Labs, participants spoke of a number of benefits and insights gained through using the simulation model:

- As with the CMDT's experience in developing the model, stakeholders spoke of the process of using the model as valuable, extremely important, and different from anything that they have experienced before. They attributed this to the process of bringing people together who have different experiences and perspectives and who come from diverse sectors of the system. For example, attendees of the Learning Lab included policy-makers, front-line staff, and people with lived experience from different parts of the system, including schools/education, criminal/juvenile justice, mental health, employment, child welfare, homelessness crisis response, and housing. Some of these system stakeholders had worked together, but many had not. Additionally, young people with lived experience of homelessness and housing instability both contributed to the development of the model and also co-led some of the Learning Labs. Their engagement and unique perspectives were greatly valued by other stakeholders, resulting in a rich dialogue and new understanding of why programs may or may not be working.
- A big "ah-ha" moment for stakeholders was a shift in thinking about the time it takes to see their desired changes in outcomes after implementing an intervention. They realized that they may not see the positive effect of interventions until several years down the line. This realization brought about some reflection regarding how they may be shifting strategies too early because they had believed the strategies to be ineffective when reviewing short-term performance metrics that indicated no change. In fact, those strategies may actually be working, and anticipating a longer-term view of change was important. One of the stakeholders commented: "I'm telling other people about the model. It is really groundbreaking if we can think this way. It made me think differently about time—how it might take more time for an intervention to have its effect." This insight also resulted in a dialogue about how to communicate with policymakers and funders that some programs will take time before seeing the desired effect so that funding is maintained over the necessary period.
- Stakeholders were able to test a widely-held theory that youth homelessness could be significantly reduced by targeting funding and resources to increase the capacity of the current crisis response system (e.g., outreach, diversion, and housing programs). They were surprised to see that this strategy was both expensive and had only a limited impact. When they added prevention efforts to this strategy, they observed a significant cost reduction and much higher impact on reducing youth homelessness. The insight that 'housing helped less than prevention' was not what they had expected. They learned that a balance of preventive programs with crisis response interventions was most effective in reducing youth homelessness. They also learned that some interventions may be redundant, and adding interventions may achieve diminishing

returns. This led to the insight that it is important to be very selective in crafting combined strategies when resources are limited and coordinating programs from different agencies is a challenge. The model provides a framework for experimenting with different combinations of interventions to find the most efficient one for reaching a particular goal.
- They learned there are unintended consequences to some strategies that can result in greater, rather than fewer, young people experiencing homelessness. For example, when screening and referrals of minors and young adults to Systems of Care (SOCs) were increased, more youth/young adults experienced homelessness than in the baseline simulation. They discovered that this was the result of having more young people leaving those Systems of Care without adequate discharge planning and falling into unstable housing and homelessness. Increased referrals to SOCs had to be combined with expanded discharge planning in order to avoid that negative effect.
- Finally, the stakeholders using the model learned that youth homelessness could not be driven to zero regardless of how many resources are applied. Experience across a large number of simulations suggested that the maximum reduction in homelessness was around 67%. When the number of youths experiencing homelessness is significantly reduced, the ones remaining will be those with more significant problems that will make them more difficult to house.

There are naturally some limitations to the work. One is that the model is a learning environment, not a program planning or predictive tool. The state-level model lacks the precision and explicit variables to plan the implementation of programs. Insights gained from using the model can guide planning, but other tools are required to plan the implementation of indicated interventions. Taking the model down to the regional level will still face the same limitation. Using data specific to each region will adjust the model parameters so that the simulation results will be on a scale familiar to regional users. However, the use of the model will still be for learning rather than planning the specific details of interventions.

Another limitation is the baseline assumption that the rates of youth experiencing unstable housing and homelessness will remain constant in the absence of new or stronger interventions. This is an assumption that may have to be revisited periodically to see if those rates are remaining stable or if they are trending upward or downward. Those trends could be the result of changes in the state's environment (e.g., economic stresses) or as a result of programmatic interventions that have an impact on youth homelessness. The model's parameters would have to be adjusted to reflect the causes of those trends.

5. Conclusions

The System Dynamics simulation model has achieved its initial goal of engaging Connecticut stakeholders in the search for leverage points for reducing youth homelessness. A large number of people participated, including representatives of agencies and organizations dealing with various causes and consequences of youth homelessness and young people with lived experience with the problem. Their participation has produced shared insights that enable them to pursue solutions in a more coherent manner. There is now an extensively tested decision-support tool in place that enables additional stakeholders to explore combinations of interventions for reducing youth homelessness.

The Learning Labs using the statewide model have continued. The Learning Labs have focused on: (a) the CMDT building their capacity and confidence in using the simulation model and sharing the model with others; (b) learning and identifying key system insights from using the model; and (c) developing a plan for engaging key system stakeholders in using the model as a learning- and decision-support tool. For example, some initial model insights highlight a need for engaging stakeholders in changing policies and practices concerning discharge planning from Systems of Care, as well as advocating for potential reallocation or leveraging of resources. Future Learning Labs would engage important decision makers on these issues. In addition, the CMDT plans to facilitate regional use of the model at the level of Connecticut's eight regions. Each region will be given a spreadsheet to enter its own data and have the model simulate the results of various strategies for its region.

Supplementary Materials: The following supporting information can be downloaded at: https://www.mdpi.com/article/10.3390/systems11030163/s1, Table S1: Initial Values of Statuses (Stocks) in the Model; Table S2: Flow Rates and Intervention Assumptions, (A): Minors at Risk (Including in SOC's), (B): Young Adults at Risk (Including in SOC's), (C): Minors Unstably Housed or Homeless, (D): Young Adults Unstably Housed or Homeless, (E): Formerly Homeless Stably Housed Minors, (F): Formerly Homeless Stably Housed Young Adults; Table S3: Flow Variables Developed by Model Calibration or from Data Dashboards; Table S4: Cost Data Used on the Youth Homelessness Model.

Author Contributions: The phase 1 model building process was facilitated by H.I.M.; Model conceptualization in phase 2 was done by both G.B.H. and H.I.M.; literature review and data acquisition were done by H.I.M.; H.I.M. managed interactions with the CMDT advisory panel and other key stakeholders; G.B.H. developed the quantitative model; the interface was designed by both G.B.H. and H.I.M.; both G.B.H. and H.I.M. wrote sections of the article. All authors have read and agreed to the published version of the manuscript.

Funding: Melville Charitable Trust, New Haven, CT, USA (https://melvilletrust.org/); Hartford Foundation for Public Giving, Hartford, CT, USA (https://www.hfpg.org/); US Department of Housing & Urban Development, Washington, DC, USA (https://www.hud.gov/).

Institutional Review Board Statement: The study was approved by the Institute for Community Research Institutional Review Board (No. 2017-01).

Data Availability Statement: All relevant data and their sources are cited in the Supplementary Materials.

Acknowledgments: The Core Modeling and Data Team (CMDT) played an essential role in developing and using the model. Membership organizations are listed in Appendix A. Rebecca Niles led a number of the Learning Labs based on the simulation model.

Conflicts of Interest: The authors declare no conflict of interest.

Appendix A

Connecticut Organizations Represented on the Core Modeling and Data Team

1. Career Resources/Capital Workforce Partners
2. Center for Children's Advocacy
3. CT Court Support Services Division
4. CT Department of Children & Families
5. CT Department of Housing
6. CT DMHAS—Young Adult Services
7. Journey Home
8. Partnership for Strong Communities
9. The Connection, Inc.
10. Tow Youth Justice Institute
11. University of New Haven
12. Youth Action Hub/Institute for Community Research

Appendix B

Intervention Descriptions

Prevention	Legislation, Policy and Investment Strategies That Build Assets and Address System Gaps That Increase the Risk of Homelessness.
School Counseling and Academic Support for Minors	Improves graduation rates and academic performance, reduces fraction of minors at risk by 20%, and increases later employability of young adults, also by 20%.

Prevention	Legislation, Policy and Investment Strategies That Build Assets and Address System Gaps That Increase the Risk of Homelessness.
Diagnostic and Behavioral Services for Minors	Reduces the fraction of minors at risk by 20% by identifying and providing services for various conditions.
Family Mediation and Counseling for Minors	Reduces fraction of minors at risk by 20% and increases ability of young adults to remain with family.
Screening and Referral of Minors to Systems of Care	Increases the fraction of minors at risk entering Systems of Care by 20%.
Young Adult Screening and Referral to Systems of Care	Increases fraction of at-risk young adults entering Systems of Care and receiving services by 50%.
Juvenile Justice Diversion for Minors	Reduces likelihood of juvenile justice involvement of minors and later criminal justice involvement as young adults by 50%.
Criminal Justice Diversion of Young Adults	Halves likelihood of young adults' involvement with criminal justice system and affects employability and ability to remain with family and, in turn, reduces the fraction at risk by 17%.
Pregnancy Prevention	Reduces fraction of both minors and young adults at risk due to pregnancy and parenting by 20%.
Remedial Education and Job Training	Doubles employability of young adults and reduces fraction at risk by 17% (Impact will depend on job creation intervention).
Job Creation	Will increase availability of jobs and is necessary for job training to have its full impact on fraction of young adults at risk.
Transition/Permanency Planning from Systems of Care for Minors	Doubles the fraction of minors aging out of Systems of Care going into appropriate programs as young adults.
Young Adult Discharge Planning in Systems of Care	Reduces fraction of young adults leaving Systems of Care becoming unstably housed or homeless by half.
Crisis Response	Policies and Practice to Identify Young People Experiencing Housing Instability or Homelessness and to Intervene Early by Connecting Them to Housing and Supportive Services.
Systems of Care Outreach to Unstably Housed Minors	Increases flow of unstably housed minors into Systems of Care that can provide services by 50%.
Outreach to Homeless Minors	Connects 50% more minors experiencing homelessness to housing.
Outreach to Homeless Young Adults	Connects 50% more young adults experiencing homelessness to housing, preventing persistent homelessness.
Outreach to Repeatedly Homeless Young Adults	Outreach with special emphasis on young adults who have experienced repeated homelessness to connect them to housing.
Diversion Programs	Increases the number of young adults who can receive diversion funds that keep unstably housed young adults from experiencing homelessness, reduces fraction of unstably housed who might experience homelessness by 20%. Examples: financial, utility, and/or rental assistance, short-term case management, conflict mediation, connection to jobs and mainstream services, and housing search.
Expand Access to Emergency Housing and Services	Increases the number of emergency beds/apartments to serve a larger number of young adults experiencing first time and repeated homelessness.
Mental Health and Substance Abuse Services for Homeless Young Adults	Services that reduce cumulative trauma of being homeless by half and thereby reduce the fraction of young adults who experience repeated homelessness. Examples: Mental health services and substance use programs delivered by agencies or community providers.

Housing Stability	Initiatives and Support for People Who Have Experienced Homelessness That Allows Them to Exit Homelessness Quickly and Never Experience It Again.
Expand Temporary Housing Capacity	Increase the capacity of temporary housing programs to serve a larger number of young adults experiencing first time and persistent homelessness. Examples: Transitional housing, host homes, DMHAS Young Adult Services' supervised apartments, and rapid re-housing programs that are time-limited and aim to stably rehouse young people by providing them with housing/rental assistance and supports for health and well-being, education, and employment.
Expand Long-Term Supportive Housing	Make additional housing units available for young adults experiencing persistent homelessness who require extensive additional services to keep them stably housed. Examples: Permanent supportive housing that combines affordable housing assistance with voluntary support services.
Preventing Returns to Homelessness	Reduce the flow of young adults by half who had achieved stable housing and fell back to unstable housing with short-term rental assistance and other supports. Examples: Temporary housing programs that offer short-term assistance to young adults who experience a housing crisis (loss of job/roommate, increased rent, etc.) within a year of exiting their programs.

References

1. Morton, M.H.; Dworsky, A.; Matjasko, J.L.; Curry, S.R.; Schlueter, D.; Chávez, R.; Farrell, A.F. Prevalence and Correlates of Youth Homelessness in the United States. *J. Adolesc. Health* **2018**, *62*, 14–21. [CrossRef] [PubMed]
2. USICH. *Key Federal Terms and Definitions of Homelessness among Youth*; United States Interagency Council on Homelessness: Washington, DC, USA, 2018. Available online: https://www.usich.gov/resources/uploads/asset_library/Federal-Definitions-of-Youth-Homelessness.pdf (accessed on 4 September 2022).
3. Fraser, B.; Pierse, N.; Chisholm, E.; Cook, H. LGBTIQ+ Homelessness: A Review of the Literature. *Int. J. Environ. Res. Public Health* **2019**, *16*, 2677. [CrossRef] [PubMed]
4. Ecker, J.; Aubry, T.; Sylvestre, J. Pathways Into Homelessness Among LGBTQ2S Adults. *J. Homosex.* **2019**, *67*, 1625–1643. [CrossRef] [PubMed]
5. Britton, L.; Pilnik, L. Preventing Homelessness for System-Involved Youth. *Juv. Fam. Court J.* **2018**, *69*, 19–33. [CrossRef]
6. Edidin, J.P.; Ganim, Z.; Hunter, S.J.; Karnik, N.S. The mental and physical health of homeless youth: A literature review. *Child Psychiatry Hum. Dev.* **2012**, *43*, 354–375. [CrossRef]
7. Auerswald, C.L.; Lin, J.S.; Parriott, A. Six-year mortality in a street-recruited cohort of homeless youth in San Francisco, California. *PeerJ* **2016**, *4*, e1909. [CrossRef]
8. Kulik, D.M.; Gaetz, S.; Crowe, C.; Ford-Jones, E. Homeless youth's overwhelming health burden: A review of the literature. *Paediatr. Child Health* **2011**, *16*, e43–e47. [CrossRef]
9. Roy, É.; Haley, N.; Leclerc, P.; Sochanski, B.; Boudreau, J.-F.; Boivin, J.-F. Mortality in a cohort of street youth in Montreal. *Jama* **2004**, *292*, 569–574. [CrossRef]
10. Srivastava, A.; Rusow, J.A.; Holguin, M.; Semborski, S.; Onasch-Vera, L.; Wilson, N.; Rice, E. Exchange and Survival Sex, Dating Apps, Gender Identity, and Sexual Orientation Among Homeless Youth in Los Angeles. *J. Prim. Prev.* **2019**, *40*, 561–568. [CrossRef]
11. Santa Maria, D.; Hernandez, D.C.; Arlinghaus, K.R.; Gallardo, K.R.; Maness, S.B.; Kendzor, D.E.; Reitzel, L.R.; Businelle, M.S. Current Age, Age at First Sex, Age at First Homelessness, and HIV Risk Perceptions Predict Sexual Risk Behaviors among Sexually Active Homeless Adults. *Int. J. Environ. Res. Public Health* **2018**, *15*, 218. [CrossRef]
12. Walls, N.E.; Bell, S. Correlates of Engaging in Survival Sex among Homeless Youth and Young Adults. *J. Sex Res.* **2011**, *48*, 423–436. [CrossRef] [PubMed]
13. Rosenthal, D.; Rotheram-Borus, M.J.; Batterham, P.; Mallett, S.; Rice, E.; Milburn, N.G. Housing stability over two years and HIV risk among newly homeless youth. *AIDS Behav.* **2007**, *11*, 831–841. [CrossRef] [PubMed]
14. Perlman, S.; Willard, J.; Herbers, J.E.; Cutuli, J.; Eyrich Garg, K.M. Youth homelessness: Prevalence and mental health correlates. *J. Soc. Soc. Work Res.* **2014**, *5*, 361–377. [CrossRef]
15. Rosenberg, R.; Kim, Y. Aging out of foster care: Homelessness, post-secondary education, and employment. *J. Public Child Welf.* **2018**, *12*, 99–115. [CrossRef]
16. Manfra, L. Impact of Homelessness on School Readiness Skills and Early Academic Achievement: A Systematic Review of the Literature. *Early Child. Educ. J.* **2019**, *47*, 239–249. [CrossRef]
17. Samuels, G.M.; Cerven, C.; Curry, S.; Robinson, S.R.; Patel, S. *Missed Opportunities in Youth Pathways through Homelessness*; Chapin Hall at the University of Chicago: Chicago, IL, USA, 2019. Available online: https://voicesofyouthcount.org/wp-content/uploads/2019/05/ChapinHall_VoYC_Youth-Pathways-FINAL.pdf (accessed on 7 September 2022).

18. Fowler, P.J.; Toro, P.A.; Miles, B.W. Pathways to and from homelessness and associated psychosocial outcomes among adolescents leaving the foster care system. *Am. J. Public Health* **2009**, *99*, 1453–1458. [CrossRef] [PubMed]
19. Census. *Population Projections for CT*; Connecticut Data Collaborative: Hartford, CT, USA, 2015.
20. CCEH. *Connecticut Counts: Annual Point-In-Time Count and Youth Outreach and Count*; Connecticut Coalition to End Homelessness: Hartford, CT, USA, 2019. Available online: https://cceh.org/wp-content/uploads/2019/06/PIT_2019.pdf (accessed on 21 August 2022).
21. CTDOH. *Opening Doors for Youth 2.0: An Action Plan to Provide All Connecticut Youth and Young Adults with Safe, Stable Homes and Opportunities*; Connecticut Department of Housing: Hartford, CT, USA, 2017. Available online: https://cca-ct.org/wp-content/uploads/2012/07/OpeningDoorsforYouth_FullPlan_03-25-2015.pdf (accessed on 14 September 2022).
22. USICH. *Criteria and Benchmarks for Achieving the Goal of Ending Youth Homelessness*; United States Interagency Council on Homelessness: Washington, DC, USA, 2018. Available online: https://www.usich.gov/resources/uploads/asset_library/Youth-Criteria-and-Benchmarks-revised-Feb-2018.pdf (accessed on 22 August 2022).
23. Andersen, D.F.; Vennix, J.A.; Richardson, G.P.; Rouwette, E.A. Group model building: Problem structuring, policy simulation and decision support. *J. Oper. Res. Soc.* **2007**, *58*, 691–694. [CrossRef]
24. Hovmand, P.S. *Group Model Building and Community-Based System Dynamics Process*; Springer: New York, NY, USA, 2014.
25. Gullett, H.L.; Brown, G.L.; Collins, D.; Halko, M.; Gotler, R.S.; Stange, K.C.; Hovmand, P.S. Using community-based system dynamics to address structural racism in community health improvement. *J. Public Health Manag. Pract.* **2022**, *28*, S130–S137. [CrossRef]
26. Wong, N.T.; Zimmerman, M.A.; Parker, E.A. A Typology of Youth Participation and Empowerment for Child and Adolescent Health Promotion. *Am. J. Community Psychol.* **2010**, *46*, 100–114. [CrossRef]
27. Cuppen, E. Stakeholder analysis. In *Foresight in Organizations*; van der Duin, P., Ed.; Routledge: New York, NY, USA, 2016; pp. 208–214.
28. Hovmand, P.S.; Andersen, D.F.; Rouwette, E.; Richardson, G.P.; Rux, K.; Calhoun, A. Group model building scripts as a collaborative planning tool. *Syst. Res. Behav. Sci.* **2012**, *29*, 179–193. [CrossRef]
29. Luna-Reyes, L.F.; Martinez-Moyano, I.J.; Pardo, T.A.; Cresswell, A.M.; Andersen, D.F.; Richardson, G.P. Anatomy of a group model-building intervention: Building dynamic theory from case study research. *Syst. Dyn. Rev. J. Syst. Dyn. Soc.* **2006**, *22*, 291–320. [CrossRef]
30. Hovmand, P.; Rouwette, E.; Andersen, D.; Richardson, G. *Scriptapedia*; Wikibooks: San Francisco, CA, USA, 2015. Available online: https://en.wikibooks.org/wiki/Scriptapedia (accessed on 7 March 2023).
31. ISEE Systems. Stella Architect. 2017. [Computer Software]. Available online: https://www.iseesystems.com/Store/Products/Stella-Architect.Aspx (accessed on 7 March 2023).
32. Stemler, S.E. Content analysis. In *Emerging Trends in the Social and Behavioral Sciences: An Interdisciplinary, Searchable, and Linkable Resource*; Scott, R.A., Kosslyn, S.M., Eds.; John Wiley & Sons, Inc.: Hoboken, NJ, USA, 2015; pp. 1–14. [CrossRef]
33. Andersen, D.F.; Richardson, G.P. Scripts for group model building. *Syst. Dyn. Rev. J. Syst. Dyn. Soc.* **1997**, *13*, 107–129. [CrossRef]
34. Larkin, H.; Park, J. Adverse childhood experiences (ACEs), service use, and service helpfulness among people experiencing homelessness. *Fam. Soc.* **2012**, *93*, 85–93. [CrossRef]
35. Herman, D.B.; Susser, E.S.; Struening, E.L.; Link, B.L. Adverse childhood experiences: Are they risk factors for adult homelessness? *Am. J. Public Health* **1997**, *87*, 249–255. [CrossRef]
36. Oppenheimer, S.C.; Nurius, P.S.; Green, S. Homelessness history impacts on health outcomes and economic and risk behavior intermediaries: New insights from population data. *Fam. Soc.* **2016**, *97*, 230–242. [CrossRef]
37. Anda, R.F.; Felitti, V.J.; Bremner, J.D.; Walker, J.D.; Whitfield, C.; Perry, B.D.; Dube, S.R.; Giles, W.H. The enduring effects of abuse and related adverse experiences in childhood. *Eur. Arch. Psychiatry Clin. Neurosci.* **2006**, *256*, 174–186. [CrossRef]
38. Crouch, E.; Strompolis, M.; Bennett, K.J.; Morse, M.; Radcliff, E. Assessing the interrelatedness of multiple types of adverse childhood experiences and odds for poor health in South Carolina adults. *Child Abus. Negl.* **2017**, *65*, 204–211. [CrossRef]
39. Dong, M.; Anda, R.F.; Felitti, V.J.; Dube, S.R.; Williamson, D.F.; Thompson, T.J.; Loo, C.M.; Giles, W.H. The interrelatedness of multiple forms of childhood abuse, neglect, and household dysfunction. *Child Abus. Negl.* **2004**, *28*, 771–784. [CrossRef]
40. Dupre, M.E. Educational differences in health risks and illness over the life course: A test of cumulative disadvantage theory. *Soc. Sci. Res.* **2008**, *37*, 1253–1266. [CrossRef]
41. Rich-Edwards, J.W.; Mason, S.; Rexrode, K.; Spiegelman, D.; Hibert, E.; Kawachi, I.; Jun, H.J.; Wright, R.J. Physical and sexual abuse in childhood as predictors of early-onset cardiovascular events in women. *Circulation* **2012**, *126*, 920–927. [CrossRef]
42. Roy, A.; Janal, M.N.; Roy, M. Childhood trauma and prevalence of cardiovascular disease in patients with type 1 diabetes. *Psychosom. Med.* **2010**, *72*, 833–838. [CrossRef] [PubMed]
43. Waite, R.; Davey, M.; Lynch, L. Self-rated health and association with ACEs. *J. Behav. Health* **2013**, *2*, 197–205. [CrossRef]
44. Roos, L.E.; Mota, N.; Afifi, T.O.; Katz, L.Y.; Distasio, J.; Sareen, J. Relationship between adverse childhood experiences and homelessness and the impact of axis I and II disorders. *Am. J. Public Health* **2013**, *103*, S275–S281. [CrossRef] [PubMed]
45. Sacks, V.; Murphey, D. *The Prevalence of Adverse Childhood Experiences, Nationally, by State, and by Race or Ethnicity*; Child Trends: Bethesda, MD, USA, 2018. Available online: https://www.childtrends.org/publications/prevalence-adverse-childhood-experiences-nationally-state-race-ethnicity (accessed on 23 August 2022).

46. Sacks, V.; Murphey, D.; Moore, K. *Adverse Childhood Experiences: National and State-level Prevalence*; Child Trends: Bethesda, MD, USA, 2014. Available online: https://www.childtrends.org/wp-content/uploads/2014/07/Brief-adverse-childhood-experiences_FINAL.pdf (accessed on 23 August 2022).
47. Tucciarone, J.T., Jr. Adverse Childhood Experiences, Homeless Chronicity, and Age at Onset of Homelessness. *Electron. Diss.* **2019**, 3534. Available online: https://dc.etsu.edu/etd/3534 (accessed on 23 August 2022).
48. Turner, H.A.; Merrick, M.T.; Finkelhor, D.; Hamby, S.; Shattuck, A.; Henly, M. *The Prevalence of Safe, Stable, Nurturing Relationships Among Children and Adolescents*; US Department of Justice: Washington, DC, USA, 2017. Available online: https://ojjdp.ojp.gov/sites/g/files/xyckuh176/files/pubs/249197.pdf (accessed on 23 August 2022).
49. Radcliff, E.; Crouch, E.; Strompolis, M.; Srivastav, A. Homelessness in childhood and adverse childhood experiences (ACEs). *Matern. Child Health J.* **2019**, *23*, 811–820. [CrossRef] [PubMed]
50. Brakenhoff, B.; Jang, B.; Slesnick, N.; Snyder, A. Longitudinal predictors of homelessness: Findings from the National Longitudinal Survey of Youth-97. *J. Youth Stud.* **2015**, *18*, 1015–1034. [CrossRef] [PubMed]
51. Heerde, J.A.; Bailey, J.A.; Kelly, A.B.; McMorris, B.J.; Patton, G.C.; Toumbourou, J.W. Life-course predictors of homelessness from adolescence into adulthood: A population-based cohort study. *J. Adolesc.* **2021**, *91*, 15–24. [CrossRef] [PubMed]
52. Martijn, C.; Sharpe, L. Pathways to youth homelessness. *Soc. Sci. Med.* **2006**, *62*, 1–12. [CrossRef]
53. Thompson, S.J.; Pillai, V.K. Determinants of runaway episodes among adolescents using crisis shelter services. *Int. J. Soc. Welf.* **2006**, *15*, 142–149. [CrossRef]
54. Van den Bree, M.B.; Shelton, K.; Bonner, A.; Moss, S.; Thomas, H.; Taylor, P.J. A longitudinal population-based study of factors in adolescence predicting homelessness in young adulthood. *J. Adolesc. Health* **2009**, *45*, 571–578. [CrossRef]
55. Courtney, M.E.; Dworsky, A.; Brown, A.; Cary, C.; Love, K.; Vorhies, V. *Midwest Evaluation of the Adult Functioning of Former Foster Youth: Outcomes at Age 26*; Chapin Hall Center for Children: Chicago, IL, USA, 2011.
56. Hail-Jares, K.; Vichta-Ohlsen, R.; Butler, T.; Dunne, A. Psychological distress among young people who are couchsurfing: An exploratory analysis of correlated factors. *J. Soc. Distress Homelessness* **2021**, 1–5. [CrossRef]
57. Hail-Jares, K.; Vichta-Ohlsen, R.; Nash, C. Safer inside? Comparing the experiences and risks faced by young people who couch-surf and sleep rough. *J. Youth Stud.* **2021**, *24*, 305–322. [CrossRef]
58. McLoughlin, P.J. Couch surfing on the margins: The reliance on temporary living arrangements as a form of homelessness amongst school-aged home leavers. *J. Youth Stud.* **2013**, *16*, 521–545. [CrossRef]
59. Moore, S.; Landvogt, K. Couch-surfing limbo: 'Your life stops when they say you have to find somewhere else to go'. *Parity* **2016**, *29*, 17.
60. Petry, L.; Hill, C.; Milburn, N.; Rice, E. Who Is Couch-Surfing and Who Is on the Streets? Disparities Among Racial and Sexual Minority Youth in Experiences of Homelessness. *J. Adolesc. Health* **2022**, *70*, 743–750. [CrossRef] [PubMed]
61. Gultekin, L.E.; Brush, B.L.; Ginier, E.; Cordom, A.; Dowdell, E.B. Health risks and outcomes of homelessness in school-age children and youth: A scoping review of the literature. *J. Sch. Nurs.* **2020**, *36*, 10–18. [CrossRef] [PubMed]
62. Castellow, J.; Kloos, B.; Townley, G. Previous Homelessness as a Risk Factor for Recovery from Serious Mental Illnesses. *Community Ment. Health J.* **2015**, *51*, 674–684. [CrossRef]
63. Toros, H.; Flaming, D.; Burns, P. *Early Intervention to Prevent Persistent Homelessness: Predictive Models for Identifying Unemployed Workers and Young Adults Who Become Persistently Homeless*; SSRN: Rochester, NY, USA, 2019. [CrossRef]
64. Zerger, S.; Strehlow, A.J.; Gundlapalli, A.V. Homeless Young Adults and Behavioral Health: An Overview. *Am. Behav. Sci.* **2008**, *51*, 824–841. [CrossRef]
65. Shinn, M.; Schteingart, J.S.; Williams, N.C.; Carlin-Mathis, J.; Bialo-Karagis, N.; Becker-Klein, R.; Weitzman, B.C. Long-term associations of homelessness with children's well-being. *Am. Behav. Sci.* **2008**, *51*, 789–809. [CrossRef]
66. Nyamathi, A.; Hudson, A.; Greengold, B.; Slagle, A.; Marfisee, M.; Khalilifard, F.; Leake, B. Correlates of substance use severity among homeless youth. *J. Child Adolesc. Psychiatr. Nurs.* **2010**, *23*, 214–222. [CrossRef]
67. Rosenthal, D.; Mallett, S.; Gurrin, L.; Milburn, N.; Rotheram-Borus, M.J. Changes over time among homeless young people in drug dependency, mental illness and their co-morbidity. *Psychol. Health Med.* **2007**, *12*, 70–80. [CrossRef]
68. Whitbeck, L.B.; Hoyt, D.R.; Johnson, K.D.; Chen, X. Victimization and posttraumatic stress disorder among runaway and homeless adolescents. *Violence Vict.* **2007**, *22*, 721–734. [CrossRef] [PubMed]
69. Russell, M.; Soong, W.; Nicholls, C.; Griffiths, J.; Curtis, K.; Follett, D.; Smith, W.; Waters, F. Homelessness youth and mental health service utilization: A long-term follow-up study. *Early Interv. Psychiatry* **2021**, *15*, 563–568. [CrossRef] [PubMed]
70. Davis, J.P.; Diguiseppi, G.; De Leon, J.; Prindle, J.; Sedano, A.; Rivera, D.; Henwood, B.; Rice, E. Understanding pathways between PTSD, homelessness, and substance use among adolescents. *Psychol. Addict. Behav.* **2019**, *33*, 467. [CrossRef] [PubMed]
71. Cohen-Cline, H.; Jones, K.; Vartanian, K. Direct and indirect pathways between childhood instability and adult homelessness in a low-income population. *Child. Youth Serv. Rev.* **2021**, *120*, 105707. [CrossRef]
72. Brothers, S.; Lin, J.; Schonberg, J.; Drew, C.; Auerswald, C. Food insecurity among formerly homeless youth in supportive housing: A social-ecological analysis of a structural intervention. *Soc. Sci. Med.* **2020**, *245*, 112724. [CrossRef]
73. Schneider, M.; Brisson, D.; Burnes, D. Do We Really Know how Many Are Homeless?: An Analysis of the Point-In-Time Homelessness Count. *Fam. Soc.* **2016**, *97*, 321–329. [CrossRef]

74. Hallett, R.E. Living doubled-up: Influence of residential environment on educational participation. *Educ. Urban Soc.* **2012**, *44*, 371–391. [CrossRef]
75. Pergamit, M.; Cunningham, M.K.; Burt, M.R.; Lee, P.; Howell, B.; Bertumen, K.D. Counting homeless youth: Promising practices from the Youth Count! initiative. Urban Institute: Washington, DC, USA, 2013. Available online: https://www.urban.org/sites/default/files/publication/23871/412876-Counting-Homeless-Youth.PDF (accessed on 7 September 2022).

Disclaimer/Publisher's Note: The statements, opinions and data contained in all publications are solely those of the individual author(s) and contributor(s) and not of MDPI and/or the editor(s). MDPI and/or the editor(s) disclaim responsibility for any injury to people or property resulting from any ideas, methods, instructions or products referred to in the content.

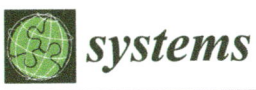

Article

Use of System Dynamics Modelling for Evidence-Based Decision Making in Public Health Practice

Abraham George [1,*], Padmanabhan Badrinath [1], Peter Lacey [2], Chris Harwood [2], Alex Gray [2], Paul Turner [2] and Davinia Springer [1]

1. Public Health Department, Kent County Council, Sessions House, County Road, Maidstone ME14 1XQ, Kent, UK; Padmanabhan.badrinath@kent.gov.uk (P.B.); davinia.springer@kent.gov.uk (D.S.)
2. Whole Systems Partnership, 8 York Place, Knaresborough HG5 0AA, North Yorkshire, UK; peter.lacey@thewholesystem.co.uk (P.L.); chris.harwood@thewholesystem.co.uk (C.H.); alex.gray@thewholesystem.co.uk (A.G.); paul.turner@thewholesystem.co.uk (P.T.)
* Correspondence: abraham.george@kent.gov.uk; Tel.: +44-300-041-6137

Abstract: In public health, the routine use of linear forecasting, which restricts our ability to understand the combined effects of different interventions, demographic changes and wider health determinants, and the lack of reliable estimates for intervention impacts have limited our ability to effectively model population needs. Hence, we adopted system dynamics modelling to forecast health and care needs, assuming no change in population behaviour or determinants, then generated a "Better Health" scenario to simulate the combined impact of thirteen interventions across cohorts defined by age groups and diagnosable conditions, including "no conditions". Risk factors for the incidence of single conditions, progression toward complex needs and levels of morbidity including frailty were used to create the dynamics of the model. Incidence, prevalence and mortality for each cohort were projected over 25 years with "do nothing" and "Better Health" scenarios. The size of the "no conditions" cohort increased, and the other cohorts decreased in size. The impact of the interventions on life expectancy at birth and healthy life expectancy is significant, adding 5.1 and 5.0 years, respectively. We demonstrate the feasibility, applicability and utility of using system dynamics modelling to develop a robust case for change to invest in prevention that is acceptable to wider partners.

Keywords: system dynamics; public health; decision making; prevention; long-term conditions; resource allocation; complex systems

Citation: George, A.; Badrinath, P.; Lacey, P.; Harwood, C.; Gray, A.; Turner, P.; Springer, D. Use of System Dynamics Modelling for Evidence-Based Decision Making in Public Health Practice. *Systems* **2023**, *11*, 247. https://doi.org/10.3390/systems11050247

Academic Editor: Andreas Größler

Received: 22 March 2023
Revised: 9 May 2023
Accepted: 12 May 2023
Published: 14 May 2023

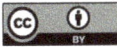

Copyright: © 2023 by the authors. Licensee MDPI, Basel, Switzerland. This article is an open access article distributed under the terms and conditions of the Creative Commons Attribution (CC BY) license (https://creativecommons.org/licenses/by/4.0/).

1. Introduction

In any local health system, data and intelligence are essential for service planning and investment/disinvestment decision making for a defined population. This will invariably include forecasting demographics, health determinants, disease distribution and health status. At present, most attempts at forecasting the future health and care needs of local populations rely on linear extrapolations, which use a series of limited assumptions to estimate the likely burden of a specific health condition or demand for a service. These assumptions include trends in population change as well as in the condition or service under investigation [1]. This method of forecasting can be described as predictive analytics, where historical data are used to make predictions about future events [2]. Prevention is a key activity in public health, and this requires robust evidence to convince decision makers to invest in prevention where the gains may not be immediately apparent.

A variety of tools explaining the public health cost-effectiveness of individual interventions have been published, providing evidence for implementing them or not [3]. However, the use of such tools may not be feasible when it comes to extrapolating directly to local systems and contexts for financial and capacity planning, and decision making for investing in prevention. While this provides a baseline estimate, it does not consider the complexities and interdependencies within populations and systems. For example, the onset of multimorbidity, the effect of intersectionality [4] and the interaction between social and economic factors. Historically, evidence-based public health relied upon estimating the health impacts of interventions separately. However, in local health systems, health planners are routinely expected to calculate the combined effect of multiple interventions to make robust decisions on resource allocation. Due to the current limitations of evidence in the field of public health, this is not always feasible. Moreover, estimates of the effectiveness of interventions are from varied populations and may not be externally valid. Traditional public health approaches are limited by our inability to assess the combined effects of multiple interventions and their interdependencies, the issues of external validity, i.e., applying the results of peer-reviewed external research to a given local population, and the use of linear extrapolation in forecasting. Hence, we need an evidence-based approach that overcomes the above limitations and addresses the key properties of complex systems, such as systems dynamics modelling (SDM). SDM is a powerful tool for assessing the impact of multiple interventions within a complex and dynamic system [5]. Jadeja et al. [6] conducted a recent systematic review that found at least 29 studies that used SDM approaches that incorporate health economic efficiency analyses for decision making, either as embedded sub-models or as cost calculations based on SDM outputs, across a variety of themes ranging from communicable diseases to behavioural and wider health determinants.

There have been previous attempts to use SDM "to align prevention efforts and maximise the effect of limited resources" [7]. A prevention impacts simulation model [8] was employed in the field of cardiovascular disease prevention to simulate the medium- and long-term impact of the various interventions. However, the simulation and the application of the SDM approach here were disease-specific. From a complex adaptive system perspective, population health needs are dynamic, and are shaped by socio-economic risk factors as well as the level of access to health and care services. Rutter et al. [9] describe the following properties of complex systems: emergence is defined as "properties of a complex system which cannot be directly predicted from the elements within it and are more than just the sum of its parts", feedback where "a change reinforces, or balances further change" and adaptation, which refers to "adjustments in behaviour in response to interventions". Such properties are the basis on which public health practice operates within a local health system. As such, it is essential that we move towards an approach that takes these complexities into account to help to answer the key questions in public health of what can be done and how it can be done in practice. Prescriptive analytics is the process of using data to determine an optimal course of action [2]. This would not only provide more accurate estimates of future health need but enable the system to better plan services and to ultimately reduce health inequalities. There are many evaluations of the use of SDM in health policy and planning; however, recent reviews [10,11] in this area have highlighted the lack of research prior to 2013. Reviews also highlighted the importance of stakeholder involvement [12], which was highly valued in our study.

Cohort modelling using SDM is an accepted methodology in improving health policy making in complex systems, using qualitative and quantitative approaches. One such international example is the "Rethink health dynamics model" developed by the Rippel Foundation [13]. The model simulates a range of scenarios for a combination of preventive interventions, including reducing health risks and improving healthcare, on a defined US population over a 40-year period. This has generated evidence on the value of these interventions, which informs the planning and decision making, including investment in prevention. To our knowledge, such an approach has not been employed across multiple programme areas within a local health system in the United Kingdom to inform policy and decision making.

The Joint Strategic Needs Assessment (JSNA) uses a range of health indicators to identify the current health and care needs of the population and is a mandatory requirement for all local authority public health departments in England. Using the JSNA [14], local system leaders can work together to understand and agree on the needs of all local people, setting the priorities for collective action. Our aim is to demonstrate and apply the use of simulation modelling in the area of routine public health intelligence, analysis and inference. In this regard, our objective is to create a population cohort model using SDM to generate necessary evidence on the value of various preventive interventions for local priority setting within the current Kent JSNA development process and intelligence tools.

2. Materials and Methods

This study was carried out in the county of Kent, positioned in the southeast of England, with a diverse population of approximately 1.6 million [15] that varies considerably in terms of deprivation and ethnicity. Like other local areas in England, Kent exhibits wide health inequalities by geography and different vulnerable groups [16]. The model outputs were presented at the level of three sub-geographical regions, which aligned with existing commissioning boundaries—West Kent, East Kent and North Kent—and for this communication, we present selected examples from North Kent.

The prototype model was co-produced with the local council public health team, and was conceptualised, tested, populated and validated over a period of 9–12 months. Two parallel group model building workshops were run alongside each other, one for adults and one for children and young people (CYP). A series of three dedicated engagement sessions were carried out for each cohort and involved between 8 and 12 experts from across health and care settings as appropriate, as well as regular contact, dialogue and checking in with group participants in between sessions. These two groups were brought together at the Better Health Workshop in 2018. The model conceptualisation was socialised and developed, followed by scenario generation and testing, which was an iterative process. Stakeholders explored the key factors that influenced better health outcomes for population health within the Kent system. Variables, interactions and feedback loops were identified and informed the design of the causal loop diagram. We discussed key interventions impacting population health outcomes, identified cohorts of interest, selected relevant peer-reviewed evidence and agreed on appropriate data sources to input into the model. Data sources are described in Table S1 [17–27]. Cohorts were based on the health or disease status of the individuals, and disease status is further broken down into individual long-term conditions (LTCs). The Kent County Council (KCC) senior team of public health specialists met to identify a combined scenario in which thirteen prevention/public health measures were achieved, including, for example, the rates of breastfeeding, the presence of adverse childhood experiences and the levels of smoking and obesity in the population. This has resulted in a 'Better Health' scenario being created that forecasts potential changes in the prevalence of a range of conditions, and, as a result, the prospects for increasing healthy life expectancy and the potential demand for health and care services. This exercise took place in January 2019 within days of the release of the NHS Long Term Plan [28] blueprint, in which many of the prevention strategies included in the model were heralded. This gave the public health specialists a 'real-time' opportunity to evidence the benefit of the Long Term Plan in our local context.

Population segmentation: Segmentation aims to categorise the population according to their health status, healthcare needs and priorities. According to this approach, groups of people share characteristics that influence the way they interact with health and care services. There is value in segmenting patients by need, complexity and severity of conditions. Segmentation was performed differently for children and adults. Segmentation for the CYP cohort was based on earlier work from the Derbyshire local health system [29]. Adult segmentation was based the work carried out by Outcome Based Health Care on behalf of NHS England [30].

For CYP, the population aged under 25 years was initially segmented into 8 cohorts and 6 age groups using a local person-level longitudinally linked population dataset known as the Kent Integrated Dataset (KID) [17]. The hierarchy for segmentation is illustrated in

Figure 1. The eight cohorts for CYP were physical enduring, mental health enduring, learning disability, physical non-enduring, mental health non-enduring, autism and attention deficit hyperactivity disorder and no identified condition. This list is comprehensive and includes 100% of all people within the KID. These cohorts are described in Table S2.

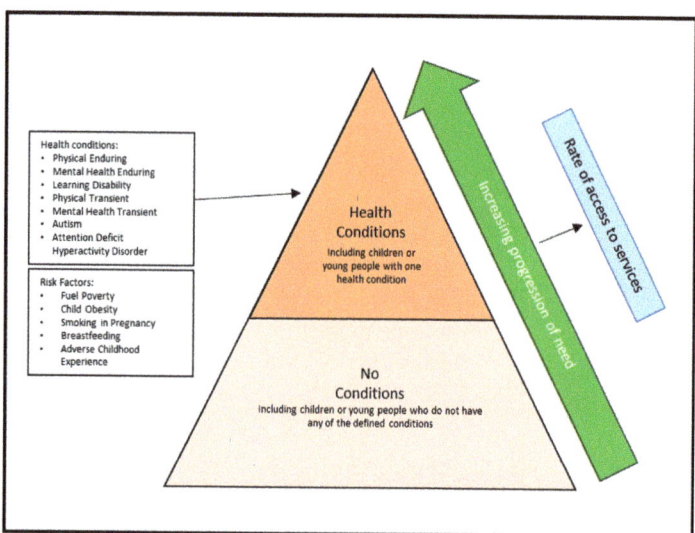

Figure 1. Children and young people (CYP) population segmentation. This figure shows the logic tree for segmentation and its relationship to cohort modelling, progression of need and service utilisation for children and young people. If a CYP is eligible for more than one cohort, they are placed within the highest need cohort. The long-term conditions included within the health conditions segment and the risk factors are outlined in text boxes.

For adults, the population was segmented using the English Longitudinal Study of Ageing (ELSA) [31] to gain insight about the progression of need and mortality. The hierarchy of segmentation is illustrated in Figure 2. The KID was also accessed in the same hierarchy to extract local prevalence and rates of access to health and care services.

The modelled adult population was segmented into five cohorts based on the presence of pre-defined health conditions or frailty. These cohorts are (1) severely frail, (2) single conditions with high/complex needs, (3) multiple conditions, (4) single conditions and (5) no conditions. In Figure 2, cohorts (2) and (3) are combined into "Multiple and Complex needs". These cohorts have an increasing progression of need, with cohort (5) as the lowest and cohort (1) as the highest need, and if an individual meets the requirements for more than one cohort, they are assigned to the highest need cohort. Cohort (1) includes those who are severely frail, which is defined as a score of 6 or more disabilities equivalent to moderate and severe frailty within the electronic frailty index [32]. Cohort (2) includes individuals with high-needs serious mental illness, severe learning disability, dementia or neurological conditions. Cohort (3) includes individuals with more than one of the following conditions: asthma, coronary heart disease, chronic obstructive pulmonary disease, type 2 diabetes, heart failure, stroke or moderate frailty. Cohort (4) includes individuals who have one of the conditions listed for cohort (3). Cohort (5) includes individuals who do not meet the requirements for cohorts (1–4). These cohorts are described in Table S3.

Model building: The model was split into two sections, CYP (under 18 years and under 25 years for selected health conditions) and adults (18 years and over). The CYP section and adult section have different structures, and the CYP section provides projected populations at age 18 years (and 25 years for selected health conditions), which form inputs to the adult section. The starting point for the model used the incidence, prevalence and mortality for each cohort in 2012 and projects forward to 2037. Initial prevalence as well as incidence and mortality for CYP and adults are shown in Tables S4–S10 [17,19,31]. This was calculated using local data analysis from the KID and nationally published longitudinal studies [17–20] The approach used epidemiological information to estimate the contributions of changes in population-level risk factors relating to health and wellbeing where the impacts were mainly on the incidence of individual conditions and cohorts. Changes in the uptake of evidence-based interventions were subsequently applied and the impacts of these interventions were mainly measured using case fatality rates over time. The model scope incorporated additional risk factors relating to socioeconomic circumstances. Tables S11 and S12 [21,31] provide details about the sources and methods that were used to accommodate socio-economic circumstances. We used socio-economic status as a proxy indicator of socioeconomic circumstances. This model examined the effects of changes in treatment uptake and risk factor trends on changes in cohort incidence, prevalence and mortality. It also explored the extent to which prevention strategies impact the incidence and mortality of cohorts.

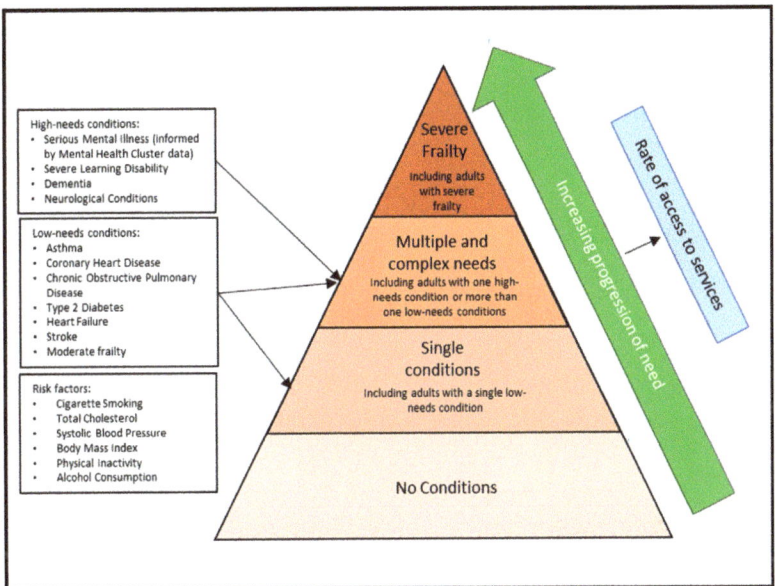

Figure 2. Adult population segmentation. This figure shows the logic tree for segmentation of the adult population and its relationship to cohort modelling, progression of need and service utilisation for adults. If an adult is eligible for more than one cohort, they are placed within the highest need cohort. The long-term conditions included within each segment and the risk factors are outlined in text boxes.

The model estimated changes in incidence and deaths related to changes in adult risk factor levels in the population. The risk factors considered were cigarette smoking, total cholesterol (TC), systolic blood pressure (SBP), body mass index (BMI), physical inactivity and alcohol consumption, and these are listed in Table S13 [21]. The Health Survey for England was used to calculate trends in the prevalence (or mean values) of each risk factor. In both the CYP and adult sections of the model, two approaches to calculating relative risk reductions from changes in risk factors were used: the regression approach and change in the population attributable fraction (PAF). In the regression model for adults, the incidences of cohorts in 2012 (the start year) were multiplied by the absolute change in risk factor level and by a regression coefficient ('beta') quantifying the estimated relative change in cohort incidence and mortality that would result from a one-unit change in risk factor level. The regression (beta) coefficients used in these analyses for key risk factors are listed in Tables S14–S16 [33–36]. A 'fixed gradient' approach was used to stabilise the estimates of risk factor change across the quintiles. Natural logarithms were used, as is conventional, in order to best describe the log-linear relationship between absolute changes in risk factor levels and relative change in incidence and mortality. The PAF approach can be interpreted as the proportion by which the incidence or mortality would be reduced if the exposure were eliminated. Worked examples for the two approaches are presented in Figures S1 and S2. Relative risks are displayed in Tables S17–S23 [37–43]. The CYP section included 5 interventions, as shown in Table 1, which were activated to test projected future impact. For each of the CYP cohorts, we estimated the proportions of incidence that were attributable to various treatments or interventions. We adopted the general approach of calculating the risk reduction from an intervention among a particular cohort by multiplying the change in the proportion of people exposed to a risk factor by the incidence rate and by the relative reduction due to the change in intervention or exposure. The approach to measuring the impact of interventions or risk factors for children was exactly the same as for adults using the PAF in most cases. The only difference was the application of a delay if the impact of an intervention in childhood occurs in adulthood. For example, the impact of changes in adverse childhood experience upon serious mental illness in adults is delayed by an average of 10 years. However, changes in smoking during pregnancy impact upon stillbirths immediately, similarly for breastfeeding upon child obesity.

Table 1. Population-level interventions to achieve "Better Health" scenario. Impacts were applied proportionally or absolutely to the baseline to achieve the target.

Intervention	Title	Baseline	Impact (%)	Number	Start	End	Target	Implementation
1	Increase breastfeeding at 6–8 weeks	45.2	20	NA	2019	2024	65.2	absolute
2	Reduce smoking in pregnancy	13.9	6	NA	2019	2025	7.9	absolute
3	Reduce child obesity	16.5	20	NA	2019	2025	13.2	proportional
4	Reduce fuel poverty in children	17.4	20	NA	2019	2022	13.9	proportional
5	Reduce ACE in childhood	24	20	NA	2020	2030	19.2	proportional
6	Improve recognition and treatment of hypertension	40	30	NA	2020	2025	28	proportional
7	Improve recognition and treatment of CVD risk	50	30	NA	2020	2025	65	proportional
8	Improve smoking cessation	20	8	NA	2019	2024	28	absolute
9	Increase weight management	25	10	NA	2019	2024	27.5	proportional
10	Alcohol screening	NA	Screening	50,000	2019	2025	NA	absolute
11	Alcohol treatment	NA	Treatment	5000	2019	2030	NA	absolute
12	Reduce fuel poverty for older people	11.5	20	NA	2019	2024	9.2	proportional
13	Reduce ACE at 15 years	7.5	20	NA	2020	2030	6	proportional

The primary outcome measures of the model were cohort incidence, prevalence and deaths projected over the model timescale and the impacts of cohort incidence and prevalence on potential demand for health and wellbeing services. The calculation of the modelled impacts of change on incidence and mortality was based on utilising two well-studied relationships. The first is a change in risk factor against a relative change in incidence and mortality, and the second is changes in intervention uptake resulting in mortality reductions. Estimates in relative risk reduction for both relationships were derived from previous randomised controlled trials and meta-analyses, as shown in Tables S17–S23 [37–43]. The incidence and mortality benefits from the risk factor reduction in the population and the treatment and intervention benefits in patient groups were then summed. This summing used a cumulative approach rather than an additive approach [44] to avoid double-counting benefits in the same individual. This sum represents the changes in incidence and mortality 'explained' by policy changes made within the model.

Model structure: SDM was chosen for this project due to the complex interactions and dynamic nature of the system. An example of the causal loop diagrams used to investigate and visualise relationships in the system prior to model building is demonstrated in the Supplementary Materials (Figure S3). As the final SDM model has a total of 63 stocks, 170 flows and 869 converters, which generated 9024 variables including multiple element arrays and graphical functions, a simplified model structure is illustrated in Figure 3. The first five interventions in Table 1 apply to CYP section of the model and the others apply to the adult section. The left of the figure shows the CYP model structure and illustrates the movement of the population from birth through an aging chain (0–1, 2–4, 5–10, 11–15, 16–17 and 18–24 years) whilst also moving between different health cohorts, represented by the vertical arrows. The aging chain arrows represent the natural flow of the population from birth on to different age groups and flowing to the adult model at 18 and 25 years. The physical and mental enduring and LD cohorts move to the adult model at 25 years and progress to the same cohort group. For all other cohorts, they enter the adult model at 18 years and progress to the healthy cohort. Risk factors for CYP do carry a rate of risk across to the adult cohorts (e.g., child obesity and adult diabetes). The vertical arrows represent the progression or recovery of CYP who are flowing from different cohorts or health states over time (incidence). Adults flow from one cohort to another cohort without an aging chain, e.g., from healthy to a single condition. People flowing into or out of the geography are included in the model via net migration per cohort and people flowing out of a cohort due to death are represented by the red arrows. These rates of flow were determined by the data outlined in Tables S4–S12 [17,19,31]. Tables S2 and S3 outline the cohorts used in the model and illustrate the SD model structure in more detail.

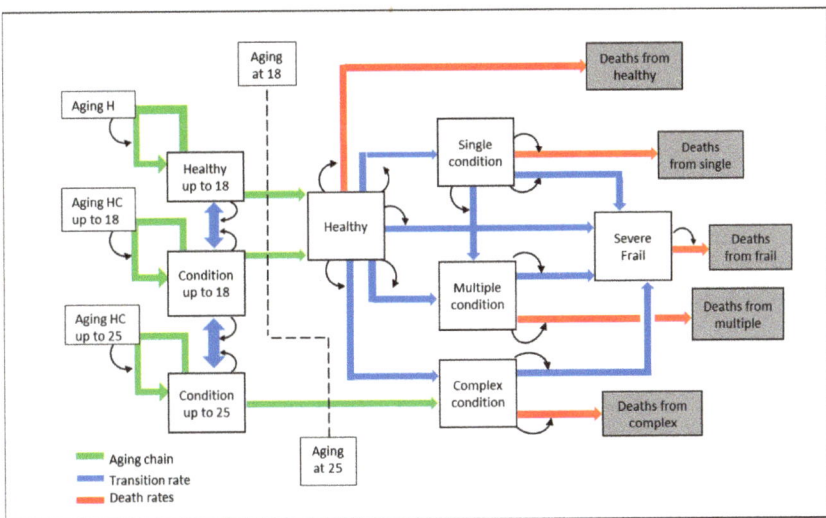

Figure 3. Conceptualisation of the system dynamics model. This figure shows a basic conceptualisation of the stocks and flows in the System Dynamics cohort model. Blue arrows show flows between cohorts, green arrows show ageing chains and red arrows show flow out of the stock due to death.

Model calibration: To initiate the model with population cohorts through incidence, prevalence and mortality, we used various data sources, which are outlined in Tables S4–S12 [17,19,31]. Additionally, population-level risk factors were used to influence the impacts across cohorts, which are listed in Tables S17–S23 [37–43]. In the first instance, we used local data to initiate the model to consider differences in demographics and risk factors. The process of calibration involved importing baseline data and projections from various national sources including the Office for National Statistics and KCC housing forecast [18] to carry out validation of general outcome measures such as population and mortality. Locally, further validation took place to check against known outcome measures such as the Quality Outcome Framework [45] and health and care activity data.

The model validation process followed the framework outlined by Yarnoff et al. [46], and the five validation stages were undertaken in accordance with this. Face validation, involving assessment by subject matter experts (public health consultants from the locality), was achieved through model development in group model building workshops and through ongoing testing. This included continual one-way sensitivity analysis in order to validate input factors and the ranges of variables with their associated effect. Internal validation, verifying the model's code and calculations, involved a secondary modeller and analyst, who had not participated in the model development, reviewing model logic and calculations and evaluating the sensitivities. In cross validation, which compared the model output to other available models, we reviewed all of the available evidence of comparable models. Due to the novel nature and aims of this project, we were unable to find models with a similar magnitude and scope; however, individual sources of evidence were used in calibration and sensitivity testing. We encountered a similar challenge with external validation, which compares modelled outputs to surveillance data, and predictive validation, which compares modelled impacts to actual observations resulting from interventions. Although surveys were not available for the local health population and limited intervention and actual data could be retrieved, consensus amongst public health experts and healthcare providers along with the triangulation of academic literature was used where data were not available. Where appropriate, proxies for comparable regions or national average data were used in agreement with subject matter experts. Due to the complexity of the model and high number of variables, including graphical functions and arrayed elements, a small number of key prevalence percentages were selected for single output-level validation through discussion with subject matter experts and ongoing sensitivity testing throughout development. Similarly to Zhang et al., [47] relative deviation rate and average relative deviation rate were used to demonstrate the deviation between simulated outputs and surveillance data or externally modelled data (calculations for these are available in Figure S4). Single output and population validation results are shown in Figures S5 and S6 and Tables S24 and S25. The model represented the time trends in the population for CYP (0–17) and adults (18+) well when compared to ONS 2018 [48] population projections, with the largest average relative deviation of 1.12% (Table S25 and Figure S6). Validation against external data sources was difficult because the base population of the model included major longitudinal studies. However, there was good agreement between modelled condition prevalence for CHD, COPD, stroke and diabetes compared to quality and outcomes framework (QoF) data (Table S24 and Figure S5) [45]. The relative deviation for these variables ranges from 0.01% to 10.35%, and the average relative deviation ranges from 3.77% to 4.84%.

Sensitivity testing was based on Hekimoğlu and Barlas' behaviour sensitivity analysis algorithm [49]. The initial screening of key input factors was created during development, where sensitivities and ranges of input values, practical for public health planning and policy, were agreed on by experts. As noted above, sensitivities were further tested during internal validation. The regression model of behaviours was undertaken using ranges around selected input values (for example, input variables for healthy life expectancy at 18 are shown in Table S26), and five runs for each variable based on incremental steps were run through Stella Architect's model analysis tool (including all combinations). For the healthy life expectancy at 18 output, this resulted in 625 runs and the behaviour shown in Figure S7. However, selecting a dependent variable value that represents the behaviour did not fall within the examples of Hekimoğlu and Barlas' work [49]. Firstly, this model can not be defined as an inherently oscillating or tipping point. Secondly, our model is significantly more complex and has a far greater number of elements, including graphical interface variables and multiple arrays. The regression-dependent variable selected was based on the difference between the start and end values of the outputs, representing the change in health over the modelled period. The results of the regression in this example based on this calculation showed an R^2 adjusted >80 and significance at $p < 0.05$ of all included variables.

The model was developed using a software platform known as Stella Architect developed by Isee Systems, which is accessible via Isee exchange [50]. Following calibration of the model, outputs were viewed and extracted.

Model interventions: Thirteen public health interventions were agreed on by Kent County Council public health professionals to achieve "Better Health" for their population. They were selected based on the latest published evidence and national policy [27] of these interventions in improving health. The interventions are listed in Table 1. The level of change and the target to be achieved were also agreed on by local professionals in the better health workshop by mutual consensus.

The CYP section of the model included interventions 1–5 in Table 1, and relative risk is shown in Table S27 [51–57]. The adult section of the model included interventions 6–13 in Table 1, which could be activated to test the projected future impact. For each cohort, we estimated the proportion of incidence and deaths that were attributable to various treatments or interventions. Data sources used to estimate the percentage at risk from the included interventions are displayed in Table S1 [17–27]. The general approach to calculating the risk reduction from an intervention among a particular cohort was to multiply the change in the proportion of people exposed to a risk factor by the incidence rate and by the relative reduction due to the change in intervention or exposure. Sources for current risk factors and treatment uptake are shown in Table S1 [17–27]. Sources for estimates of treatment efficacy (relative risk reductions) are shown in Tables S17–S23 and S27 [37–57]. When multiple risk factors impacted simultaneously on incidence and mortality, they were jointly estimated by calculating cumulative risk reduction. Examples of the calculations to find treatment or incidence impacts, cumulative risk factor impact and proportional changes in incidence and mortality over time are shown in Figures S8–S11. This accounts for risk factor prevalence overlap but assumes independence of effects [44].

3. Results

We present the outputs of the model using North Kent as an example, which covers 22% of the Kent population and 27% of Kent County's land mass.

The children's section was primarily used for setting appropriate assumptions on interventions and other factors within the children age group, and the model scenarios were run to determine the consequential impact in the adult population over time. Hence, results are presented for the adult population of the model (Figures 4–6). Table 2 shows the prevalence of long-term conditions in 2012 and 2037 and demonstrates the percentage difference between no interventions and "Better Health" scenarios.

Table 2. Modelled changes in the prevalence of long-term conditions due to no interventions or "Better Health" scenario.

Long-Term Condition	2012	No Interventions		Better Health		Difference between Better Health and No Interventions
		2037	Percentage Difference	2037	Percentage Difference	
Asthma	6.83%	5.95%	−12.90%	5.88%	−13.90%	−1.00%
CHD	1.92%	1.59%	−17.23%	1.51%	−21.48%	−4.25%
COPD	0.75%	0.63%	−15.79%	0.57%	−23.92%	−8.13%
Diabetes	2.76%	3.25%	18.02%	3.07%	11.35%	−6.66%
HF	0.02%	0.02%	−10.74%	0.02%	−10.96%	−0.22%
Stroke	0.67%	0.59%	−12.52%	0.49%	−27.56%	−15.04%
Frail moderate	1.30%	1.53%	17.88%	1.55%	19.27%	1.39%
Multiple	3.89%	3.51%	−9.61%	3.42%	−12.01%	−2.40%
SE MI	0.54%	0.46%	−14.18%	0.44%	−18.27%	−4.09%
Neuro	0.18%	0.19%	4.82%	0.19%	5.17%	0.35%
Dementia	0.32%	0.34%	8.12%	0.34%	7.60%	−0.52%
LD	0.28%	0.26%	−7.46%	0.26%	−7.59%	−0.13%
Frail severe	2.96%	3.35%	13.21%	3.27%	10.45%	−2.76%

4. Discussion

Main Finding

We have described an SD simulation model for the population of Kent in southeast England, showing the impacts of a range of prevention interventions on life expectancy, the prevalence of long-term conditions, healthcare utilisation and cost. The model was initialised from 2012 and closely matches the historical data up till 2018. Of the 13 evidence-based prevention interventions that were simulated, 5 were applied to children and young people and 8 to the adult section. The application of the "Better Health" scenario in the model resulted in changes to the size of the four cohorts over the model period (Figure 4). The size of the no-condition cohort increased, and the other three cohorts decreased in size. This shows the marginal benefit of the combined effect of the interventions across the course of life, at pace and scale. The impact of the interventions on both life expectancy at birth and healthy life expectancy is significant, adding 5.1 and 5.0 years, respectively (Figure 5). This is significant from an individual perspective in terms of adding years to life and life to years, but the increase in the overall proportion and size of the healthy living population is moderated due to the dynamic properties of complex systems. Any improvement in the health status of the population leads to a productive workforce and its associated positive impact on the wider economy and society as a whole.

Using the modelling approach, we have also demonstrated the impact on healthcare utilisation in terms of emergency admissions and attendance at accident and emergency centres. Although the reduction in activity appears insignificant, the estimated accrued cost savings calculated using the unit price of activity over the model period is noteworthy, as for one area of Kent, it is GBP 7.8 million (GBP (Pound Sterling) 1 = USD (United States Dollar) 1.22) (Figure 6). In the "Better Health" scenario, the modelling shows a significant reduction in most of the long-term conditions over the course of the model. All thirteen conditions except neurological conditions and moderate frailty show varying levels of reduction. Three conditions show a reduction well over 5% when compared to no interventions—stroke (15.04%), COPD (8.13%) and diabetes (6.66%). This demonstrates the robustness of the evidence base behind the included interventions (Table 2).

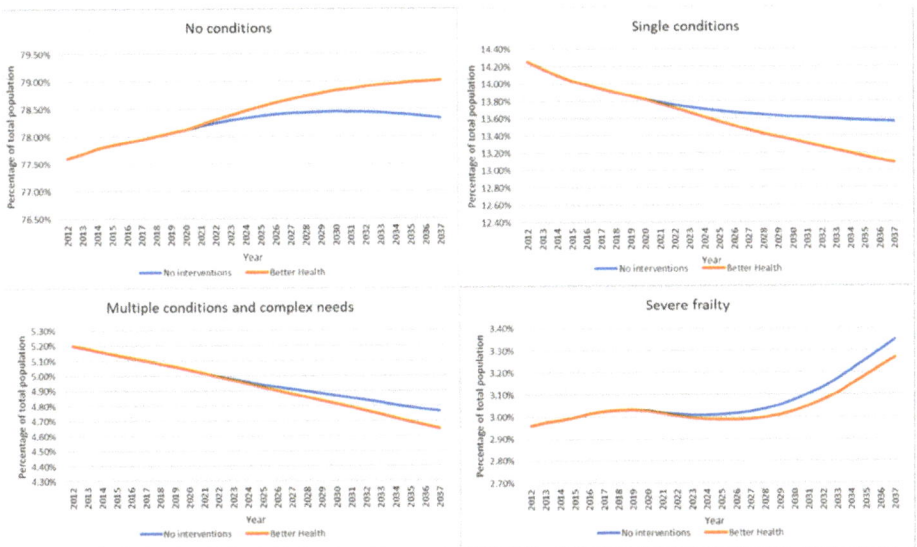

Figure 4. Population changes in the four cohorts due to no interventions or "Better Health" scenario. This shows the four cohorts and the difference in percentage of the population of that cohort at the end of the model period from the do nothing (no interventions) or "Better Health" scenarios.

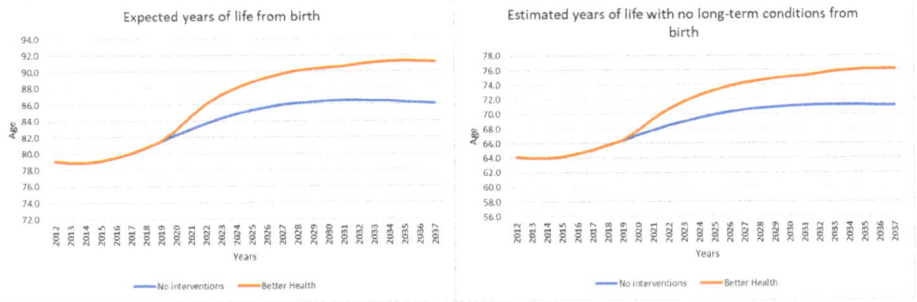

Figure 5. Output of the model showing change in life expectancy and healthy life expectancy from birth due to no interventions or "Better Health" scenario.

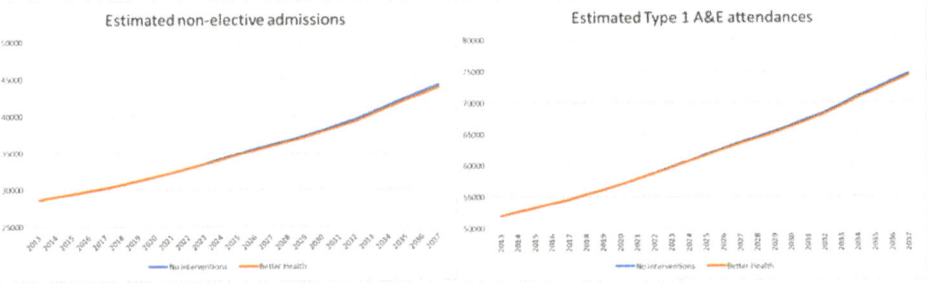

Figure 6. Model output of non-elective admissions and accident and emergency attendance due to no interventions or "Better Health" scenario.

The result of our study aligns with broader research in this area that uses SDM to address the complexities of preventing chronic diseases and other associated conditions. By creating "do nothing" versus "do something" scenarios, important distinctions are revealed, showing the long-term gains by investing in preventative actions [58]. To our knowledge, the systematic review by Wang et al. is the first attempt to evaluate the application of SDM to chronic diseases, which included 34 studies. Surprisingly, there were no studies from the UK, and the majority were from the USA. This represents a gap in the literature in the UK and the relevance of this research. Studies analysed differences between upstream and downstream prevention measures for chronic conditions. Upstream interventions include wider determinants such as improving income and community cohesion, whereas downstream interventions include behaviour-related interventions. Although only downstream interventions were found to significantly reduce chronic disease and mortality, the resources to fund them would need to be redirected from upstream allocations to meet these pressures. Upstream interventions, however, would reduce the prevalence of chronic illness but would have the added value of an increased impact on economic productivity. This demonstrated how SDM analyses health challenges as a whole, rather than taking a less reliable, simplistic view. Homer and Hirsh [7] explain the conditions that are best suited for the application of SDM to public health actions. They state that prevention models should incorporate all the elements of the ecological approach, incorporating disease outcomes, health and risk behaviour, environmental factors and health-related resources and delivery systems. There were notably very few examples of studies that simulated wider determinants, including employment, socioeconomic status and community cohesion, in the literature. This is one of the limitations of our model, as explained in the limitations section. Some studies focus on the qualitative process of engaging thought leaders and health planners in prioritising actions. Loyo et al. [59] demonstrated that SD modelling and local expertise were valuable tools in reprioritising community issues, obtaining community buy-in and determining the best use of community resources.

Further steps and future direction: The model provided the basis for conversations with health leaders, particularly in the North Kent system, where this needs-led approach to forecasting future demand became the subject of healthy debate. The approach was distinct from the extant 'big consultancy' solutions that projected future demand based on recent trends, sometimes also 'adding on' demographic changes, making the relationship between need and demand opaque. This led to a significant over-estimation of future demand, to the point that local plans to invest in community alternatives to inpatient care became unaffordable, thus undermining the confidence of local leaders in their ability to achieve a sustainable long-term solution. The use of the cohort model outputs formed the basis of a blended approach to demand forecasting that used trend analysis in the short term, gradually being replaced in a blended fashion using a needs-led approach. Cohort modelling is seen as complementary to population health management approaches [60] that are also based on segmentation but are designed to enable targeted interventions by professionals rather than strategic prospective modelling. Population health management represents the population segmented at a particular point in time. In SDM, the segmentation data are used to produce a dynamic projection of the population across segments and cohorts. Thus, both approaches complement each other. Going forward, investment is required to build up local research infrastructure to undertake evaluation studies in order to generate reliable evidence for model inputs. Currently, the cohort model does not include wider determinants. However, we are in the process of expanding the model by including wider determinants such as income, housing and education. This is likely to simulate much more pronounced health effects on the population than behavioural and healthcare determinants [61].

Strengths and limitations: SDM is a better approach than the traditional linear modelling and forecasting as it is able to deal with complex and dynamic systems and their interactions. For example, the draining of a stock through the application of incidence rates based on the presence of risk factors feeds back to reduce the absolute size of the stock and, therefore, the relationship between relative and absolute rates of flow, i.e., absolute rates of flow will reduce as a result of this feedback. These complex relationships are easily represented and calculated at each model time-step using the stock–flow characteristics of SDM, making these explicit and transparent to a model user. During the development of the model, we involved key stakeholders, including subject matter experts, in conceptualising the model, testing and developing the various inputs, and validated the selected scenarios. We also used validated, up-to-date local data to inform model assumptions and calibrate the model outputs.

In terms of the reliability of the results of the model, SDM is deterministic and, hence, the scenario run outputs will remain the same, assuming model inputs and assumptions remain constant, which is the case in our study.

Consideration of possible lag time and our approach: As the model is operating at a population level, the concept of considering lag at an individual patient level is not directly applicable. In the 'no intervention' scenario, disease incidence is routinely applied as an annual rate, which is converted into a monthly rate. Changes in risk factors in the Better Health scenario are applied to the incidence to increase or decrease this rate. Secondly, the specification of a timescale for each intervention is displayed in Table 1. This also affects disease incidence rates and is applied over the model timeframe.

Our model did not include an aging chain for the adult model and, hence, age-level assumptions could not be used. This led to the model being more generic. As set out in the Main Finding section, our initial model also did not incorporate wider determinants, and we are addressing all the identified limitations in the future version of the model, which is currently under development. Additionally, in regard to the sensitivity analysis performed, the significance of the input values on change in health over the model period are meaningful. However, the understanding of behaviour patterns and the ability to compute the simulation runs needed to test the model based on the behaviour sensitivity analysis algorithm [48] mentioned above require further study.

5. Conclusions

We have demonstrated the feasibility, applicability and utility of using system dynamics modelling to simulate the impacts of various preventive interventions on health status and healthcare utilisation in the local population. We created a "Better Health" scenario based on 13 interventions and were able to produce outputs through the model compared to the "no intervention" scenario. From the model conception stage to selecting interventions, we worked with stakeholders and subject matter experts, which further strengthened and added value to our approach. Through our modelling, we were able to demonstrate to the decision makers that investing in these prevention interventions will lead to an increase in the proportion of healthy people in the local population, a reduction in those with one or more health conditions and frailty, an increase in life expectancy, reduced urgent healthcare utilisation and reduced expenditure to the local health services, and will prevent the occurrence of many long-term conditions. If these results are scaled up to a wider geography, this could be potentially very significant. This modelling approach has helped us to have informed conversations backed by evidence with local healthcare leaders in our attempt to provide a realistic view of prevention impact on population health and reducing demand on local health services and cost.

Supplementary Materials: The following supporting information can be downloaded at: https://www.mdpi.com/article/10.3390/systems11050247/s1. The Supplementary Materials include Table S1: Data inputs and sources, Table S2: Children and young people cohort definitions, Table S3: Adult cohort definitions, Table S4: Prevalence of children and young people long-term conditions, Table S5: Prevalence of adult long-term conditions, Table S6: Adult percentage prevalence of single-condition long-term conditions within multiple and frail cohorts, Table S7: Incidence per 1000 people aged 18 and over, Table S8: Incidence and mortality rates per 1000 people aged 18 and over, Table S9: Cause of death percentage aged 50 and over, Table S10: ONS mortality by main cause of death, Table S11: Adult percentage prevalence of long-term conditions by social group, Table S12: Observed risk factor levels in 1999 and 2009 by social class, Table S13: Variable definitions for adult risk factors, Table S14: Beta coefficients for major risk factors: systolic blood pressure, Table S15: Beta coefficients for major risk factors: body mass index, Table S16: Beta coefficients for major risk factors: cholesterol, Table S17: Relative risk for underlying risk, incidence and mortality: smoking in adults, Table S18: Relative risk for underlying risk, incidence and mortality: physical inactivity in adults, Table S19: Relative risk for underlying risk, incidence and mortality: obesity and overweight in adults, Table S20: Relative risk for underlying risk, incidence and mortality: dementia in adults, Table S21: Relative risk for underlying risk, incidence and mortality: hypertension and hypercholesterolaemia in adults, Table S22: Relative risk reduction for CHD and stroke, Table S23: Relative risk for underlying risk, incidence and mortality: alcohol consumption in adults, Table S24: Single prevalence validation through relative deviation rates for Kent, Table S25:Population validation through relative deviation rates for Kent, Table S26: Sensitivity analysis testing ranges, Table S27: Relative risk for underlying risk, incidence: breastfeeding, smoking in pregnancy, child obesity, fuel poverty and ACE in Children and Young People, Figure S1: Estimation of risk factor changes using regression method, Figure S2: Estimation of incidence and mortality changes from risk factor changes using the PAF method, Figure S3: Causal Loop Diagram, Figure S4: Relative deviation, Figure S5: Visual single prevalence model validation for Kent, Figure S6: Visual population model validation for Kent, Figure S7: Sensitivity analysis variation for Healthy Life Expectancy (HLE) at 18, Figure S8: Model validation, Figure S4: Estimation of incidence and mortality changes from a specific treatment, Figure S9: Estimation of incidence changes from fuel poverty changes, Figure S10: Cumulative risk-reduction and Figure S11: Proportional change in cohort incidence and mortality rate over time.

Author Contributions: All authors have met authorship requirements. Specifically, all authors substantially contributed to manuscript development across the following inputs: conception and design (A.G. (Abraham George), A.G. (Alex Gray), P.B., C.H., P.T., P.L., D.S.), acquisition of data (A.G. (Abraham George)., A.G. (Alex Gray), C.H., P.T., P.L.), analysis (A.G. (Alex Gray), C.H., P.T., P.L.) and interpretation of data (A.G. (Abraham George), A.G. (Alex Gray), D.S., C.H., P.B., P.T., P.L.), drafting the article (A.G. (Abraham George), A.G. (Alex Gray), D.S., C.H., P.B., P.T., P.L.), data visualization (A.G. (Alex Gray), CH.) and reviewing the article and revising it critically (A.G. (Abraham George), A.G. (Alex Gray), D.S., C.H., P.B., P.T., P.L.) All authors have read and agreed to the published version of the manuscript.

Funding: This research received no specific external funding. Kent County Council commissioned the Whole Systems Partnership to develop a system modelling tool for the local Joint Strategic Needs Assessment.

Data Availability Statement: All data presented in this article were extracted from local and publicly available data sources.

Acknowledgments: The authors are grateful to Natalie Adams for her contributions in the development of the manuscript in its early stages.

Conflicts of Interest: A.G., C.T., P.T. and P.L. are part of the Whole Systems Partnership, who provide support for partnership development and system redesign in health and social care, and one of the approaches they use is systems dynamic modelling. A.G., D.S. and P.B. have no conflicts of interest to declare.

References

1. Oxford Brookes University: Protecting Older People Population Information. Available online: https://www.poppi.org.uk (accessed on 23 March 2023).
2. Lepenioti, K.; Bousdekis, A.; Apostolou, D.; Mentzas, G. Prescriptive analytics: Literature review and research challenges. *Int. J. Inf. Manag.* **2020**, *50*, 57–70. [CrossRef]
3. Public Health England: Health Economics: Evidence Resource. Available online: www.gov.uk/government/publications/health-economics-evidence-resource (accessed on 23 March 2023).
4. Bauer, G.R. Incorporating intersectionality theory into population health research methodology: Challenges and the potential to advance health equity. *Soc. Sci. Med.* **2014**, *110*, 10–17. [CrossRef] [PubMed]
5. McGill, E.; Er, V.; Penney, T.; Egan, M.; White, M.; Meier, P.; Whitehead, M.; Lock, K.; de Cuevas, R.A.; Smith, R.; et al. Evaluation of public health interventions from a complex systems perspective: A research methods review. *Soc. Sci. Med.* **2021**, *272*, 113697. [CrossRef] [PubMed]

6. Jadeja, N.; Zhu, N.J.; Lebcir, R.M.; Sassi, F.; Holmes, A.; Ahmad, R. Using system dynamics modelling to assess the economic efficiency of innovations in the public sector—A systematic review. *PLoS ONE* **2022**, *17*, e0263299. [CrossRef] [PubMed]
7. Homer, J.B.; Hirsch, G.B. System dynamics modeling for public health: Background and opportunities. *Am. J. Public Health* **2006**, *96*, 452–458. [CrossRef]
8. Yarnoff, B.; Bradley, C.; Honeycutt, A.A.; Soler, R.E.; Orenstein, D. Estimating the relative impact of clinical and preventive community-based interventions: An example based on the Community Transformation Grant Program. *Prev. Chronic Dis.* **2019**, *16*, 180594. [CrossRef]
9. Rutter, H.; Savona, N.; Glonti, K.; Bibby, J.; Cummins, S.; Finegood, D.T.; Greaves, F.; Harper, L.; Hawe, P.; Moore, L.; et al. The need for a complex systems model of evidence for public health. *Lancet* **2017**, *390*, 2602–2604. [CrossRef]
10. Currie, D.J.; Smith, C.; Jagals, P. The application of system dynamics modelling to environmental health decision-making and policy—A scoping review. *BMC Public Health* **2018**, *18*, 402. [CrossRef]
11. Davahli, M.R.; Karwowski, W.; Taiar, R. A System Dynamics Simulation Applied to Healthcare: A Systematic Review. *Int. J. Environ. Res. Public Health* **2020**, *17*, 5741. [CrossRef]
12. Király, G.; Miskolczi, P. Dynamics of participation: System dynamics and participation—An empirical review. *Syst. Res. Behav. Sci.* **2019**, *36*, 199–210. [CrossRef]
13. Apostolopoulos, Y.; Lich, H.K.; Lemke, M.K. *Complex Systems and Population Health: A Primer*; Oxford University Press: New York, NY, USA, 2020.
14. Department of Health and Social Care. Joint Strategic Needs Assessment and Joint Health and Wellbeing Strategies Explained. 2011. Available online: www.gov.uk/government/publications/joint-strategic-needs-assessment-and-joint-health-and-wellbeing-strategies-explained (accessed on 23 March 2023).
15. Statistical Bulletin. 2021 Mid-Year Population Estimates: Age and Sex Profile. Kent Analytics. January 2023. Available online: https://www.kent.gov.uk/__data/assets/pdf_file/0019/14725/Mid-year-population-estimates-age-and-gender.pdf (accessed on 23 March 2023).
16. ONS. Census 2021: Total Population Change between 2011 and 2021. Available online: https://www.ons.gov.uk/peoplepopulationandcommunity/populationandmigration/populationestimates (accessed on 23 March 2023).
17. Data Resource: The Kent Integrated Dataset (KID). Available online: https://ijpds.org/article/view/427 (accessed on 23 March 2023).
18. Kent County Council (KCC) Housing Led Forecasts 2021. Available online: www.kent.gov.uk/__data/assets/pdf_file/0010/59806/KCC-housing-led-summary.pdf (accessed on 12 March 2023).
19. ONS, Deaths Broken Down by Age, Sex, Area and Cause of Death. Available online: https://www.ons.gov.uk/peoplepopulationandcommunity/birthsdeathsandmarriages/deaths (accessed on 23 March 2023).
20. ONS, General Lifestyle Survey: 2011. Available online: www.ons.gov.uk/peoplepopulationandcommunity/personalandhouseholdfinances/incomeandwealth/compendium/generallifestylesurvey/2013-03-07 (accessed on 23 March 2023).
21. Health Survey for England. Available online: https://digital.nhs.uk/data-and-information/publications/statistical/health-survey-for-england (accessed on 3 March 2023).
22. General Household Survey. Available online: https://www.data.gov.uk/dataset/138ca035-a90c-4e37-80f5-4c73eeb6ae04/general-household-survey (accessed on 23 March 2023).
23. Maternity and Breastfeeding. Available online: https://www.england.nhs.uk/statistics/statistical-work-areas/maternity-and-breastfeeding/ (accessed on 23 March 2023).
24. Statistics on Women's Smoking Status at Time of Delivery: England. Available online: https://digital.nhs.uk/data-and-information/publications/statistical/statistics-on-women-s-smoking-status-at-time-of-delivery-england (accessed on 23 March 2023).
25. National Child Measurement Programme. Available online: https://www.gov.uk/government/collections/national-child-measurement-programme (accessed on 23 March 2023).
26. English Indices of Deprivation 2010. Available online: https://www.gov.uk/government/statistics/english-indices-of-deprivation-2010 (accessed on 23 March 2023).
27. Millennium Cohort Study. Available online: https://cls.ucl.ac.uk/cls-studies/millennium-cohort-study/ (accessed on 23 March 2023).
28. NHS Long Term Plan 2019. Available online: www.longtermplan.nhs.uk (accessed on 23 March 2023).
29. Lacey, P. Strategic Workforce Planning (SWiPe) Derbyshire Re-shaping Community Workforce, Child health and wellbeing services Draft report—July 2016. (Unpublished report July 2016). 20 July 2016.
30. Outcomes Based Healthcare. Available online: https://outcomesbasedhealthcare.com/segmentation-approaches (accessed on 23 March 2023).
31. English Longitudinal Study of Ageing (ELSA). Available online: www.elsa-project.ac.uk (accessed on 23 March 2023).
32. NHS Electronic Frailty Index (EFI). Available online: www.england.nhs.uk/ourwork/clinical-policy/older-people/frailty/efi/ (accessed on 23 March 2023).
33. Lewington, S.; Clarke, R.; Qizilbash, N.; Peto, R.; Collins, R.; Prospective Studies Collaboration. Age specific relevance of usual blood pressure to vascular mortality: A meta-analysis of individual data for one million adults in 61 prospective studies. *Lancet* **2002**, *360*, 1903–1913. [CrossRef] [PubMed]

34. Bogers, R.P.; Hoogenveen, R.T.; Boshuizen, H.; Woodward, M.; Knekt, P.; Van Dam, R.M.; Hu, F.B.; Visscher, T.L.S.; Menotti, A.; Thorpe, R.J.; et al. Overweight and obesity increase the risk of coronary heart disease: A pooled analysis of 30 prospective studies. *Eur. J. Epidemiol.* **2006**, *21*, 107.
35. James, W.P.T.; Jackson-Leach, R.; Mhurchu, C.N.; Kalamara, E.; Shayeghi, M.; Rigby, N.J.; Nishida, C.; Rodgers, A. Overweight and obesity (high body mass index). In *Comparative Quantification of Risk Global and Regional Burden of Disease Attributable to Selected Major Risk Factors*; Ezatti, M., Lopez, A.D., Rodgers, A., Murray, C.J.L., Eds.; World Health Organization: Geneva, Switzerland, 2004; pp. 497–596.
36. Lewington, S.; Whitlock, G.; Clarke, R.; Sherliker, P.; Emberson, J.; Halsey, J.; Qizilbash, N.; Peto, R.; Collins, R. Blood cholesterol and vascular mortality by age, sex, and blood pressure: A meta-analysis of individual data from 61 prospective studies with 55000 vascular deaths. *Lancet* **2007**, *370*, 1829–1839. [CrossRef] [PubMed]
37. Statistics on Smoking, England—2013. Available online: https://digital.nhs.uk/data-and-information/publications/statistical/statistics-on-smoking/statistics-on-smoking-england-2013 (accessed on 23 March 2023).
38. Bull, F.; Armstrong, T.P.; Dixon, T.; Ham, S.; Neiman, A.; Pratt, M. Physical inactivity. In *Comparative Quantification of Risk Global and Regional Burden of Disease Attributable to Selected Major Risk Factors*; Ezatti, M., Lopez, A.D., Rodgers, A., Murray, C.J.L., Eds.; World Health Organization: Geneva, Switzerland, 2004; pp. 729–881.
39. Joubert, J.; Norman, R.; Lambert, E.V.; Groenewald, P.; Schneider, M.; Bull, F. Estimating the burden of disease attributable to physical inactivity in South Africa in 2000. *SAMJ S. Afr. Med. J.* **2007**, *97*, 725–731. [PubMed]
40. Mathers, C.; Vos, T.; Stevenson, C. The Burden of disease and injury in Australia, (AIHW Catalogue No. PHE 17). In *Comparative Quantification of Risk Global and Regional Burden of Disease Attributable to Selected Major Risk Factors*; Ezatti, M., Lopez, A.D., Rodgers, A., Murray, C.J.L., Eds.; World Health Organization: Geneva, Switzerland, 2004.
41. Tackling Obesity in England. Available online: https://www.nao.org.uk/reports/tackling-obesity-in-england/ (accessed on 23 March 2023).
42. Livingston, G.; Sommerlad, A.; Orgeta, V.; Costafreda, S.G.; Huntley, J.; Ames, D.; Ballard, C.; Banerjee, S.; Burns, A.; Cohen-Mansfield, J.; et al. Dementia prevention, intervention, and care. *Lancet Comm.* **2017**, *390*, 2673–2734. [CrossRef]
43. Ezatti, M.; Lopea, A.D.; Rodgers, A.; Murray, C.J.L. (Eds.) *Comparative Quantification of Risk. Global and Regional Burden of Disease Attributable to Selected Major Risk Factors*; World Health Organization: Geneva, Switzerland, 2004.
44. Unal, B.; Critchley, J.A.; Capewell, S. Explaining the Decline in Coronary Heart Disease Mortality in England and Wales Between 1981 and 2000. *Circulation* **2004**, *109*, 1101–1107. [CrossRef]
45. Public Health England, QoF Data: Public Health Profiles—OHID. Available online: www.phe.org.uk (accessed on 5 May 2023).
46. Yarnoff, B.; Honeycutt, A.; Bradley, C.; Khavjou, O.; Bates, L.; Bass, S.; Kaufmann, R.; Barker, L.; Briss, P. Validation of the prevention impacts simulation model (PRISM). *Prev. Chronic Dis.* **2021**, *18*, 200225. [CrossRef]
47. Zhang, Y.; Zhang, M.; Hu, H.; He, X. Research on supply and demand of aged services resource allocation in China: A system dynamics model. *Systems* **2022**, *10*, 59. [CrossRef]
48. ONS, Population Projections. Available online: https://www.ons.gov.uk/peoplepopulationandcommunity/populationandmigration/populationprojections (accessed on 23 March 2023).
49. Hekimoğlu, M.; Barlas, Y. Sensitivity analysis for models with multiple behavior modes: A method based on behavior pattern measures. *Syst. Dyn. Rev.* **2016**, *32*, 332–362. [CrossRef]
50. Isee Systems, Stella Architect. Available online: https://www.iseesystems.com/store/products/stella-architect.aspx (accessed on 23 March 2023).
51. Victora, C.G.; Bahl, R.; Barros, A.J.; França, G.V.; Horton, S.; Krasevec, J.; Murch, S.; Sankar, M.J.; Walker, N.; Rollins, N.C.; et al. Breastfeeding in the 21st century: Epidemiology, mechanisms, and lifelong effect. *Lancet* **2016**, *387*, 475–490. [CrossRef]
52. Gaysina, D.; Fergusson, D.M.; Leve, L.D.; Horwood, J.; Reiss, D.; Shaw, D.S.; Elam, K.K.; Natsuaki, M.N.; Neiderhiser, J.M.; Harold, G.T. Maternal Smoking During Pregnancy and Offspring Conduct Problems. Evidence From 3 Independent Genetically Sensitive Research Designs. *JAMA Psychiatry* **2013**, *70*, 956–963. [CrossRef] [PubMed]
53. Langley, K.; Heron, J.; Smith, G.D.; Thapar, A. Maternal and Paternal Smoking During Pregnancy and Risk of ADHD Symptoms in Offspring: Testing for Intrauterine Effects. *Am. J. Epidemiol.* **2012**, *176*, 261–268. [CrossRef] [PubMed]
54. Oken, E.; Levitan, E.B.; Gillman, M.W. Maternal smoking during pregnancy and child overweight: Systematic review and meta-analysis. *Int. J. Obes.* **2008**, *32*, 201–210. [CrossRef] [PubMed]
55. Barnes, M.; Butt, S.; Tomaszewski, W. *The Dynamics of Bad Housing: The Impact of Bad Housing on the Living Standards of Children*; National Centre for Social Research: London, UK, 2008.
56. Boardman, B. *Fixing Fuel Poverty: Challenges and Solutions*; Earthscan: London, UK, 2010.
57. Public Health Wales. *Welsh Adverse Childhood Experiences (ACE) Study: Adverse Childhood Experiences and Their Impact on Health-Harming Behaviours in the Welsh Adult Population*; Public Health Wales: Cymru, UK, 2016.
58. Wang, Y.; Hu, B.; Zhao, Y.; Kuang, G.; Zhao, Y.; Liu, Q.; Zhu, X. Applications of system dynamics models in Chronic disease prevention: A systematic review. *Prev. Chronic Dis.* **2021**, *18*, 210175. [CrossRef] [PubMed]
59. Loyo, H.K.; Batcher, C.; Wile, K.; Huang, P.; Orenstein, D.; Milstein, B. From model to action. *Health Promot. Pract.* **2012**, *14*, 53–61. [CrossRef] [PubMed]

60. NHS England. Population Health and the Population Health Management Programme. Available online: https://www.england.nhs.uk/integratedcare/what-is-integrated-care/phm (accessed on 23 March 2023).
61. Interdisciplinary Association for Population Health Science. County Health Ranking Model. Available online: https://iaphs.org/institutional-member-highlight-university-of-wisconsin (accessed on 23 March 2023).

Disclaimer/Publisher's Note: The statements, opinions and data contained in all publications are solely those of the individual author(s) and contributor(s) and not of MDPI and/or the editor(s). MDPI and/or the editor(s) disclaim responsibility for any injury to people or property resulting from any ideas, methods, instructions or products referred to in the content.

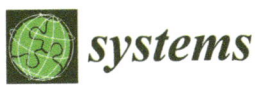

Article

Dynamics of Medical Screening: A Simulation Model of PSA Screening for Early Detection of Prostate Cancer

Özge Karanfil [1,2,3]

1 College of Administrative Sciences and Economics, Koç University, Istanbul 34450, Turkey; okaranfil@ku.edu.tr
2 Research Center for Translational Medicine (KUTTAM), Koç University, Istanbul 34450, Turkey
3 School of Medicine, Koç University, Istanbul 34450, Turkey

Abstract: In this study, we present a novel simulation model and case study to explore the long-term dynamics of early detection of disease, also known as routine population screening. We introduce a realistic and portable modeling framework that can be used for most cases of cancer, including a natural disease history and a realistic yet generic structure that allows keeping track of critical stocks that have been generally overlooked in previous modeling studies. Our model is specific to prostate-specific antigen (PSA) screening for prostate cancer (PCa), including the natural progression of the disease, respective changes in population size and composition, clinical detection, adoption of the PSA screening test by medical professionals, and the dissemination of the screening test. The key outcome measures for the model are selected to show the fundamental tradeoff between the main harms and benefits of screening, with the main harms including (i) overdiagnosis, (ii) unnecessary biopsies, and (iii) false positives. The focus of this study is on building the most reliable and flexible model structure for medical screening and keeping track of its main harms and benefits. We show the importance of some metrics which are not readily measured or considered by existing medical literature and modeling studies. While the model is not primarily designed for making inferences about optimal screening policies or scenarios, we aim to inform modelers and policymakers about potential levers in the system and provide a reliable model structure for medical screening that may complement other modeling studies designed for cancer interventions. Our simulation model can offer a formal means to improve the development and implementation of evidence-based screening, and its future iterations can be employed to design policy recommendations to address important policy areas, such as the increasing pool of cancer survivors or healthcare spending in the U.S.

Keywords: simulation model; early detection of cancer; mass screening; decision-making; dissemination; chronic disease; prevention; clinical practice guidelines; evidence-based guidelines; policy decision thresholds; prostate cancer; natural history of disease; dissemination; biomarker; prostate cancer; PSA

Citation: Karanfil, Ö. Dynamics of Medical Screening: A Simulation Model of PSA Screening for Early Detection of Prostate Cancer. *Systems* **2023**, *11*, 252. https://doi.org/10.3390/systems11050252

Academic Editor: Vladimír Bureš

Received: 3 March 2023
Revised: 2 May 2023
Accepted: 10 May 2023
Published: 16 May 2023

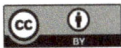

Copyright: © 2023 by the author. Licensee MDPI, Basel, Switzerland. This article is an open access article distributed under the terms and conditions of the Creative Commons Attribution (CC BY) license (https://creativecommons.org/licenses/by/4.0/).

1. Introduction and Motivation

Decades after routine medical screening became common, our understanding of screening and its consequences remains limited. Over the last few decades, the criteria for screening for several disorders have changed significantly, including thresholds dividing positive from negative test results and the recommended ages for routine screening. Major health organizations have recommended changes in several common disease definitions, often resulting in the expansion of the criteria for screening, diagnosis, and treatment, generally leading to increases in reported incidence and prevalence [1,2].

PCa is the second most frequently diagnosed cancer in men, and about two-thirds of these are diagnosed in high-income countries where 18% of the world's male population resides, with much of the variation reflecting differences in the use of PSA testing [3]. In the U.S., approximately 90% of PCa is detected by means of screening. The lifetime risk of receiving a diagnosis of PCa nearly doubled after the introduction of prostate-specific antigen (PSA) testing and increased from approximately 9% in 1985 [4] to 16% in 2007 [5]. The value of PSA screening to reduce deaths from PCa while balancing potential harms remains controversial, and routine screening is not recommended in many European countries [6,7]. In the U.S., the U.S. Preventive Services Task Force (USPSTF) recommends that average-risk men aged 55–69 have a conversation with their healthcare provider about the benefits and limitations of PSA testing to make an informed decision about whether to be tested based on their personal values and preferences [8]. Based on 2017–2019 data, approximately 12.6 percent of U.S. men will be diagnosed with PCa at some point during their lifetime, with an estimated 3.3 million men living with PCa [9].

In this study, we present an extended case study specific to the PSA screening for PCa, with the end goal of building a sound dynamic theory firmly grounded in empirical evidence and data to explain both the core harm-and-benefit issues and the natural disease progression and dissemination of the PSA screening practice among clinicians and the general population. The PSA case study includes a natural history disease progression model for PCa and a behavioral theory explaining how guidelines change over time in response to changes in the evidence. These in turn depend on the fundamental tradeoff between test sensitivity and specificity, the natural progression of the disease, and changes in population size and composition. While PSA screening is not specific to the U.S., we mainly treat the problem within the U.S. context where early detection of disease is most controversial. Our model has a natural history disease model at its core as well as a classical evidence-based dynamic theory for evolving screening indications, and interventions such as screening are superimposed on the natural history model based on available evidence. The natural history model has two stages, locoregional (M0) and distant (M1), and three grades (high, low, and indolent) of disease can both be screen- or clinically detected. The fundamental approach and assumptions for screening and its adoption/dissemination are explained, while the various assumptions and propositions are supported by reference to the modeling and medical literature. Model behavior shows reasonable correspondence to historical screening trends in the U.S.

2. Methodology and Background of Systems Models for Cancer

We use the system dynamics (SD) modeling approach to complex systems to explain the dissemination of medical screening for cancer within the U.S. context, supported by qualitative data [10,11]. Modeling of PCa in this study draws on an extensive body of SD work on healthcare issues across various domains and SD has been increasingly used to model many public health and healthcare issues [12–21]. A full recent account on SD applications in health and medicine can be found in Darabi and Hosseinichimeh [22]. Problems around early detection of disease are particularly suited to SD modeling because of the presence of many time-related phenomena, delayed feedback, and nonlinearities, such as varying trends in screening dissemination and population structure, and the delays associated with disease progression, translation of evidence, and policy-making efforts. SD methodology employs a series of guidelines for the model-building process, and a variety of tests and types of evidence organized around the purpose of the model that serve to increase confidence in model structure and dynamic theory [11,23,24].

The first attempt at a systems model of cancer was undertaken by Richmond, demonstrating a structural model for cancer development [25]. Fett built two SD models to examine breast cancer screening for public health policy analysis [26,27]. Fett et al. [27] represented a model with multiple stages of breast cancer that could be used to examine the Australian breast cancer screening program. There have been a few other SD studies involving population health screening: chlamydia, cervical cancer, or diabetes screening, and decision/referral thresholds in developmental and behavioral screening such as autism [28–30]. Royston et al. [28] used SD models to test alternative policies for cervical cancer and chlamydia screening. The U.K. Department of Health found the results to be useful for the development of screening guidelines. Policy questions included the optimal screening interval and coverage. The results suggested that it is more effective to increase the screening coverage than to decrease the screening interval. More recently, Palma and Lounsbury et al. [31] built an SD model for PCa that replicates the Prostate, Lung, Colorectal, and Ovarian (PLCO) cancer screening trial to assess the benefits of PSA screening for PCa-specific mortality.

Karanfil and Sterman [32] provide the foundations for the development of evidence-based screening guidelines for the early detection of disease. They develop and test an endogenous theory for population screening and present a stylized model to explore and formalize the guideline formation process. In this study we are expanding the boundaries of this classical evidence-based model for screening to create a more realistic life setting and present a case study for cancer, particularly focusing on the adoption and diffusion dynamics of PSA screening for PCa in the U.S. context. We tie the generic model presented by [32,33] to a natural history model for PCa that simulates the population-level changes in screening and dissemination. The range of screening indications in the model includes the biopsy referral threshold and the recommended starting age.

3. Overview of the PSA Screening Model

We demonstrate correspondence to historical data on various metrics including population counts, death rates, and some metrics on disease progression. Then, policy-relevant factors and analysis in the base run will be shown, which replicates history and shows the future trajectory. The case study model for PSA screening consists of six fundamental sectors, including the dynamics of the U.S. male population and natural history of disease; screening and clinical detection; treatment; screening dissemination; harm reduction technology; and the PSA screening harms and benefits. The fundamental approach, sector diagrams, and assumptions for each sector with critical formulations are explained in the Supplementary Materials. The various assumptions and propositions are supported by references to the modeling and medical literature.

3.1. Data Types and Inputs

Data used in this study are from multiple sources. Some are secondary data based on the literature, such as medical articles and reports we accessed directly. Others are composite data, which we obtained by combining several data points to support the model design. Most of the historical population and PCa trends are widely available on organization websites such as the NCI, CDC, NHANES, U.S. mortality files by the NCHS, NCI-SEER database, and NHIS. Complementary data were gathered from a literature review of the history of PSA screening in the U.S. To bring the model assumptions and findings closer to the real trends and to support the emerging model structure, we collected additional data through interviews with domain experts from medical and healthcare professions [33]. Figure 1 presents the conceptual framework used for modeling PCa's natural history, screening, adoption, utilization, harms, and benefits. Table 1 lists important model inputs and references used throughout the paper with the range used for sensitivity analysis, as well as associated data sources.

3.2. Population and Natural History of Disease
3.2.1. Population Increase and Aging

The target population of interest is U.S. males (all races) 50–80-year-olds; however, we also model younger ages (35–50-year-olds) to improve the quality of model calibration to target population trends. We define nine age groups by five-year intervals starting from 35, and another age group that represents the 80$^+$ male population. Different age groupings are used to represent simulation results, including the most used 50$^+$ or 65$^+$ populations. Other subpopulations include the 35 to 44, 45 to 54, 55 to 64, 65 to 75, and 75+-year-old age groups, for which mortality data and population counts were made available by the National Center for Health Statistics (NCHS) at the CDC [34]. The aging structure comprises one inflow that indicates the rate of entering the indicated age category, for nine age groups, and one outflow that indicates the rate of leaving the age category. The inflow-of-male-population-turning-35 time series is provided exogenously for the years 1980–2040, based on U.S. census data history and future projections. The age cohort-specific all-cause death rates and projections for the decrease in all-cause mortality were derived from sex- and age-specific data. The all-cause death rates for all age groups are then compared to the death counts specified by the CDC WONDER- [34,35]. Net immigration (migration to and from a country) is another component that influences the historical and future population counts in the U.S. that we considered.

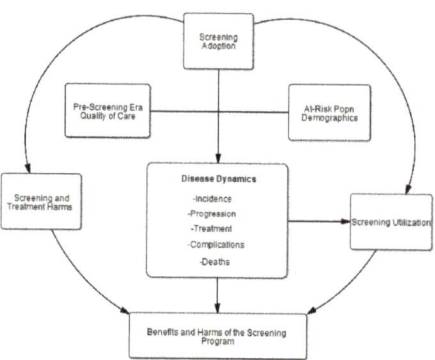

Figure 1. Framework for modeling of PSA screening for prostate cancer (PCa).

3.2.2. Natural History of Disease

Figures 2–4 gradually illustrate the sectors or the main stock-flow structure for the natural history of PCa and its diagnosis, including the health states and transitions, the asymptomatic onset of screen-detectable cancer, and disease progression through stages. The model design (onset and progression through disease stages) and assumptions were inspired by the PCa natural history diagnosis and history models developed by the NCI-sponsored Cancer Intervention and Surveillance Modeling Network (CISNET) group and other modeling studies published previously [36–40].

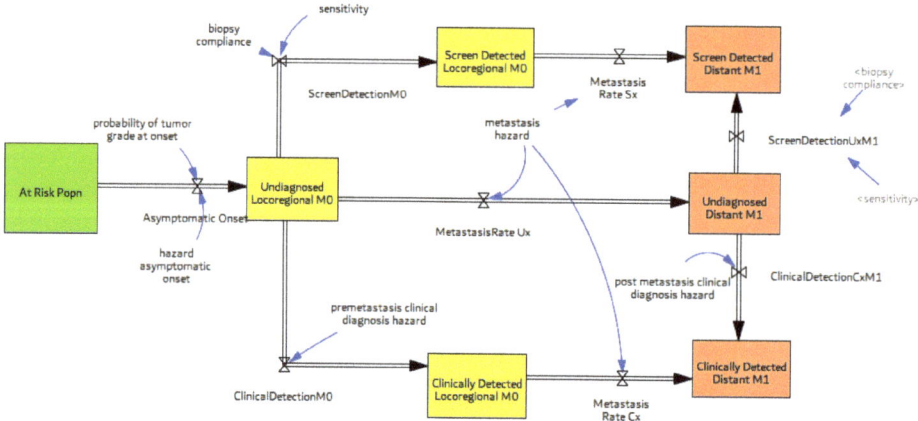

Figure 2. Simplified structure for natural disease progression, screen- and clinical detection.

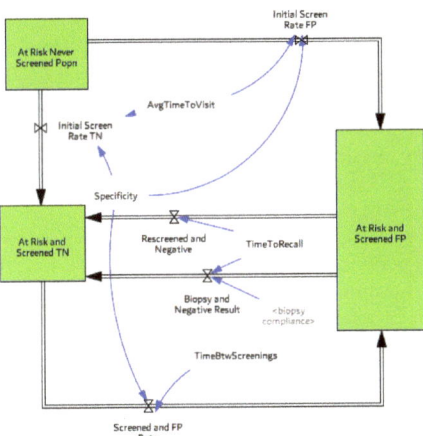

Figure 3. Generic structure of cancer screening for the general (at-risk) population—simplified.

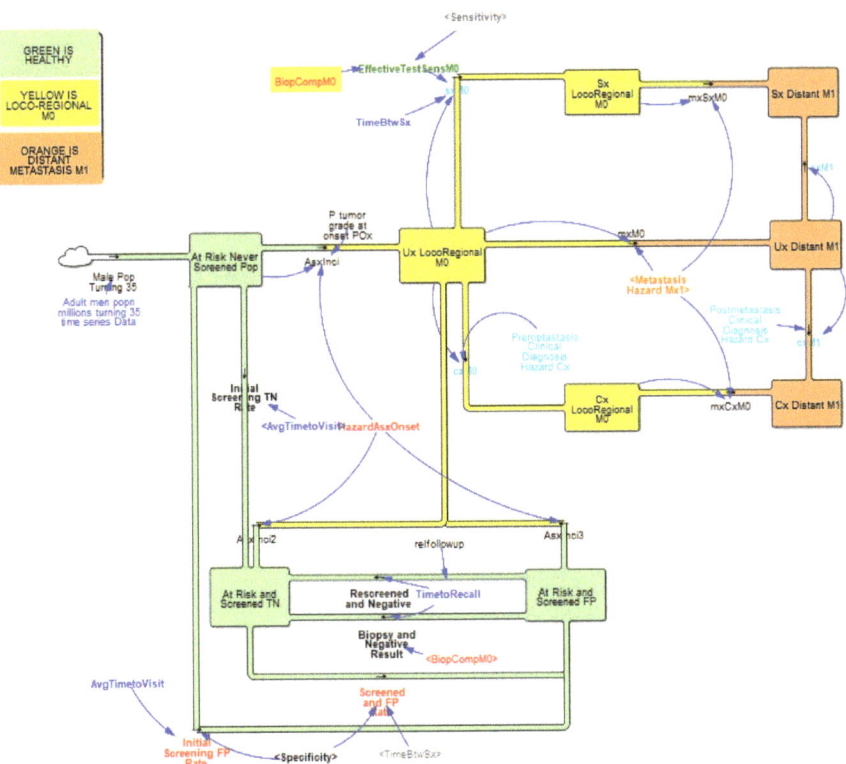

Figure 4. Combined sector diagram for natural disease progression, screen detection and clinical detection (net immigration, aging, all cause and cancer death flows, and other parameters not shown).

Figure 2 shows the model sector for natural disease progression, where screen-detectable cancers progress from the loco-regional (M0) to the distant-metastatic stage (M1). "At Risk" populations with different screening results are lumped into one group here for simplicity. People with undiagnosed disease may get both screening and clinical detection, or progress to metastatic disease before being diagnosed. Cancers are localized at onset and may be either low-grade (Gleason score 2–7), high-grade (Gleason score 8–10), or indolent (any Gleason). High- and low-grade cancers represent those that are of a progressive type and may get metastasized, while the indolent class tumors represent the non-progressive or latent tumors, including regressive tumors which are, by definition, destined to stay confined to the prostate and not metastasize or kill the patient. The model assumes stage durations to be distributed independently according to exponential distributions and not correlated with each other. Disease progression rates are independent of patient age or disease onset, as with other studies.

Asymptomatic onset used in the model is estimated from autopsy studies and previously published models [36,41–43]. The model assumes that these adequately reflect the real prevalence of disease in the U.S., although that may be an underestimation of the true amount of latent disease in the population. Biopsy studies using better techniques find a higher age-specific prevalence. The present model assumes a constant secular trend in incidence, in line with other modeling studies. The probabilities of tumor grade at onset determine the fraction of disease in each grade category (high, low, indolent) at the onset. The metastasis hazard for men with cancer depends on the grade, and the hazard of transition to metastatic disease from the loco-regional to distant stage is selected based on the medical literature [44]. Mortality of PCa from loco-regional and distant disease stages is represented with death fractions defined by grade. The death fraction and metastasis hazard of indolent tumors are zero, by its definition.

3.3. Screening, Clinical Detection, Dissemination of Screening

3.3.1. Screening Structure and Test Specifics

We introduce a more realistic screening stock-flow structure for the at-risk population compared to the available literature, which includes an explicit demonstration of all potential pathways a subject can go through during the screening process (Figure 3). Subjects in all the three at-risk stocks (at-risk and never screened, at risk and screened true negative-TN, or at risk and screened false positive-FP) may eventually develop a disease based on their age-specific onset. Note that subjects who are at risk and never screened may get an initial screening test with an TN test result or an FP test result. Subjects with an FP test result may then have a follow-up test or get a biopsy to confirm that they do not have the disease.

The model estimates an effective test sensitivity that combines test sensitivity, biopsy compliance, and biopsy detection rate. The endogenous PSA test sensitivity of loco-regional, stage M0 disease is determined by the evidence-based model structure [32,33]. The sensitivity of stage M1 disease is assumed to be 100% accurate, as the test sensitivity increases substantially when the disease has progressed beyond M0. The standard for biopsy referral in the U.S. from 1990 to 2005 was a PSA level greater than 4 ng/mL, yet lower thresholds were suggested and used in the 1990s, including 3, or even 2.5 ng/mL. In this model, men are eligible for biopsy after screening if their PSA exceeds this endogenously changing threshold. The screen detection rate of disease is given by age and grade. For the average time between two consecutive screening tests; a testing interval of 2 years is found to be reasonably consistent [39].

Not all men with positive test results submit to a follow-up biopsy. The model base biopsy compliance rate following a positive PSA test is taken as 0.5, which is lower than in Europe, where estimates range around 0.8–0.9. In the PLCO trial of the U.S., 40% of men with a PSA between 4 and 7, 53% of men with a PSA between 7 and 10, and 69% of men with a PSA greater than 10 had a follow-up biopsy [45]. Biopsy detection rate (or biopsy accuracy) represents the ability of biopsy to detect men with the disease. Its value has increased with the dissemination of extended biopsy schemes over time. Before 1990, 4-core biopsies were standard, 6-core biopsies were by 1995, and 8- to 12-core biopsies were standard by the early 2000s. A 6-core biopsy is 80% accurate, 4-core biopsy accuracy is 2/3 of this amount, and extended-core biopsies, which are presently used, are 100% accurate. The biopsy detection rate varied from 0.6 to 1, based on estimates provided in previous studies [46]. Cancer can also be clinically detected at any stage and the clinical detection hazard by grade is assumed to be much higher after metastasis of the disease [39]. We do not model digital rectal exam (DRE) testing explicitly and assume that the clinical detection hazard stays constant after the PSA era. This is an important assumption that may lead to an overestimation of the value of the PSA test since we do not capture possible increases in the frequency of the DRE test rate. In fact, DRE detections are also likely to increase because of disease awareness, which has increased over the years. Figure 4 illustrates the final and simplified sector stock-flow structure for the natural history of disease including disease progression and its detection by screening or clinical detection.

3.3.2. Screening Dissemination

The screening dissemination sector stock/flow structure is given in Figure 5. In our model, the doctor's adoption of PSA screening is modeled as adoption fraction A that ranges between 0 and the maximum adoption fraction. Screening dissemination takes place after 1985, the year PSA screening is introduced and rapidly diffuses in the medical community after that. Adoption and dissemination parameters are estimated by the first and repeat PSA screening data [46]. Screen eligibility is determined by the formally recommended starting and stopping ages in guidelines and the standard eligibility fraction, which indicates the maximum eligibility or the reference market for the PSA practice. The effects of starting/stopping ages on screening-eligible fractions are modeled by using graphical functions for an S-shaped curve. Accordingly, the screen-eligible fraction F is closer to the maximum between the recommended starting and stopping ages, yet it fails to reach its maximum within this range and extends beyond the formal ranges. Both the screen-eligible fraction and the currently screened fraction are given for 5-year age groups between the defined age ranges of 35–80+. Critical equations, graphical functions, and other supporting assumptions are provided in Supplementary Materials.

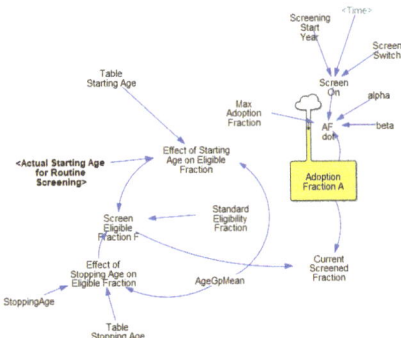

Figure 5. Screening Adoption Sector.

Table 1 lists important model inputs and symbols used with the range used for sensitivity analysis, and associated data sources. The key selected outcome measures for the model are selected to show the fundamental tradeoff between the harms and benefits of screening. These include proxy variables for the most common harms and benefits of screening and detection, mainly screen vs. clinical detection fractions, the fraction of overdiagnosed cases, the number of unnecessary biopsies, the metastasized fraction of cancer at initial detection, and men with FP test results. The main harms of screening include (i) false positives, (ii) unnecessary biopsies, and (iii) overdiagnosis (and, hence, overtreatment). The main benefit is saving lives, or early detection of cancer (before it gets metastasized).

Table 1. List of Important Model Inputs.

Name	Parameter [Unit]	Sensitivity Range	Source(s) for Base Case
Probability of indolent tumor at onset	pOx [dmnl]	0.2–0.6	Expert judgement [36,41,42]
Hazard Asymptomatic Onset (by age group)	Oxi [1/year]	0.0–0.05	SEER survival curves by stage, [37,47,48]
PCa specific mortality fraction (by grade)	dfM0, dfM1 [1/year]	0.07–0.37	
Pre-metastasis clinical diagnosis hazard (by age, grade)	Cx1, Cx2 [1/year]	0–0.03	[37,39]
Multiplier for Hazard of Clinical Diagnosis (by age group)	MCx [dmnl]	15–25	[39]
Time between screenings	TimeBtwSx [year]	1.5–2.5	[39]
Biopsy compliance (by stage)	BiopCompM0/M1 [dmnl]	0.3–0.7; 0.9	[39,45]
Time to act	τ [year]	0.25–0.5	[49]
alpha	α [1/year]	0.015–0.03	Based on PSA curve [46]
beta	β [1/year]	0.45–0.65	Based on PSA curve [46]
Max adoption fraction	A^{max} [dmnl]	0.25–0.9	Expert judgement
Stopping age to screen	Age^{stop} [years]	70–85	Expert judgement
HBR Translation Delay	λt [year]	2–10	Expert judgement

4. Simulation Results

4.1. Basic Dynamics and Model Validation

The model is implemented using Vensim^{TM} software (Ventana Systems Inc., Harvard, MA, USA), initialized in 1980, in the pre-PSA era, and simulates forward by increments of a 1/8th of a year through 2040; all output variables are calculated at every increment. The time horizon is selected as 1980–2040, about 60 years, to capture the dynamic trends in the diffusion of screening and compliance with recommendations and the potential trajectories for selected policy variables. Detailed documentation of the model is available upon request from the authors. We demonstrated correspondence to historical data on various metrics including population counts, crude and death rates by age group, disease prevalence, and some metrics on disease progression.

We conducted structurally oriented behavior validation experiments throughout the model-building process to test the validity of the model with respect to its intended purpose. First, we tested the model's response to a series of extreme conditions to check its robustness. For example, the latent disease cannot get detected in the absence of PSA screening. After screening gets introduced, the loco-regional fraction of indolent disease at detection becomes 100%, as an indolent disease cannot get metastasized by definition. Table 2 provides a summary of the qualitative behavior of the PSA model under selected extreme conditions and various logic tests, e.g., the indolent disease cannot get detected in the absence of PSA screening and cannot get metastasized. Experiments prove that model behavior matches the behavior expected from the model for the listed conditions and passes all logic and extreme condition tests. Throughout the model-building process, we also tested the model's mass balance for the population counts by calculating the sum of all the stocks in the model and comparing it against the integration of the net inflow over the simulation horizon. The only inflow to the population stocks is the male-population-turning-35 exogenous time series, and the net immigration flows.

Table 2. Extreme condition tests with the corresponding (expected and confirmed) qualitative behavior.

Extreme Condition Test	Qualitative Behavior
Screening switch turned off	PSA screening tests go to zero, % Ever had PSA goes to zero, % of Screen detected cancer goes to zero, % of Clinically detected cancer goes to 100%, Reported PCa prevalence goes down, % of men healthy with a FP goes to zero, no detection, and treatment of latent (indolent) disease
Clinical detection switch turned off	% of Cancer clinically detected goes to zero, All cancer detection is through PSA screening
Both screen and clinical detection switches turned off	Reported PCa incidence goes to zero, Reported PCa prevalence goes to zero, no new PCa cancer survivors
Treatment switch turned off	% Ever treated goes to zero, There are no survivors with primary treatment
Treatment is 100% effective	No one dies of prostate cancer, M0 and M1 PCa deaths go to zero
Metastasis switch turned off	M0 loco-regional disease doesn't get metastasized, no distant M1 cases, no M1 prostate cancer deaths
All-cause mortality turned off	Mean population age increases, only deaths are PCa deaths
Decrease in mortality trend is removed	Overall deaths increase, population's mean age goes down
All disease is indolent	No prostate cancer deaths, 100% overdiagnosis
Other logic tests	
% PSA detected	% of disease detected by screening is 100% for indolent disease (Latent cancer cannot get detected clinically)
PCa incidence/prevalence	Reported PCa incidence is higher for older age groups
% Loco-regional at detection	100% for latent disease, as latent disease cannot get metastasized to M1 disease
% Distant at detection	0% for latent disease, higher for higher grade cancer

We provide a summary of simulation results to show the correspondence of the model to historical data and future projections for the population stocks, including the total population, percent above 65 years old, and for various age groups in Supplementary Materials. The death rate is in terms of millions of deaths per year, and as a crude death rate, expressed as the number of deaths reported each calendar year per factor selected. The default factor at the CDC compressed mortality file is per 100,000 of the population, reporting the death rate per 100,000 persons. Rates are for three age groups, 35–55, 55–75, and 75+. Model behavior shows reasonable correspondence to historical behavior of the total population counts and deaths.

4.1.1. Cancer Prevalence

The main and most important risk factor affecting all types of cancer, except cervical cancer, is getting older. Autopsy studies indicate that prevalence of PCa is an increasing function of age [41–43]. Since the real underlying prevalence of PCa is unknown, we use estimates from autopsy studies. Figure 6 shows the fraction of men with a PCa tumor at autopsy, a proxy for real underlying cancer prevalence. Prevalence estimates are from Carter et al. [50], who studied 5250 autopsies from the U.S. literature. Estimates apply to the symptom-free male population; men with a PCa diagnosis are excluded. Please note that more recently conducted autopsy studies are finding a higher age-specific prevalence [41,42], so our estimates are conservative with respect to the underlying (unknown) asymptomatic disease in the U.S. male population.

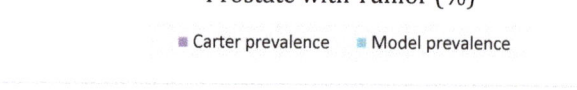
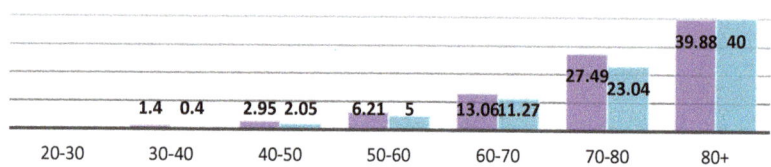

Figure 6. Age specific prevalence of asymptomatic PCa among symptom-free men based on autopsy studies [50] vs. base case simulation.

4.1.2. Screen vs. Clinical Detection and Overdiagnosis Rates

Cancer overdiagnosis is a contentious issue with various definitions and implications for policy making. Models of cancer registry data and trial results estimate that 23% to 42% of PSA-detected cancers would not be found without screening, and 42–66% of all diagnosed prostate cancers would have caused no clinical harm had they remained undetected [51]. Cancer overdiagnosis has several definitions. It refers to people diagnosed with indolent disease, and to others who die of other causes. This study uses the most conservative definition of overdiagnosis, where a screen-detected case is considered overdiagnosed if it is an indolent tumor. While existing estimates vary widely between 23–66% [1,51] our base case estimate is somewhere in this range on the conservative side, indicating 24% of all diagnosed cases, and 33% of all screen-detected cases, are overdiagnosed, once the adoption trends get stabilized. PSA screening started in 1985, before which cancer could only be detected clinically, as confirmed by the base case simulation (Figure 7).

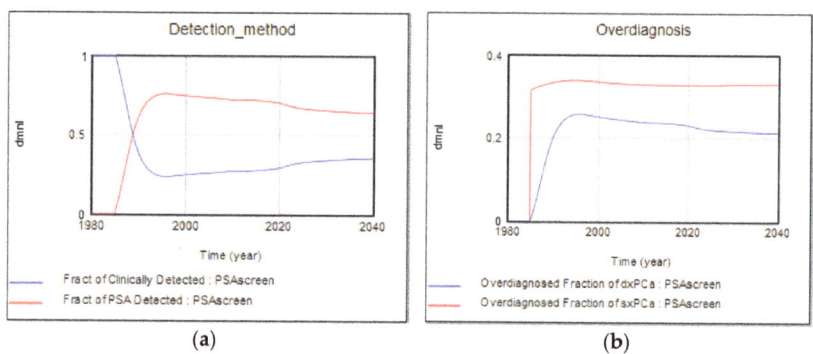

Figure 7. Base-case (**a**) fraction of screen- vs. clinically detected cancers; (**b**) overdiagnosis fraction of all diagnosed vs. screen-detected cases.

4.2. Sensitivity Testing

We conducted several types of sensitivity tests on the model by exploring the parameter space for selected key indicators, mainly overdiagnosis rates by detection method, other harms such as unnecessary biopsies due to an FP test result, and metastatic disease fraction at initial diagnosis. We chose these key outcome measures to provide insights into different system features, inform policymakers regarding each indicator's tradeoffs, and apply the notion of multiplism suggesting that essential problems should be measured in different ways.

4.2.1. Over-Diagnosis Due to Large Pool of Indolent (Latent) Disease

Experimental results summarized in Figure 8a,b demonstrate the "indolent" or "latent" fraction of disease as one of the most important underlying parameters affecting cancer overdiagnosis rates. Indolent class tumors represent the non-progressive, or latent tumors, including regressive tumors which are destined to stay confined to the prostate and not metastasize or kill the patient by definition. We varied the value of the latent fraction of disease between 20–50% (base case = 35%) to show its effect on the overdiagnosis fraction of screen-detected, or all (screen- and clinically) detected cancers. Adoption of the screening practice is another important parameter determining overdiagnosis rates. Figure 8c shows that overdiagnosis rates are also affected by the PSA screening adoption practice by medical professionals (base case value for maximum adoption fraction = 0.75). As expected, detection and overdiagnosis of indolent disease drops to zero without PSA screening, since they cannot be detected without screening.

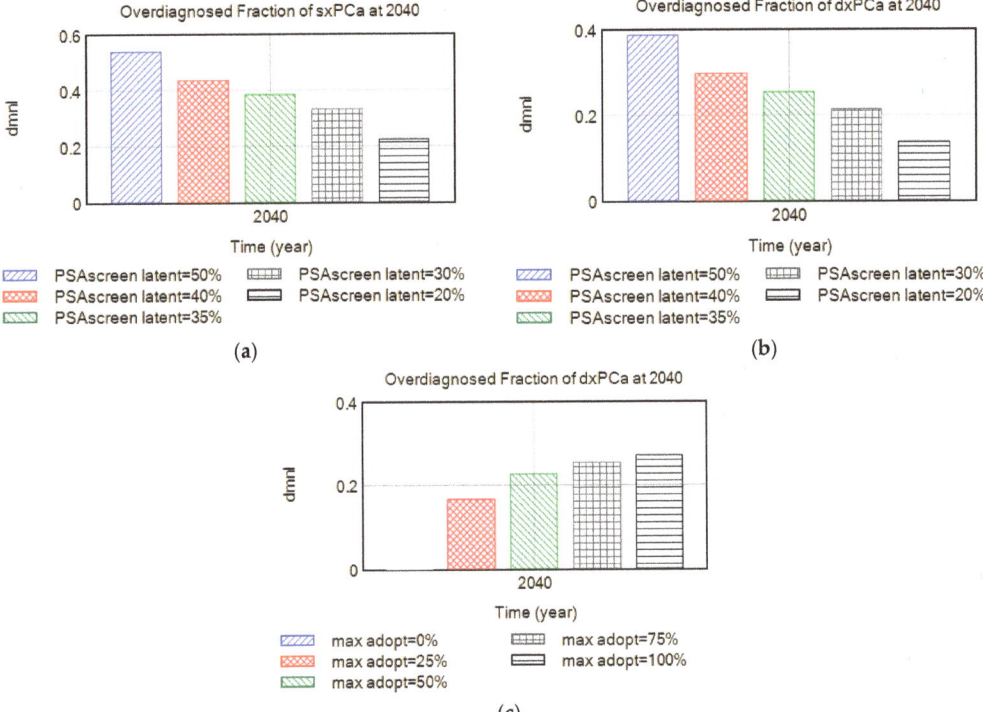

Figure 8. Overdiagnosis of (**a**) screen-detected vs. (**b**) all cases by varying latent fraction, after adoption trends are stabilized, and (**c**) overdiagnosis rates as maximum adoption fraction for the PSA practice varies between 0–100%.

4.2.2. Parameter Set Exploration for Benefits and Harms of Screening

To explore the parameter space, we ran a global sensitivity analysis with combined variations in all the parameters the model is sensitive to (as identified in Table 1). These include all the important time constants related to screening, including the harms and benefits ratio (HBR) translation delay indicating how long it takes to translate scientific evidence to clinical practice, the time between screenings, the stopping age to screen, and the time to act. Other sensitive parameters include the biopsy compliance rate (by patients with a positive test result) and the maximum adoption fraction (of the PSA test by clinicians). The experimental results, in turn, show the confidence intervals (up to 100%) of the key indicators for harms and benefits from 300 runs, sufficient to explore the state space of the harms and benefits in the screening and adoption subsystems. A Monte Carlo simulation, also known as multivariate sensitivity simulation (MVSS), was used to automate the sensitivity analysis. The experiment gives us the full range of possibilities for potential harms and benefits of screening and allows us to observe their tradeoff.

Confidence plots in Figures 9 and 10 demonstrate the common and extreme operating ranges for the main harms of medical screening, and the tradeoff between its harms and benefits. The main harms of screening include (i) false positives, (ii) unnecessary biopsies, and (iii) overdiagnosis (and, hence, overtreatment). The main benefit includes saved lives, or early detection of cancer (before it gets metastasized). We selected respective proxy variables as (1) the overdiagnosed fraction of all detected cases, (2) the cumulative number of unnecessary biopsies, (3) the fraction of healthy male population living with an FP test result, and (4) the fraction of disease already metastasized at initial detection or the fraction of M1 at detection.

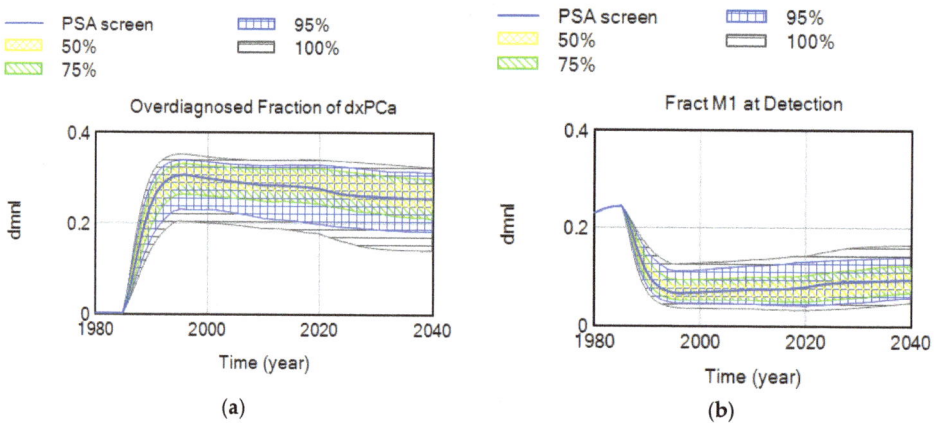

Figure 9. Confidence plot for (**a**) overdiagnosed fraction of cases; (**b**) fraction of metastasized disease at time of diagnosis.

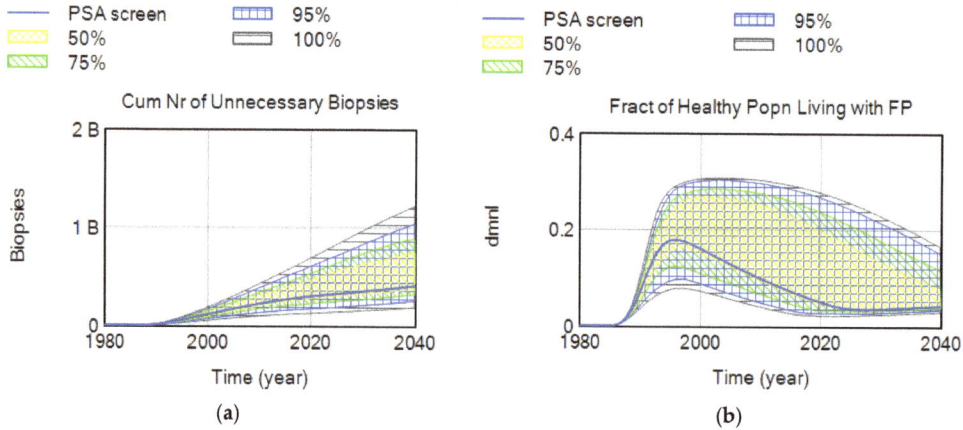

Figure 10. Confidence plot for (**a**) cumulative number of unnecessary biopsies; (**b**) fraction of healthy male population living with an FP test result.

5. Discussion

We present a generic simulation model for medical screening, and a case study specific to PSA screening for PCa, including the natural history of the disease, screening, and clinical detection of PCa; the adoption of the PSA screening test by medical professionals; and the dissemination of the test in the U.S. context. While our focus for this study is primarily on the fundamental tradeoff between the main harms and benefits of screening as exemplified by the selected key proxy variables, the model can be used for policy analysis and the estimation of potential future trajectories for other important policy variables, such as the increasing pool of cancer survivors in the U.S. The reasons for choosing these key outcome measures are to (i) keep track of the critical stocks for the cancer screening problem, (ii) provide insights into different features of the system, (iii) inform policymakers regarding the tradeoffs of each indicator, and (iv) apply the notion of multiplism suggesting that a problem should be measured in different ways.

5.1. Strategic Insights

- One of the important contributions of this study is the introduction of a more realistic yet flexible structure for routine medical screening that allows keeping track of critical stocks that have been generally overlooked in previous modeling studies. Existing modeling studies do not explicitly define some of these population stocks in the screening process, including men who currently live with an FP test result, which has implications for anxiety and depression. In this study, we use the flexibility of the SD modeling stock-flow structure to keep track and account for all critical stocks in the cancer screening problem, while their values are not readily measured in the literature. Simulations show that the fraction of healthy men who live with an FP may vary between 5 and 15% in most situations, depending on screening criteria, or breadth indications of disease, and may increase up to 30% with lower biopsy compliance rates. The value of the FP stock relative to the healthy population (i.e., "the fraction of healthy male population currently living with an FP") may be an important indicator for policy making. Another variable for which we were not able to find historical data includes the the "fraction of disease in target screening population". These metrics are potentially very important, yet not readily measured or considered in existing medical and modeling literature. Simulations show that the fraction of false positives in the healthy male population may have increased to as high as 18% in the 1990s when screening was overused. At the same time, the real diseased fraction of the target population must have dropped down to its historical minimum. We do not aim to suggest optimal estimates for these variables but would like to highlight the importance of having a better understanding of their dynamics by additional data collection, rather than excluding them from our "mental" models, or making the constancy assumption [52].

- The addition of an "indolent/latent" disease category is a novel addition in this modeling study, facilitating to make of inferences about the real (yet unknown) occult disease prevalence in the population. One aspect that increases the reported cancer prevalence is the existence of a silent pool of indolent diseases, which varies among different types of cancers. These are "TP" cases where the disease identified has uncertain significance, and where men would never become aware of their disease if they were not tested for it, as evidenced by the silent reservoirs of undetected thyroid, breast, and prostate [41] cancers. Our interview data for the PCa case study confirms the importance of the size of this latent pool of disease: " ... *If you take enough time to understand what this means, if I tell a patient, "Look I'm 47, my probability to have a prostate cancer histologically under the microscope right now as I sit here, is about 30%. Period." That's a start, so there's a pool of prostate cancer that we all carry, most of them they'll never become symptomatic, some of us have to have bad cards. Do we understand who have bad cards and who don't? No, we don't. There's a residual risk that there's something going on.* "—Peter Juni. MD-PhD, Director, Applied Health Research Centre, St. Michael's Hospital, *and Professor of Medicine, University of Toronto, Previous: University of Bern, Director of the Institute of Primary Health Care, Professor and Chair of Primary Health Care and Clinical Epidemiology in the Faculty of Medicine, Switzerland.*

- We endogenize variables that are mostly taken as constants in other studies. These include the breadth of indications of screening (including the biopsy threshold and the starting age to screen), the prevalence of disease in the screening population, the sensitivity and specificity of the test, and the harm reduction technology. It also separates the formal decision thresholds for screening from the decision thresholds that are implemented, showing their interdependency to each other as well as to the diagnostics of the test. For example, existing studies usually assume a constant PSA level as the trigger for biopsy, which stays constant over time, but this is not an accurate reflection of the clinical practice. Endogenizing such variables allows us to show how they are changing over time, affecting the target screening prevalence, and, hence, the screening diagnostics themselves which are also taken as constants in most studies. To be specific, the model endogenizes the adoption and diffusion of the screening process and defines the different components of screen detection explicitly. These include the fraction of the population that receives the screening test, the sensitivity of the test, biopsy compliance, and biopsy detection. The test sensitivity and currently screened fraction are endogenous to the model, while biopsy compliance and detection are exogenous. Subjects are eligible to receive regular screenings if their doctor adopted the PSA screening test at the time, and if they are around the age-eligible range for the test. Interview results confirm that one of the main determinants of screening is the doctor's opinion: *"Access to care, coverage, and I also think it is how the screening is presented by their doctor ... .a lot of medicine is sales, and if a doctor presents something as either optional or a bad idea like, "You don't really want to do that, do you?" the patient's going to say no. But if their doctor's enthusiastic about it and believes in it, then they're probably more likely to go ahead and get it done ... "*—MD, PhD Erin Hofstatter, Medical Oncologist, Yale School of Medicine.

- Karanfil and Sterman show that the "formal" recommended starting age to screen varies, both over time and between different guideline-issuing organizations [32]. The recommended "formal" biopsy threshold for PSA testing stayed constant at 4 ng/mL throughout the initial years of screening dissemination, after which it starts to vary in the 2000s. The informal, "practice" threshold, however, has reportedly been lower than the formal one, suggesting poor compliance with recommendations. The real pattern for the average biopsy threshold is unknown, but it is generally accepted to be 2.5 ng/mL between 1990 and 2000 [39]. In addition, Pinsky et al. [53] have shown that biopsy frequencies of men with PSAs between 2.5 and 4 ng/mL were of the same order of magnitude as for men with a PSA higher than 4 ng/mL. The actual starting age data are also not available, but they presumably follow the same pattern as the biopsy threshold, where formal indications first expand in the early years of screening and then start to narrow as harms and the evidence for harms accumulate over time.

- Since the test diagnostics are directly derived from the underlying probability distributions for diseased and healthy people, the model can as well be used to estimate the real prevalence of the disease.

5.2. Limitations and Further Research

The results of this study rest on several key assumptions. First, as with any other natural history model, we make assumptions about disease onset, progression, and diagnosis in the absence of screening. Second, we assume that disease incidence remains constant at pre-PSA levels after 1987. Third, the model assumes that baseline PCa survival remains constant in the PSA era. We use data from a variety of sources that are subject to limitations. Data on some key indicators, such as the actual starting age and the actual biopsy threshold used in clinical practice, are not available. We used data from expert opinions and published medical literature to justify model propositions.

We also assume a constant clinical detection hazard in the base case, which may lead to an overestimation of screening benefits. In fact, clinical detection rates may also have increased over time because of increased disease awareness in the PSA era. Immigration data was not available by age group and was assumed to be distributed proportionally between age groups, yet it may have implications for population aging. No historical data were available for some other variables we identified as important, including the fraction of healthy men with a false positive or true negative, or the progress of harm reduction technology. However, the focus of this study was on building the most reliable and flexible model structure for medical screening, rather than point prediction for policy variables.

This model is not primarily designed for making inferences about optimal screening policies but can inform modelers and policymakers about potential levers in the system and complement other modeling and interactive studies designed for cancer interventions [54]. Simulation models like ours are flexible tools that can aid healthcare professionals and policymakers in making complex decisions. They can provide constructive insights and dynamic intuition to supplement the typical empirical evidence for updating cancer screening recommendations and can offer a formal means to improve the development and implementation of evidence-based screening.

Future iterations of our simulation model can be employed to design policy recommendations and address important problem areas, such as policy making for cancer survivors, cost of care, or quality of life considerations. Particularly, the increasing pool of cancer survivors in the U.S. is an important consideration, as their numbers in the U.S. are at a record high. The AACR Cancer Progress Report 2022 reports that there are 18 million cancer survivors in the U.S., up from 3 million in 1971, and the number is expected to increase to 26 million by 2040 [55].

The aging of the U.S. population and the increase in life expectancy has serious implications for chronic disease incidence and prevalence since cancer is an age-related disease and the aging of the male population implies more PCa survivors in the future. As more and more men are given a cancer diagnosis by screening, the natural perception of each "survivor" is that screening "saved" his life. However, a portion of these survivors have a type of PCa that could have been treated as effectively when found later, or that might not have caused problems. The problem is that for each "survivor", there is no way to know whether screening and the treatment "caused" survival, as there is no counterfactual. Thus, the number of men who perceive benefits from screening may be substantially greater than the actual number who receive benefits, and the impression of benefit may get exaggerated.

Existing studies primarily focus on the medical evidence supporting different screening guidelines but usually neglect the broad boundary processes that condition the adoption of and adherence to evidence-based guidelines by clinicians and the public. This simulation study is part of a continuing line of research in our investigation of the universal problem of evidence-based development of sound and reliable clinical practice guidelines (CPGs). Despite their importance especially in high-risk conditions, guidelines are far from optimal in practice. While there is a proliferation of modeling studies to inform CPGs, not many are addressing the actual guideline-making process itself. The scientific community also recently recognized the inherent complexity of the guideline formation process itself and invited researchers to explore the potential implications of this complexity that is inherent in complex decision-making environments. In line with this motivation, we aim to come up with empirically grounded theoretical frameworks and provide formal simulation models to document the long-term effects and unintended consequences of changing disease definitions on published screening guidelines and, consequently, on the actual practice, the specific mechanisms that influence different implementations of these guidelines, and the mechanisms which account for the gaps between the scientific evidence and the actual practice of screening.

Eventually, we aim to expand the boundaries of this case study model to create a more realistic life setting, including the influence of the socio-political environment where the actual screening decision is embedded. More specifically, we aim to look at how medical professional societies—including radiologists, patient advocacy groups, and other principal actors—influence the adoption and diffusion dynamics of medical screening in the U.S. context.

Supplementary Materials: The following supporting information can be downloaded at: https://www.mdpi.com/article/10.3390/systems11050252/s1, Figure S1: Supplementary PSA; Table S1: Supplementary PSA.

Funding: The project was funded by the BIDEB 2232 International Fellowship for Outstanding Researchers Program of TUBITAK (Project No: 118C327) supporting Dr. Özge Karanfil. However, all scientific contributions made in this project are owned and approved solely by the author/s.

Data Availability Statement: Data presented in this article were extracted from publicly available data sources. See Table 1 for data sources. Interview data and consent was obtained from the MIT Committee on the Use of Humans as Experimental Subjects (COUHES) Protocol # 1412006813 Study Title: Dynamics of Routine Screening.

Acknowledgments: The author gratefully thanks John D. Sterman, Hazhir Rahmandad, and Jack Homer for their review of earlier iterations of this work, and to the referees for their constructive and helpful comments and recommendations.

Conflicts of Interest: The authors declare no conflict of interest.

Abbreviations

AACR	American Association for Cancer Research
CDC	Centers for Disease Control and Prevention
CISNET	Intervention and Surveillance Modeling Network
COUHES	Committee on the Use of Humans as Experimental Subjects
CPG	Clinical Practice Guidelines
DRE	Digital Rectal Exam
FN	False Negative
FP	False Positive
HBR	Harms and Benefits Ratio
HRT	Harm Reduction Technology
NCHS	National Center for Health Statistics
NCI	National Cancer Institute
NHANES	National Health and Nutrition Examination Survey.
NHIS	National Health Interview Survey
PCa	Prostate Cancer
PLCO	Prostate, Lung, Colorectal and Ovarian Trial
PSA	Prostate Specific Antigen
SEER	Surveillance, Epidemiology, and End Results
USPSTF	U.S. Preventive Services Task Force
TP	True Positive
TN	True Negative

References

1. Hoffman, J.R.; Cooper, R.J. Overdiagnosis of Disease. *Arch. Intern. Med.* **2012**, *172*, 1123–1124. [CrossRef] [PubMed]
2. Esserman, L.J.; Thompson, I.M.; Reid, B.; Nelson, P.; Ransohoff, D.F.; Welch, H.G.; Hwang, S.; Berry, D.A.; Kinzler, K.W.; Black, W.C.; et al. Addressing overdiagnosis and overtreatment in cancer: A prescription for change. *Lancet Oncol.* **2014**, *15*, e234–e242. [CrossRef] [PubMed]
3. *Global Cancer Facts & Figures*, 4th ed.; American Cancer Society: Atlanta, GA, USA, 2018; Available online: https://www.cancer.org/research/cancer-facts-statistics/global.html (accessed on 12 April 2023).
4. Seidman, H.; Mushinski, M.H.; Gelb, S.K.; Silverberg, E. Probabilities of Eventually Developing or Dying of Cancer–United States, 1985. *CA Cancer J. Clin.* **1985**, *35*, 36–56. [CrossRef] [PubMed]
5. Altekruse, S.F.; Kosary, C.L.; Krapcho, M.; Neyman, N.; Aminou, R.; Waldron, W.; Ruhl, J.; Howlader, N.; Tatalovich, Z.; Cho, H.; et al. SEER Cancer Statistics Review, 1975–2007. 2010. Available online: http://seer.cancer.gov/csr/1975_2007/ (accessed on 12 April 2023).

6. Faiena, I.; Holden, S.; Cooperberg, M.R.; Soule, H.R.; Simons, J.; Morgan, T.M.; Penson, D.; Morgans, A.K.; Hussain, M. Prostate Cancer Screening and the Goldilocks Principle: How Much Is Just Right? *J. Clin. Oncol.* **2018**, *36*, 937–941. [CrossRef] [PubMed]
7. Ebell, M.H.; Thai, T.N.; Royalty, K.J. Cancer screening recommendations: An international comparison of high income countries. *Public Health Rev.* **2018**, *39*, 7. [CrossRef]
8. US Preventive Services Task Force. Screening for Prostate Cancer: US Preventive Services Task Force Recommendation Statement. *JAMA* **2018**, *319*, 1901–1913. [CrossRef]
9. SEER. Cancer of the Prostate—Cancer Stat Facts. Available online: https://seer.cancer.gov/statfacts/html/prost.html (accessed on 3 March 2023).
10. Sterman, J.D. *Business Dynamics: Systems Thinking and Modeling for a Complex World*; Irwin/McGraw-Hill: Boston, MA, USA, 2000.
11. Homer, J.B.; Hirsch, G.B. System Dynamics Modeling for Public Health: Background and Opportunities. *Am. J. Public Health* **2006**, *96*, 452–458. [CrossRef]
12. Sterman, J.D. Learning from Evidence in a Complex World. *Am. J. Public Health* **2006**, *96*, 505–514. [CrossRef]
13. Homer, J.B. A diffusion model with application to evolving medical technologies. *Technol. Forecast. Soc. Change* **1987**, *31*, 197–218. [CrossRef]
14. Hirsch, G.; Trogdon, J.; Wile, K.; Orenstein, D. Using Simulation to Compare 4 Categories of Intervention for Reducing Cardiovascular Disease Risks. *Am. J. Public Health* **2014**, *104*, 1187–1195. [CrossRef]
15. Milstein, B.; Homer, J.; Hirsch, G. Analyzing National Health Reform Strategies with a Dynamic Simulation Model. *Am. J. Public Health* **2010**, *100*, 811–819. [CrossRef]
16. Yarnoff, B.; Honeycutt, A.; Bradley, C.; Khavjou, O.; Bates, L.; Bass, S.; Kaufmann, R.; Barker, L.; Briss, P. Validation of the Prevention Impacts Simulation Model (PRISM). In *Prev. Chronic Dis.*; 2021; 18, p. E09. Available online: www.cdc.gov/pcd/issues/2021/20_0225.htm (accessed on 12 April 2023). [CrossRef]
17. Atun, R.A.; Lebcir, R.M.; McKee, M.; Habicht, J.; Coker, R.J. Impact of joined-up HIV harm reduction and multidrug resistant tuberculosis control programmes in Estonia: System dynamics simulation model. *Health Policy* **2006**, *81*, 207–217. [CrossRef]
18. Burns, W.J.; Slovic, P. The Diffusion of Fear: Modeling Community Response to a Terrorist Strike (2006). Available online: https://ssrn.com/abstract=912736; http://dx.doi.org/10.2139/ssrn.912736 (accessed on 12 April 2023).
19. Ghaffarzadegan, N.; Rahmandad, H. Simulation-based estimation of the early spread of COVID-19 in Iran: Actual versus confirmed cases. *Syst. Dyn. Rev.* **2020**, *36*, 101–129. [CrossRef]
20. Rahmandad, H.; Sterman, J. Quantifying the COVID-19 endgame: Is a new normal within reach? *Syst. Dyn. Rev.* **2022**, *38*, 329–353. [CrossRef]
21. Lim, T.Y.; Stringfellow, E.J.; Stafford, C.A.; DiGennaro, C.; Homer, J.B.; Wakeland, W.; Eggers, S.L.; Kazemi, R.; Glos, L.; Ewing, E.G.; et al. Modeling the Evolution of the US Opioid Crisis for National Policy Development. *Proc. Natl. Acad. Sci. USA* **2022**, *119*, e2115714119. [CrossRef]
22. Darabi, N.; Hosseinichimeh, N. System dynamics modeling in health and medicine: A systematic literature review. *Syst. Dyn. Rev.* **2020**, *36*, 29–73. [CrossRef]
23. Rahmandad, H.; Sterman, J.D. Reporting guidelines for simulation-based research in social sciences. *Syst. Dyn. Rev.* **2012**, *28*, 396–411. [CrossRef]
24. Martinez-Moyano, I.J. Documentation for model transparency. *Syst. Dyn. Rev.* **2012**, *28*, 199–208. [CrossRef]
25. Richmond, B. Towards a Structural Theory of Cancer. D-Memos. D-4151. MIT Sloan School of Management, Cambridge, MA, USA, 1990. Available online: https://systemdynamics.org/d-memos-4000-4499/ (accessed on 12 April 2023).
26. Fett, M.J. Developing Simulation Dynamic Models of Breast Cancer Screening; Wellington, New Zealand, 1999. Available online: https://proceedings.systemdynamics.org/1999/PAPERS/PARA47.PDF (accessed on 12 April 2023).
27. Fett, M. Computer modelling of the Swedish two county trial of mammographic screening and trade offs between participation and screening interval. *J. Med. Screen.* **2001**, *8*, 39–45. [CrossRef]
28. Royston, G.; Dost, A.; Townshend, J.; Turner, H. Using System Dynamics to Help Develop and Implement Policies and Programmes in Health Care in England. *Syst. Dyn. Rev.* **1999**, *15*, 293–313. [CrossRef]
29. Sheldrick, R.C.; Breuer, D.J.; Hassan, R.; Chan, K.; Polk, D.E.; Benneyan, J. A System Dynamics Model of Clinical Decision Thresholds for the Detection of Developmental-Behavioral Disorders. *Implement. Sci.* **2016**, *11*, 156. [CrossRef]
30. Sheldrick, R.C.; Garfinkel, D. Is a Positive Developmental-Behavioral Screening Score Sufficient to Justify Referral? A Review of Evidence and Theory. *Acad. Pediatr.* **2017**, *17*, 464–470. [CrossRef] [PubMed]
31. Palma, A.; Lounsbury, D.W.; Schlecht, N.F.; Agalliu, I. A System Dynamics Model of Serum Prostate-Specific Antigen Screening for Prostate Cancer. *Am. J. Epidemiol.* **2015**, *183*, 227–236. [CrossRef] [PubMed]
32. Karanfil, Ö.; Sterman, J. "Saving lives or harming the healthy?" Overuse and fluctuations in routine medical screening. *Syst. Dyn. Rev.* **2020**, *36*, 294–329. [CrossRef]
33. Karanfil, Ö. Why Clinical Practice Guidelines Shift over Time: A Dynamic Model with Application to Prostate Cancer Screening. Ph.D. Thesis, Massachusetts Institute of Technology, Cambridge, MA, USA, 2016. Available online: http://dspace.mit.edu/handle/1721.1/107531 (accessed on 12 April 2023).
34. United States Department of Health and Human Services (US DHHS), Centers for Disease Control and Prevention (CDC), National Center for Health Statistics (NCHS), Compressed Mortality File (CMF) on CDC WONDER Online Database. Available online: https://wonder.cdc.gov/mortsql.html (accessed on 12 April 2023).

35. Life Tables for the United States Social Security Area 1900–2100. August 2025. Available online: https://www.ssa.gov/oact/NOTES/as120/TOC.html (accessed on 12 April 2023).
36. Cowen, M.E.; Chartrand, M.; Weitzel, W.F. A Markov model of the natural history of prostate cancer. *J. Clin. Epidemiol.* **1994**, *47*, 3–21. [CrossRef]
37. Etzioni, R.; Cha, R.; Cowen, M.E. Serial prostate specific antigen screening for prostate cancer: A computer model evaluates competing strategies. *J. Urol.* **1999**, *162*, 741–748. [CrossRef]
38. Tsodikov, A.; Szabo, A.; Wegelin, J. A population model of prostate cancer incidence. *Stat. Med.* **2006**, *25*, 2846–2866. [CrossRef]
39. Gulati, R.; Inoue, L.; Katcher, J.; Hazelton, W.; Etzioni, R. Calibrating disease progression models using population data: A critical precursor to policy development in cancer control. *Biostatistics* **2010**, *11*, 707–719. [CrossRef]
40. Ayer, T.; Alagoz, O.; Stout, N.K. OR Forum—A POMDP Approach to Personalize Mammography Screening Decisions. *Oper. Res.* **2012**, *60*, 1019–1034. [CrossRef]
41. Jahn, J.L.; Giovannucci, E.L.; Stampfer, M.J. The high prevalence of undiagnosed prostate cancer at autopsy: Implications for epidemiology and treatment of prostate cancer in the Prostate-specific Antigen-era. *Int. J. Cancer* **2015**, *137*, 2795–2802. [CrossRef]
42. Bell, K.J.; Del Mar, C.; Wright, G.; Dickinson, J.; Glasziou, P. Prevalence of incidental prostate cancer: A systematic review of autopsy studies. *Int. J. Cancer* **2015**, *137*, 1749–1757. [CrossRef]
43. Haas, G.P.; Delongchamps, N.; Brawley, O.W.; Wang, C.Y.; de la Roza, G. The Worldwide Epidemiology of Prostate Cancer: Perspectives from Autopsy Studies. *Can. J. Urol.* **2008**, *15*, 3866–3871.
44. Scardino, P.T.; Beck, J.R.; Miles, B.J. Conservative management of prostate cancer. *N. Engl. J. Med.* **1994**, *330*, 1831; author reply 1831–1832.
45. Andriole, G.L.; Crawford, E.D.; Grubb, R.L.; Buys, S.S.; Chia, D.; Church, T.R.; Fouad, M.N.; Isaacs, C.; Kvale, P.A.; Reding, D.J.; et al. Prostate Cancer Screening in the Randomized Prostate, Lung, Colorectal, and Ovarian Cancer Screening Trial: Mortality Results after 13 Years of Follow-up. *Gynecol. Oncol.* **2012**, *104*, 125–132. [CrossRef]
46. Mariotto, A.B.; Etzioni, R.; Krapcho, M.; Feuer, E.J. Reconstructing PSA testing patterns between black and white men in the US from Medicare claims and the National Health Interview Survey. *Cancer* **2007**, *109*, 1877–1886. [CrossRef]
47. Messing, E.M.; Manola, J.; Yao, J.; Kiernan, M.; Crawford, D.; Wilding, G.; di'SantAgnese, P.A.; Trump, D. Immediate versus deferred androgen deprivation treatment in patients with node-positive prostate cancer after radical prostatectomy and pelvic lymphadenectomy. *Lancet Oncol.* **2006**, *7*, 472–479. [CrossRef]
48. Aus, G.; Robinson, D.; Rosell, J.; Sandblom, G.; Varenhorst, E. Survival in prostate carcinoma—Outcomes from a prospective, population-based cohort of 8887 men with up to 15 years of follow-up. *Cancer* **2005**, *103*, 943–951. [CrossRef]
49. Hoffman, R.M.; Harlan, L.C.; Klabunde, C.N.; Gilliland, F.D.; Stephenson, R.A.; Hunt, W.C.; Potosky, A.L. Racial differences in initial treatment for clinically localized prostate cancer. *J. Gen. Intern. Med.* **2003**, *18*, 845–853. [CrossRef]
50. Carter, H.B.; Piantadosi, S.; Isaacs, J.T. Clinical Evidence for and Implications of the Multistep Development of Prostate Cancer. *J. Urol.* **1990**, *143*, 742–746. [CrossRef]
51. Hoffman, R.M.; Zeliadt, S.B. The Cautionary Tale of Psa Testing: Comment on 'risk Profiles and Treatment Patterns among Men Diagnosed as Having Prostate Cancer and a Prostate-Specific Antigen Level below 4.0 Ng/mL. *Arch. Intern. Med.* **2010**, *170*, 1262–1263. [CrossRef] [PubMed]
52. Forrester, J.W. 14 'Obvious Truths'. *Syst. Dyn. Rev.* **1987**, *3*, 156–159. [CrossRef]
53. Pinsky, P.F.; Andriole, G.L.; Kramer, B.S.; Hayes, R.; Prorok, P.C.; Gohagan, J.K. Prostate biopsy following a positive screen in the prostate, lung, colorectal and ovarian cancer screening trial. *J. Urol.* **2005**, *173*, 746–751; discussion 750–751. [CrossRef] [PubMed]
54. Castellano, T.; Moore, K.; Ting, J.; Washington, C.; Yildiz, Y.; Surinach, A.; Sonawane, K.; Chhatwal, J.; Ayer, T. Cervical cancer geographical burden analyzer: An interactive, open-access tool for understanding geographical disease burden in patients with recurrent or metastatic cervical cancer. *Gynecol. Oncol.* **2022**, *169*, 113–117. [CrossRef]
55. Cancer Progress Report. AACR Cancer Progress Report. Available online: https://cancerprogressreport.aacr.org/progress/ (accessed on 9 April 2023).

Disclaimer/Publisher's Note: The statements, opinions and data contained in all publications are solely those of the individual author(s) and contributor(s) and not of MDPI and/or the editor(s). MDPI and/or the editor(s) disclaim responsibility for any injury to people or property resulting from any ideas, methods, instructions or products referred to in the content.

MDPI
St. Alban-Anlage 66
4052 Basel
Switzerland
Tel. +41 61 683 77 34
Fax +41 61 302 89 18
www.mdpi.com

Systems Editorial Office
E-mail: systems@mdpi.com
www.mdpi.com/journal/systems

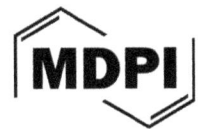

www.ingramcontent.com/pod-product-compliance
Lightning Source LLC
LaVergne TN
LVHW070728100526
838202LV00013B/1191